AF322736

Problem Based
Neurosurgery

Problem Based
Neurosurgery

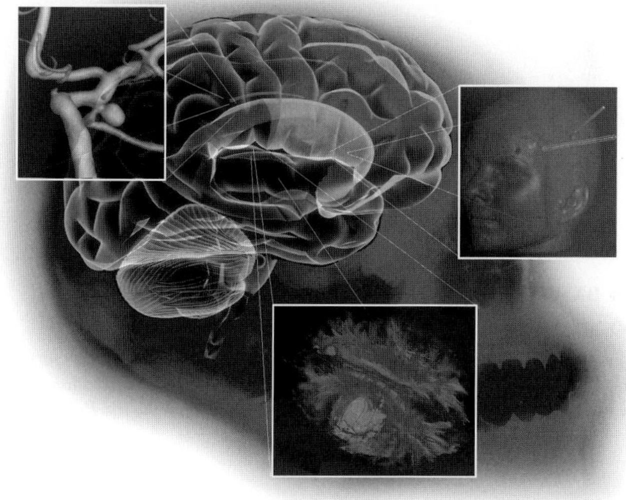

Sam Eljamel

The University of Dundee, UK

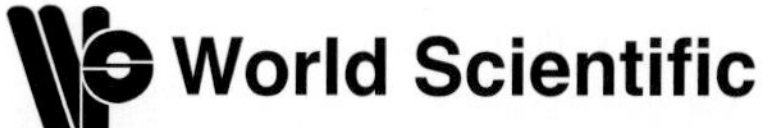

World Scientific

NEW JERSEY · LONDON · SINGAPORE · BEIJING · SHANGHAI · HONG KONG · TAIPEI · CHENNAI

Published by

World Scientific Publishing Co. Pte. Ltd.

5 Toh Tuck Link, Singapore 596224

USA office: 27 Warren Street, Suite 401-402, Hackensack, NJ 07601

UK office: 57 Shelton Street, Covent Garden, London WC2H 9HE

British Library Cataloguing-in-Publication Data
A catalogue record for this book is available from the British Library.

PROBLEM BASED NEUROSURGERY

ISBN-13 978-981-4317-07-8
ISBN-10 981-4317-07-1

Typeset by Stallion Press
Email: enquiries@stallionpress.com

Printed by FuIsland Offset Printing (S) Pte Ltd. Singapore

Disclaimer

The author provided a summary of information he thought relevant to students, doctors in training and other health care professionals learning about neurosurgical disorders. The author had made no attempt to set a standard of care and common sense should prevail. The author had made no attempt to update the information after the date of publication. The author took every precaution to accurately present the information, but errors or omissions may have occurred. Any therapeutic drug dosages or recommendations contained in this book should be verified before use and local policies, procedures, guidelines and national recommendations should be checked before use.

Dedication

I dedicate this book to my wonderful family: my supportive and loving wife "Adora", my eldest daughter "Sarah" who inspired me to do this work as she progressed through the medical course, my youngest daughter "Sana" who proof-read every word of this book on top of her busy schedule studying medicine and my son "Sam Jr" who kept me going to finish this project. To my parents who gave me the opportunity to pursue my career. To my teachers, my students, my colleagues and my patients who gave me the experience and wisdom that culminated in this project.

Contents

Preface

Problem based neurosurgery is a systematic approach to diagnosis, understanding and management of neurosurgical diseases based on symptoms and signs of disease and using common sense and the art of applying scientific knowledge to practice.

In producing this book I took the common sense approach, my patients presented me with a set of symptoms and signs creating a problem that needed diagnosis and management plans. My students and residents had asked me questions. It is these presentations and questions that formed the foundation problems in this book. I concentrated on core and common neurosurgical problems that constituted the majority of neurosurgical practice. When one's goal is to be concise, it is not possible to include every detail in this text. I envisaged that the main users of this book will be those studying neurosurgery, and neurology and those training in neurosurgery, emergency medicine, ENT, ophthalmology, general medicine, general surgery, orthopaedic surgery, and radiology and doctors in their foundation years and those practicing in the community.

Thanks for using this text.

Professor Sam Eljamel, MD, FRCS(Ed,Ir,NS)
Consultant Neurosurgeon

Chapter 1: History and Physical Exam

**Problem 1-1:   How to get the patient to tell you what is wrong.
(The smart way of taking a succinct complete history of any illness)**

The main questions on every patient's mind when (s)he walks into a doctor's office or when (s)he seeks a doctor's advice are:

What is wrong with me doctor?
What can you do about what is wrong?
and
Can you cure it?

Problem based tool box:

How to take smart history?
How to examine HMF?
How to examine cranial nerves?
How to examine motor system?
How to examine sensory
   system?

The key to unlock the mystery to these questions is to take a succinct complete history, and analyse the information you gather instantly to guide further questions and clinical examination. Throughout this book you will find examples of real life problems that patients presented with and you will learn how to take a smart history, elicit clinical signs and perform intelligent analysis of the symptoms and signs to reach a diagnosis and answer patient's questions in full, request appropriate investigations and manage the patient effectively.

To find out the cause of each symptom of the patient and manage your patient effectively, you need to collect the following essential information about each symptom. You need to know:

- *The anatomical location of the symptom (where is it coming from?),*
- *Its mode of onset (how did it start?),*
- *Its duration (how long it has been there for?), and*
- *Its course (what happened to it since it began?).*

It is important to ask *open-ended* questions to get as much accurate information from the patient as possible. Using closed-ended questions such as

1

those requiring "Yes" or "No" answers, is counterproductive and likely to lead to avoidable errors. This kind of question may become necessary to confirm the answers to open-ended questions, to narrow down the diagnosis or for systemic enquiry. Let us study few examples to understand the difference between open- and closed-ended questions.

Problem case scenario (PCS) 1-1-1:

A 35-year-old woman walks into a doctor's office and complains that she had facial pain.
As soon as such a patient turns up in my office I will be rounding two main causative suspects straightway: *idiopathic trigeminal neuralgia (ITN) or atypical facial pain syndrome caused by structural lesion inside the skull, at the skull base or in the face.*
    I will ask the patient the following four open-ended basic questions:

1. *Where exactly was this pain?* (**Exact location**)
2. *How did the pain start?* (**Mode of onset**)
3. *How long was the pain there for?* (**Duration of the pain**) and
4. *What happened to the pain since it started?* (**Course of the pain**)

Note that all my questions were open-ended questions beginning with "Where", "How", and "What". Any question that starts with a verb is a closed-ended question requiring a "Yes" or "No" answer and may lead to an incomplete history that takes longer to elicit. For example, if I had asked the patient: "Can you tell me where the pain is?" The patient may just answer: "Yes, I can", and I have to ask the patient another question: "Where is it?" or ask the patient to tell me where the pain was. It would have been much easier and quicker if I went ahead and asked the straightforward question: *Where exactly was the pain?*
    Another commonly encountered method of taking history is giving the patient a multiple choice question (MCQ). MCQ invites guessing and guessing leads to avoidable mistakes. This often leads to avoidable errors because some patients may feel that they have no option but to choose one of the choices the doctor have given. For example, instead of asking the patient the more reasonable recommended open-ended question "How did

the pain start?", you asked "Did the pain start suddenly or gradually?". If you ask such closed-ended question you are more likely to get the wrong information and miss the mode of onset.

Suppose the patient answered the four basic open-ended questions as follows: "the pain was in the right jaw, started suddenly three weeks ago and it was episodic". These answers make me think that this patient was more likely to be suffering from typical (idiopathic) trigeminal neuralgia (ITN). As I knew what the other features of ITN are, I would supplement my original four questions by the following three questions:

- *What makes this pain worse?* (**Aggravating factors**)
- *What makes this pain better?* (**Relieving factors**)
- *What was the character of the pain?* (**Description of type of pain**)

If my provisional diagnosis of ITN was correct, the patient would have said "the pain was made worse by laughing, brushing my teeth or exposure to cold wind, it was made better by carbamazepine or nothing at all and it was lancinating in nature".

Once I had finished with the facial pain symptom as above, I would go on and ask the fifth basic question:

5. *Apart from this pain, what other symptoms do you have?*

Note that I had used in my fifth question some of the information I had already gathered *(pain)*. By including the word pain in my question I am telling the patient two things: I had finished with the pain and I had listened to the patient's complaint and noted it.

For every other symptom the patient comes up with, I would use the same four basic questions again and again followed by any supplementary questions and finally by the fifth basic question and keep repeating the cycle until the patient says "No doctor, I do not have any more problems".

PCS1-1-2:

A 35-year-old woman came in with facial pain. The answers to the four basic questions were: "the pain was around my left eye, it started suddenly yesterday and it had been slowly getting worse". I had asked the fifth basic question: "apart from this pain around the left eye what other symptoms do you have?" The patient replied that her eyelid came down and she could not open her left eye. I would ask the same four basic questions about the eyelid closure: **Location:** *which eyelid?* **Onset:** *how did it start?* **Duration:** *how long was the eyelid closed for?* **Course:** *what happened to the eyelid since it closed?*

If the patient answered: "it was my left eyelid that closed suddenly at the same time as my pain started and that it remained closed since". Using this additional information I will be thinking that a painful closure of the left eyelid can be caused by left Oculomotor (III) nerve palsy caused by an intracranial aneurysm at the posterior communicating artery (PComA), left orbital cellulites or left cavernous sinus pathology. I would ask the following supplementary questions:

If you opened the left eye what happens? Looking for double vision (diplopia).

What other problems have you noticed with the left eye? Looking for redness, discharge, eye deviation or dilatation of the pupil.

The next question in the last case scenario would be: *Apart from the pain and the left eyelid closure, what else?*

If this patient comes with another symptom, e.g. double vision, I would ask the same four basic questions in the same way followed by my fifth question as described: *Which direction did you note the double vision? For how long did you have the double vision? How did it start? What happened to the double vision since it started?* If the patient said that the double vision started just before the eyelid closed, it started suddenly and was maximum looking to the right and it disappeared when the eyelid closed, this information is confirmatory of painful III nerve palsy likely to be caused by intracranial PComA aneurysm and my clinical examination would be designed to confirm this. Figure 1-1 sums up the concept of the basic questions and supplementary ones.

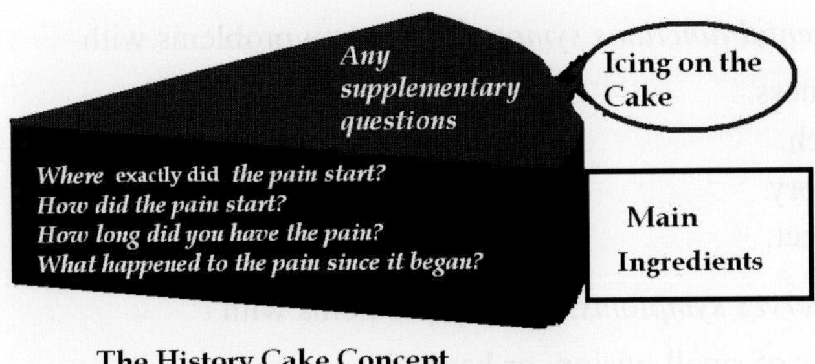

The History Cake Concept

Figure 1-1: Summary of basic and supplementary questions.

If however the patient said: "I do not have any other symptoms", the next step would be to continue the history as follows:

Step 1: *Ask questions that will narrow down the diagnosis. These are questions that will confirm or rule out other features of the diagnosis under consideration. These questions are closed-ended questions and any "Yes" answer requires going through the four basic questions for any positive symptom followed by any other supplementary questions.* For example, in the last case scenario, if I am considering orbital cellulites as a diagnosis I would ask: "Did you have discharge from the left eye?" If the answer was "Yes" then I would have asked, "What type of discharge? How long has the discharge been there for? How did it start? And what happened to the discharge since it started?"

Another example: if a patient came in with headache, I would have asked about nausea and vomiting, and blurring of vision as I would be thinking of raised intracranial pressure (ICP) as the cause of the headache.

Step 2: *Ask questions about the organ that is most likely to be involved in the illness to elicit any other symptoms the patient might have dismissed.* For example in the two previous case scenarios I would be asking questions to elicit any symptoms associated with dysfunction of the brain. These symptoms can be summarised as follows:

Symptoms of raised ICP: Any

1. Headache.
2. Nausea and vomiting.
3. Blurred vision.

Higher mental functions symptoms: Any problems with

1.   Alertness.
2.   Speech.
3.   Memory.
4.   Intellect.

Cranial nerves symptoms: Any problems with

1.   Senses of smell, vision, or hearing.
2.   Swallowing or voice change.
3.   Balance.
4.   Any vertigo or tinnitus.
5.   Facial weakness, twitching or altered sensation.

Motor functions symptoms: Any

1.   Weakness.
2.   Rigidity.
3.   Slowness.
4.   Stiffness.
5.   Tremor.
6.   Abnormal movements.

Sensory function symptoms:

1.   Any lack of or abnormal sensation anywhere in the body.

Other symptoms:

1.   Neck stiffness.
2.   Photophobia.
3.   Sphincter disturbance.

Step 3: *Ask questions about the cardinal symptoms of other systems that are likely to be affected by or implicated in the causation of the diagnosis under consideration.* For example if I am dealing with a patient likely to have suffered from cerebral infract (stroke) then I would ask questions about the cardiovascular system that is likely to be the source of thrombo-embolism: I would ask about palpitations, chest pain, ankle swelling, and shortness of breath. On the other hand if my patient had difficulty swallowing because of a stroke or tumor in the brain stem then I would be

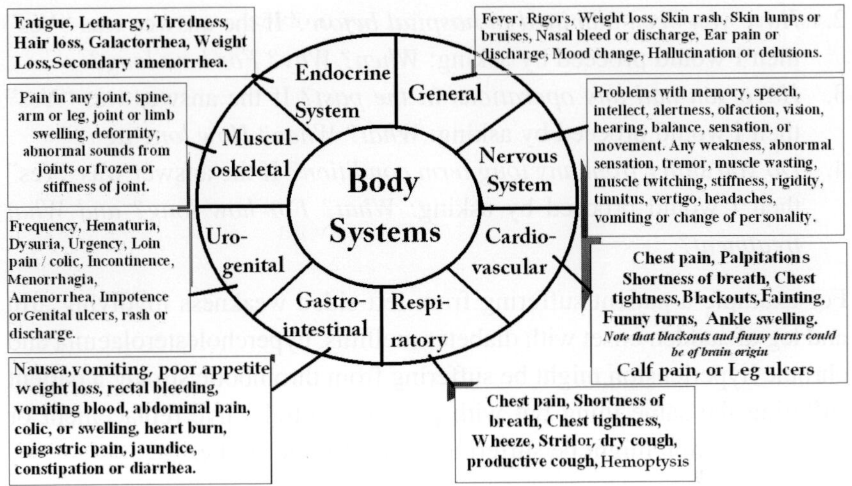

This list is not inclusive of every symptom patients bring to their doctors. You are advised to update this list as you progress in your career.

Figure 1-2: The circle of systemic review.

asking questions about the respiratory system to find out if the patient had aspirated: I would ask about cough, chest pain, and shortness of breath. A full list of the cardinal symptoms of all the body systems is listed in Figure 1-2. Imagine that the systems of the body were organised in a circle, if you start the circle at one point and follow the circle around in one direction (clockwise or anticlockwise), you will finish in the same point you have started from, without forgetting any system. Remember that the duty of care of a doctor goes beyond providing a diagnosis, treatment and prognosis. Doctors are also responsible for early detection, screening and prevention of disease as well as health promotion. The purpose of systematic systemic review is to not only narrow down the diagnosis, but is also to fulfil the doctor's obligations to patients and the community in terms of health promotion, disease prevention and early detection.

Step 4: *Elicit past history. Past history often clinches the diagnosis.* I use the following simple four opening questions:

1. *Have you had any similar symptoms in the past?* If the answer was "Yes" then I would proceed by asking: *Where? How often? How long ago?*

2. *Have you been admitted to hospital before?* If the answer was "Yes" then I would proceed by asking: *When? Why? For how long?*
3. *Have you had any operations in the past?* If the answer was "Yes" then I would proceed by asking: *What? When? How long ago?*
4. *Do you suffer from any long term condition?* If the answer was "Yes" then I would proceed by asking: *What? For how long? and What treatment?*

For example a patient suffering from left-sided weakness involving arm and leg of sudden onset with diabetes mellitus, hypercholesterolaemia and chronic hypertension might be suffering from thrombotic stroke; a patient suffering the same thing but with previous mitral valve replacement or atrial fibrillation might be suffering from embolic stroke.

Step 5: *Take drug history: Are you on any medications?* Is a very good question to start with, if the answer was "Yes" then I would proceed by asking: *What drug? What dose? How often? For how long? Who prescribed it?* For example, a patient coming in with gradual slowly progressive left-sided weakness associated with headaches and was on anticoagulants might be suffering from subdural haematoma.

Step 6: *Take family history.* Because certain diseases can run in families and may have a genetic aetiology, doctors need to explore any family history of diabetes mellitus, hypertension, strokes, heart attacks, angina, asthma or epilepsy. Some patients might go away with the wrong idea that these illnesses are transmissible or contagious and they need an explanation that they are not. I use the following questions to open this section with patients:

Did you or any of your family members suffer from chronic illness? This question combines past history with family history and saves time during history gathering. Similarly the question: *Did you or any member of your family suffer from the following illnesses: diabetes, asthma, etc.?* will save time by combining past and family histories together. It is important to explain to the patient what you mean by members of family. You are looking for family history in the patient's parents, children, brothers, sisters, grandparents, uncles and aunts, not in partners or distant relatives (Figure 1-3).

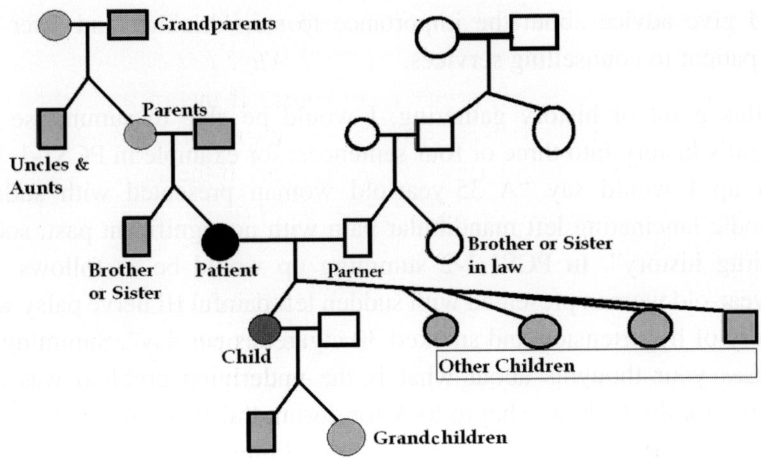

Figure 1-3: Drawing of relevant family history: illnesses in the shaded family tree of the patient are relevant, while in the unshaded is not.

Step 7: *Elicit social history. The main purpose of this section is health promotion and screening. The two main areas you wish to cover under this section are smoking and alcohol consumption. Exploring patient's lifestyles might be useful in diagnosis and management.* For example a chronic smoking patient coming with symptoms and signs of raised ICP and cough might be suffering from metastatic lung cancer in the brain. I often use the following opening questions in this section:

1. *Did you or anybody in your household smoke?* If the answer was "No", or (s)he had stopped smoking. I would use positive rein-forcement and say "Well done! That is really good for you". If the answer was "Yes", then I would ask: *How often? For how long?* Followed by: *Have you considered giving up smoking?* and direct the patient to where help for smoking cessation can be found. If the patient had stopped smoking I explore how long ago did he smoke, as that might be relevant, for example if the patient no longer smokes but had smoked heavily for 20 years, is very relevant to disease causation.

2. *Do you drink alcohol?* If the answer was "Yes", I would ask: *How much? For how long?* If I encounter an excessive drinking patient,

I give advice about the importance to stop drinking and refer the patient to counselling services.

At this point of history gathering, I would be able to summarise the patient's history into three or four sentences: for example in PCS1-1-1 to sum up I would say "A 35-year-old woman presented with sudden episodic lancinating left mandibular pain with no significant past, social or drug history". In PCS1-1-2 summing up would be as follows: "A 35-year-old woman presented with sudden left painful III nerve palsy with history of hypertension and smoked 30 cigarettes per day". Summing up focuses your thoughts about what is the underlying problem was and makes you think about what to look for during the physical examination.

Review questions:

1- What does a patient want from the healthcare provider?
   a. Diagnosis.
   b. Reassurance.
   c. Treatment.
2- What are the five basic questions in history taking?
   a. Where exactly the symptom (location)?
   b. How did it start (mode of onset)?
   c. How long it has been there for (duration)?
   d. What happened to it since it started (course)?
   e. Apart from this symptoms above, anything else?
3- What are the obligations of the healthcare provider?
   a. Make a diagnosis.
   b. Discuss all treatment options that apply to them.
   c. Inform patients if you do not know what is wrong with them.
   d. Involve the patient in the decision process.
   e. Health screening.
   f. Early diagnosis.
   g. Health promotion.

Your personal notes:

....
....
....
....
....
....
....
....
....
....

Problem 1-2:   How to elicit neurological signs effectively, demonstrate them with confidence and make a lasting impression. (The smart way of performing neurological physical examination 1)

The purpose of physical examination is to elicit clinical signs of the disease to reach or narrow down the diagnosis, order appropriate investigations, reassure the patient, and provide appropriate treatment, advice and follow-up. Smart physical examination

Problem based tool box:	
GCS	Speech assessment
MMSE	Intellect assessment
Order of physical examination	

is based on smart history. Smart physical examination will not replace or substitute poor history and vice versa. A confident clinician makes a lasting impression when (s)he performs physical examination based on smart history and performs it with confidence. Confidence can only be achieved by practice and practice (***Practice makes perfect***), so every moment and every patient in hospital wards is an educational opportunity, so practice by examining patients over and over again. Patients are your best teachers and nothing can replace or substitute this experience.

Common sense dictates that physical examination should proceed in the following order:

- *Examine the organ affected by the disease first.* It does not make any sense to the patient if the presenting complaint was left arm weakness and the doctor starts to examine the cranial nerves. Although it is essential to examine the cranial nerves at some point, it makes more sense to start the examination with the left arm first for two reasons:

  o By examining the organ or area complained of first, the doctor is in effect telling the patient that (s)he had been listened to.
  o Patients are more likely to be more cooperative and finish the examination when they know that attention was given to the organ complained of at the outset of the examination. Patients are at their best at the beginning of the physical examination.

- *Examine the system affected or implicated in the disease immediately after examining the organ affected.* In the left arm weakness case scenario I would examine the nervous system after I had examined the left arm.

- *Examine the system or systems that are more likely to be affected or implicated in the disease process next.* For example in the left arm weakness scenario I would examine the musculo-skeletal system after I had examined the left arm and the nervous system. In someone who complained of swallowing difficulty, I would examine the back of the throat and neck first, followed by the cranial nerves, the nervous system, the respiratory system, cardiovascular system and so on.

- *Examine the rest of body systems for early detection of disease, screening, or possibly detection of the source of the disease. In the case of systemic infection to detect the focus of primary infection or in the case of cancer by discovering the site of the primary cancer.*

- *Examination should begin with* **observation***, followed by* **palpation** *and then by* **special bedside tests***.* The LFT principle: Look-Feel-Test. Look before you feel, and feel before you perform special tests. For example in someone presenting with leg pain, I would observe the patient's posture, and legs looking for signs of severe pain, muscle spasm, muscle wasting or fasciculation looking for signs of severe pain, so I would be very careful not to cause more pain during the rest of physical examination.

The nervous system examination can be divided into the following sets:

1- Higher mental functions examination.
2- Cranial nerves examination.
3- Motor functions examination.
4- Sensory functions examination.
5- Other neurological signs.

1-2-1 Higher mental functions examination (HMF):

It makes a lot of sense to determine the patient's higher mental functions from the outset of any consultation, even before taking the history because impairment of consciousness, speech or memory significantly affect the conduct of history and physical examination. For example, confused patients, patients with memory problems or dysphasic patients would not be able to provide a reliable history and their physical examination needs to be modified to take account of these deficits. HMF examination includes examination of:

  i- Conscious level.
 ii- Speech and language.
iii- Memory.
iv- Intelligence.
 v- Handedness.

1-2-1i- *Assessment of level of consciousness:*

Level of consciousness is assessed at the bedside by the Glasgow Coma Scale (GCS). The GCS consists of observing the patient's responses to verbal or painful stimulation. Three responses are observed: Best Eye Opening Response (BEOR), Best Verbal Response (BVR) and Best Motor Response (BMR).

a- *Best Eye Opening Response (BEOR):*
There are four possible BEOR in any patient: 1 = no eye opening to any stimulus, 2 = eye opening to painful stimuli, 3 = eye opening to verbal stimuli, and 4 = eye opening spontaneously (Table 1-1). One drawback of the BEOR assessment is that it cannot be assessed in patients who have bilateral complete III nerve palsies or bilateral orbital haematomas. In these patients, the BEOR should be recorded as "C" for closed eyes rather than "1" for no BEOR. In patients who have either of these abnormalities in one eye only, the response of the better eye should be recorded for the purpose of level of consciousness assessment.

b- *Best Verbal Response (BVR):*
There are five possible responses under BVR: 1 = no verbal response to any stimulus, 2 = incomprehensible sounds, 3 = uttering words, 4 = confused, and 5 = oriented in time, place and person. It would not be possible to assess BVR in patients who are dysphasic and it should be recorded as "D" for dysphasia rather than "1" for no BVR. Similarly patients who are

Table 1-1: The Glasgow Coma Scale (GCS)

Score	BEOR	BVR	BMR	Definitions
1	None	None	None	Any patient within these shaded areas is in **COMA.**
2	To speech	Sounds	Extension to pain	
3	To pain	Words	Abnormal flexion to pain	
4	Spontaneous	Confused	Flexion to pain	
5		Orientated	Localising pain	
6			Obeys simple commands	Not in coma

artificially ventilated via endotracheal tube or tracheotomy cannot be assessed for BVR and it should be recorded as "T" for tube rather than "1" for no BVR (Table 1-1).

c- *Best Motor Response (BMR):*

There are six possible responses within this category: 1 = no motor response to any stimulus, 2 = extension to pain, 3 = abnormal flexion to pain, 4 = flexion to pain, 5 = localising pain, and 6 = obeying simple commands (Table 1-1). It would not be easy to assess BMR in patients with spinal cord injury leading to tetraplegia although if they can obey simple commands, BMR can be assessed by observing motor responses in the face area, e.g. closing the eyes or showing the tongue. If the BMR could not be assessed because of paralysis of the limbs due to injury or because of sedative or muscle relaxant drugs, the BMR should be recorded as "P" for paralysis rather than "1" for no BMR.

Coma is defined on the GCS as any patient who fulfils all the following three criteria: 1- no eye opening response to any stimulus (score of 1 only), 2- no comprehensible sound (score of 1 or 2) and 3- not obeying simple commands (score of 1 to 5). Therefore coma is GCS of 8 or less provided that the patient does not obey commands, does not utter any words and does not open eyes to any stimulus.

Although each response of the GCS carries a number against it, the aggregated numbers should not be used to describe patients as that leads to avoidable misunderstandings and misinterpretations of the numbers. For example a GCS of 8 could mean a patient with BEOR1,

BVR2 and BMR5 (patient is comatose) or it could mean BEO2, BVR3 and BMR3 (patient is not comatose). It would be far better to use the actual description of the patient's response in each category rather than the numbers. Aggregate numbers are useful in determining trends of progress and to perform statistical analysis in research and audit studies.

1-2-1ia *How to assess the BEOR?*

Observe the patient, if at least one eye is open without stimulation, then BEOR is spontaneous (BEOR4), if at least one eye opens only in response to speech, then the BEOR is to speech or drowsy (BEOR3), if both eyes remain closed despite verbal stimuli but at least one eye opens to painful stimulus then BEOR is open to pain (BEOR2) and if there is no BEOR to pain the BEOR is none (BEOR1). There are two ways to assess responses to pain:

1. By exerting pressure on the supra-orbital nerve by putting the thumb parallel to the eye brow, feel the supra-orbital notch and exert pressure (Figure 1-4),

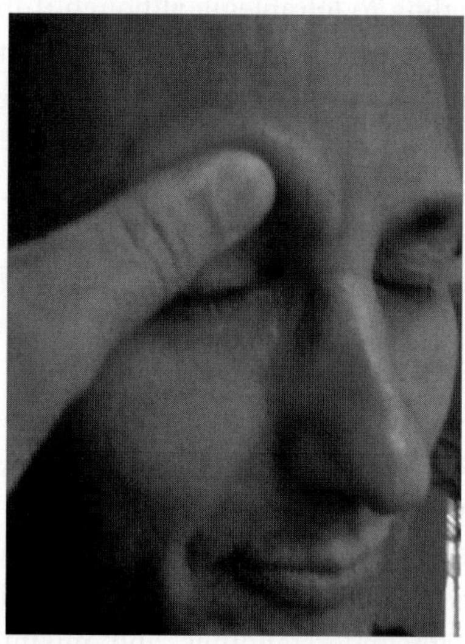

Figure 1-4: Eyebrow painful stimulus.

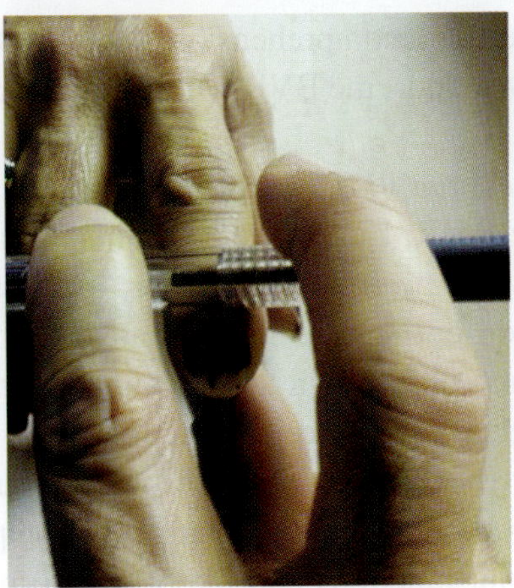

Figure 1-5: Nail bed painful stimulus.

2. By exerting pressure on the nail bed of any of the fingers using a pencil or a pen (Figure 1-5). The supra-orbital location is the preferred option as it makes the distinction of the BMR easier.

1-2-1ib *How to assess the BVR:*

To assess the BVR, I start by asking the patient the following simple questions to assess orientation in place and time: *Where are you right now? What sort of place are you in? What city are you in? And what country are you in?* If the patient could answer correctly at least two of these questions, i.e. named hospital, and city or city and country or hospital and country, then the patient is oriented in place. Then I would ask the patient: *What day of the week is today? What month of the year is it? What year is it?* If the patient got at least two of these correct (day and month, month and year or day and year) then the patient is oriented in time. If the patient was oriented in time and place their BVR is oriented (BVR5). If the patient was disoriented in place and time, but was speaking in sentences that does not make sense, then the patient is confused (BVR4). However, you have to be careful in situations where the patient has suffered from speech difficulty, particularly nominal dysphasia or aphasia. If the patient was only uttering words, then the patient is uttering words only (BVR3). If the patient was uttering sounds only and was unable to say any words then the BVR is uttering incomprehensible sounds (BVR2). If the patient was not uttering any sounds, the BVR will be no verbal response (BVR1).

1-2-1ic *How to assess the BMR:*
When assessing the BMR, I use simple commands such as: *Squeeze my fingers please, show me your tongue please, or close your eyes please.* Simple commands do not require sophisticated brain processes to carry them out and patients can perform these commands even in the presence of cognitive or higher executive dysfunctions. On the other hand the command: *Show me your little finger of the right hand please, or put your right ring finger in your left ear please,* are very complex commands that demand higher mental functions and likely to fail in patients who were fully conscious but had significant cognitive impairment. If the patient was unable to obey simple commands, then the next stage is to simulate the patient with pain as described under BEOR. By stimulating the supra-orbital nerve, the patient should be able to bring his hand up towards the stimulus to remove it. If the hand came to a level above the chin level, the BMR would be localising pain (BMR5), if the hand flexed but did not reach the level of the chin then the BMR would be flexion to pain (BMR4), if the elbow flexed, the shoulder extended and the forearm pronated then the BMR would be abnormal flexion to pain (BMR3), if the upper limb extends at shoulder and elbow and pronated then the BMR would be extension to pain (BMR2), and if there was no motor response to pain then the BMR would be none (BMR1). Figure 1-6 demonstrated the BMR from 1 to 5.

1-2-1ii- *How to assess speech and language?*

Assessment of speech should include assessments of speech perception primarily controlled in the angular gyrus of the dominant parietal lobe and speech expression primarily controlled in the frontal opercula of the dominant hemisphere (Broca's area). From the aforementioned history gathering and assessment of conscious level, one would have a good idea of whether the patient understands and expresses speech, and if the patient was fully oriented by answering the questions appropriately. If the patient was unable to respond appropriately to questions during history taking

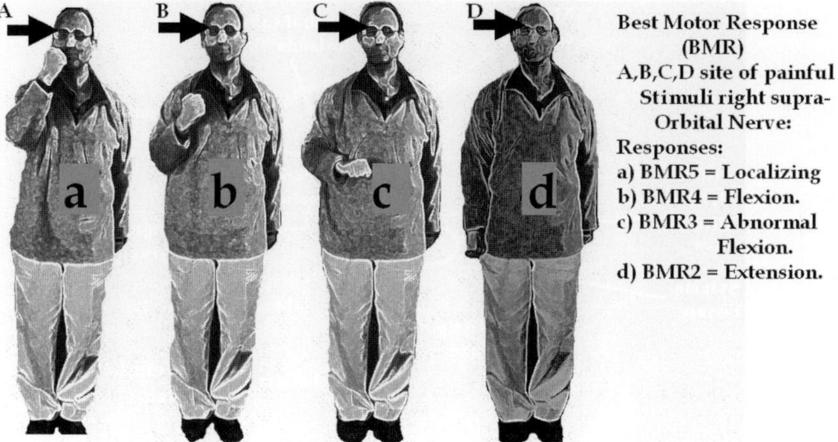

Figure 1-6: BMR to painful stimulus at the supra-orbital notch in patients not obeying simple commands.

and consciousness level assessment, then the doctor should evaluate the speech in more detail to make sure that there was no speech impairment leading to this difficulty. Simple questions such as: *What is your name? Where are you? What day of the week is it? How old are you? And how are you?*, are often sufficient to determine if the patient understands speech. In those patients who are unable to speak, one can assess understanding of speech by asking the patient to perform simple tasks, e.g. *show me your tongue, close your eyes or squeeze my hand.* If the patient was unable to understand speech altogether, the reasons could be that the patient was unable to understand the language, had receptive dysphasia or mute. *Mutism* can occur in bilateral subfrontal pathology, *receptive dysphasia* can occur due to damage of the angular gyrus on the dominant parietal lobe (*Wernike's dysphasia*) and patients who merely do not speak the language often respond in their mother tongue. If the patient can understand speech but seems to be confused or unable to respond appropriately in a verbal manner, the doctor needs to evaluate speech expression in more detail. This can be evaluated by showing the patient several objects and asking the patient to name them, e.g. *show a pen, a tie, a watch, a buckle, a strap, a spoon and a fork.* If the patient was unable to speak at all but seems to understand the language, then the

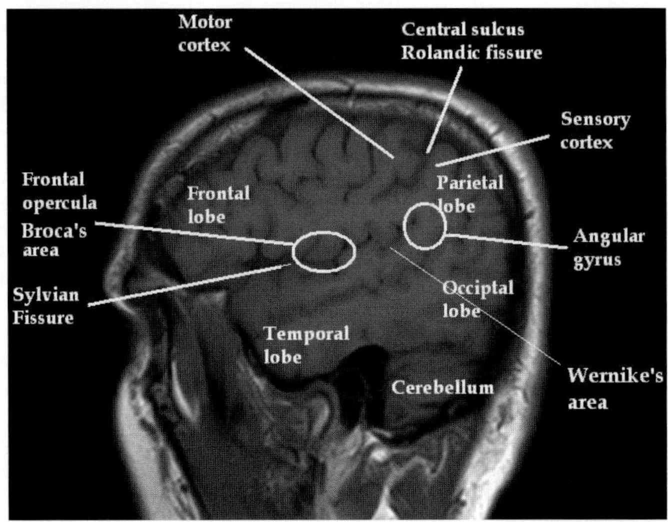

Figure 1-7: Dominant cerebral hemisphere cortex.

patient has an *expressive aphasic*. On the other hand if the patient was able to speak but unable to name objects correctly then the patient had *nominal dysphasia*. Junior clinicians often confuse nominal dysphasia with confusion, the difference is that confused patients are able to name objects presented to them, while patients with nominal dysphasia cannot (Figure 1-7).

Assessment of language should include reading and writing. Reading can be assessed by asking the patient to read simple sentences e.g. carrying a written request such as *close your eyes* or reading a written sentence aloud. Writing can be assessed by asking the patient to write his (her) name and address.

1-2-1iii- *How to assess memory?*

Memory can be divided into short- and long-term. Short-term memory includes remembering recent events and recall, and it is the most vulnerable memory after brain injury or disease. Long-term memory is more resistant to insults. Memory requires the functions of the limbic system particularly the fornix and the medial temporal structures, the hippocampus and parahippocampus. Memories can also be divided into verbal and visual memories. For simple bedside assessment of memory I often use the following questions for long-term memory: *What is your name? When were you born? What is your address or where do you live? Or factual knowledge that the patient is expected to know, e.g. date of wedding if married, names of the children if they had any, etc.*

Short-term memory assessment can be performed by giving the patient the names of three items *(spoon, ball and car)* and asking the patient to repeat them *(assessment of immediate recall)*, and asking the patient to repeat the same words after five minutes or so *(recall)* and asking patients simple questions about recent events, e.g. *When did they come to hospital? How did they come into hospital? What did they have for dinner, breakfast, etc?* A more thorough evaluation of verbal and visual memories could be performed by more sophisticated tests. For example, patients with subtle memory deficits and those who are worked up for temporal lobe surgery are examined by experts to assess their verbal and visual memories in detail.

1-2-1iv *How to assess intelligence?*

Intellect and IQ can be assessed by very sophisticated tests that are designed to assess IQ. A normal IQ should be a score of 70 or above. However, at the bedside a simple screening test such as the subtraction of 7s from 100 or spelling the word "*world*" backwards would suffice. An average patient would be able to subtract 7s from 100 fairly quickly by saying "100, 93, 86, 79, 72, 65, 58, 51…" and so on or spell the word "world" backwards as "D-L-R-O-W". Problems with calculation and spelling may indicate problems with memory, recall or pathology in the dominant parietal lobe. When dyscalculia is associated with finger agnosia and dygraphia it is said that the patient suffers from Gerstmann's syndrome and that the lesion is located in the dominant parietal lobe.[1] On the other hand a lesion in the non-dominant parietal lobe leads to disorientation in space and loss of body image.[2]

Orientation, registration, attention, concentration, recall and language can be assessed at the bedside using the mini-mental state examination (MMSE). Normal individuals score 30/30 on this scale (Appendix I).

1-2-1v *How to assess handedness?*

Assessment of handedness is very important to differentiate dominant from non-dominant hemispheric lesions. Handedness is dictated by the dominant hemisphere. In the vast majority of people, the left hemisphere is dominant.[3] To determine which hand is dominant simply ask the patient: *Are you right or left handed?* Most patients would know. If however the patient does not know, you can ask the following questions: *Which hand do you use to write? Which hand do you use to hold a knife and cut your food? Or which foot do you use to kick a football?*

Your personal notes:

....

....

....

....

....

....

....

....

....

....

Problem 1-3: How to examine the first two cranial nerves efficiently, with confidence and make a lasting impression. (The smart way of performing neurological physical examination 2)

There are 12 cranial nerves that need to be examined. To be able to examine cranial nerves effectively the doctor needs to know what each nerve does, where each cranial nerve originates from and its course from origin to destination. Knowing these anatomical and physiological facts will help the doctor localise pathological processes more precisely.

> **Problem based tool box:**
>
> **How to assess VA and CV?**
>
> **How to perform VF? Fundoscopy?**
>
> **How to examine olfaction?**
>
> **How to localise visual pathway lesion?**

1-3-1 *Where does each cranial nerve originate from?*

I use a simple formula to remind myself where each cranial nerve arises from: 2C + 2MB = 4P + 4MO. This means that the first two cranial nerves [Olfactory (I = 1st) and Optic (II = 2nd) nerves] originate in the cerebrum, the next two [Oculomotor (III = 3rd) and Trochlear (IV = 4th)] cranial nerves arise from the midbrain, the next four [Trigeminal (V = 5th), Abducens (VI = 6th), Facial (VII = 7th) and Vestibulocochlear (VIII = 8th)] cranial nerves arise from the pons and the last four [Glossopharyngeal (IX = 9th), Vagus (X = 10th), Accessory (XI = 11th) and Hypoglossal (XII = 12th)] cranial nerves arise from the medulla oblongata.

1-3-2 *What are the special features and functions of each nerve?*

I- The first cranial nerve (Olfactory nerve):
The olfactory nerve is responsible for the sense of smell, its tiny nerve fibres pass through the cribriform plate to reach the olfactory pulp on each side. Because of this fact the olfactory nerve is very susceptible at the cribriform plate to injury in anterior skull base fractures.

Symptoms:

Olfactory nerve dysfunction manifests as lack of smell (anosmia). Abnormal sensation of smell does not arise from olfactory nerve dysfunction; it originates from the temporal lobe in psychogenic seizures. Some patients with olfactory nerve dysfunction may also present with change in their taste.

1-3-2i *How to examine the first cranial nerve?*

The sense of smell can be assessed by asking patients directly if there were any problems with their sense of smell and can be confirmed by examining each nerve independently by closing one nostril at a time and asking the patient to identify the aroma of coffee, tea, an apple, cloves, or perfume.
Examination of the olfactory nerve is the most commonly omitted part of cranial nerves' examination by junior clinicians. It is however essential to assess the sense of smell in every patient requiring neurological examination because it could be the only abnormal physical sign in patients with olfactory groove meningiomas or after head injuries. Loss of sense of smell carries significant implications to patients as they would not be able to detect dangerous smells, e.g. gas leak at home and they need to be made aware of their deficit to take extra precautions.

II- The second cranial nerve (Optic nerve):
The optic nerve is responsible for vision; the optic nerve enters the orbit through the optic canal making it susceptible to compression in this region. The medial (nasal) fibres cross over in the optic chiasm. Therefore a lesion in the optic chiasm leads to bitemporal hemianopia. Some of these nasal fibres loop forwards within the distal contralateral optic nerve. As a result of this anatomical feature, a pure lesion of one optic nerve may lead to junctional scotoma in the opposite visual field. The temporal fibres of one optic nerve and the nasal fibres of the contralateral optic nerve join behind the chiasm to form the optic tract that loops around the ipsilateral cerebral peduncle and just underneath the ipsilateral globus pallidus internal (Gpi), thus over-stimulation of the Gpi may produce flashing lights in

both eyes in patients with pallidal deep brain stimulators. The optic tract in turn ends into the ipsilateral lateral geniculate body (LGB) of the thalamus before forming the optic radiation. The optic radiation is mainly located in the ipsilateral parietal lobe, except for Meyer's loop which loops anteriorly into the ipsilateral temporal lobe. The optic radiation finishes in the visual cortex in the ipsilateral occipital lobe. The visual cortex serving the central vision (the macula) has a dual blood supply and lesions in the occipital lobe often spare the macula (central vision).

What are the symptoms of optic nerve dysfunction?
The most common symptoms related to optic nerve dysfunction are *blurred vision caused by optic nerve swelling, transient obscuration of vision arising from transient ischaemic neuropathy (Amaurosis fugax), loss of vision due to visual field (VF) deficit, visual hallucinations: colours originate from the occipital lobe while well formed images originate from the temporal lobe, pain on eye movements in retrobulbar optic neuritis, and photopsia, photophobia and loss of colour vision.*

1-3-2ii *How can I localise a lesion along the visual pathways?*

The most useful test to locate the exact location of a lesion along the visual pathways is accurate and thorough VF examination:

1- VF loss in one eye means the lesion is located in the anterior segment of the optic nerve or the eye itself, *e.g. glaucoma in one eye, optic neuritis in one eye, ischaemic optic neuropathy in one eye, central retinal artery occlusion in one eye, central retinal vein occlusion in one eye, retinal detachment in one eye, or compressive optic neuropathy due to sphenoid wing meningioma (Figure 1-8, Lesions 1 and 2).*

2- VF loss involving the whole VF in one eye and junctional scotoma in the other eye means the lesion is affecting the posterior segment of the optic nerve such as that due to compressive optic neuropathy (Figure 1-8, Lesion 3).

3- Lateral chiasm lesion will cause ipsilateral nasal VF defect (Figure 1-8, Lesion 10).

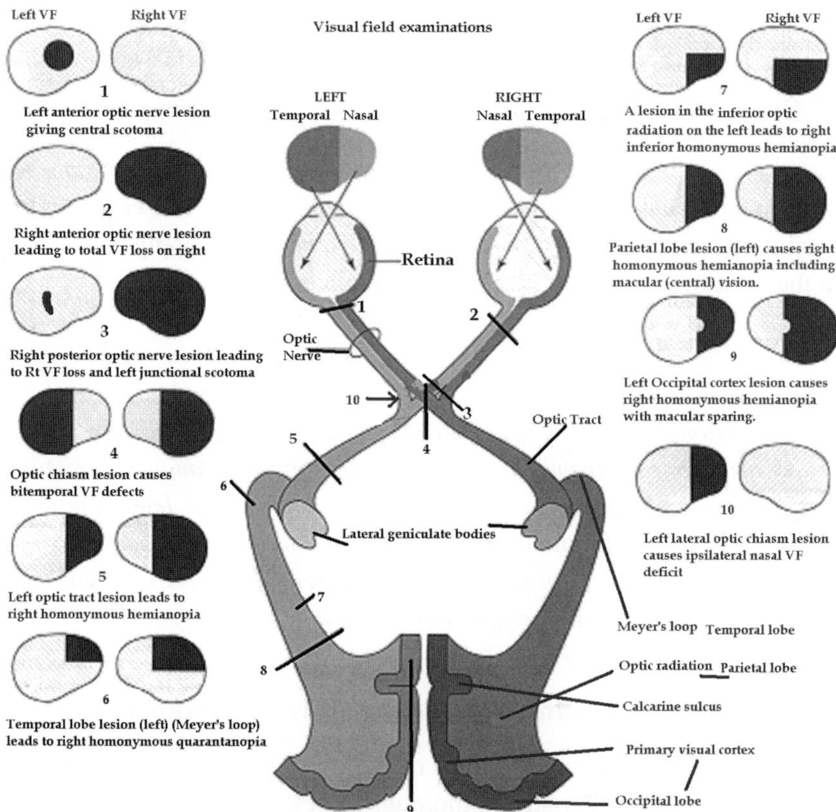

Figure 1-8: The visual pathways and visual field defects.

4- VF defect in both eyes means the lesion is located in the chiasm or behind the chiasm as follows:

 a. *Bitemporal VF defect means an optic chiasm compression from pituitary adenoma, craniopharyngioma, suprasellar meningioma, aneurysm or similar lesions in the same location (Figure 1-8, Lesion 4).*

 b. *Homonymous VF defect means the lesion lies behind the optic chiasm contralateral to the side of the VF, i.e. left sided homonymous*

VF defect means a lesion in the right visual pathways behind the optic chiasm:

i.   *Homonymous superior quadrantanopia means a lesion in the contralateral posterior temporal lobe involving Meyer's loop, sometimes described as pie in the sky (Figure 1-8, Lesion 6).*

ii. *Homonymous hemianopia without macular sparing means a lesion in the contralateral optic tract or contralateral parietal lobe (Figure 1-8, Lesions 5 and 8).*

iii. *Homonymous hemianopia sparing the central vision means a lesion in the contralateral occipital lobe (Figure 1-8, Lesion 9).*

iv. *Some parietal lobe lesions may cause contralateral homonymous inferior quadrantanopia (Figure 1-8, Lesion 7).*

1-3-2iii *How to examine the optic nerve?*

Examination of the optic nerve is not complete unless the visual acuity (VA), colour vision (CV), visual field (VF) and fundoscopy are performed. VA is assessed using Snellen's chart for distant vision and for near vision by using reading charts. CV is assessed by using Ischihara plates (Figures 1-9a and 1-9b) to detect colour blindness. VFs are

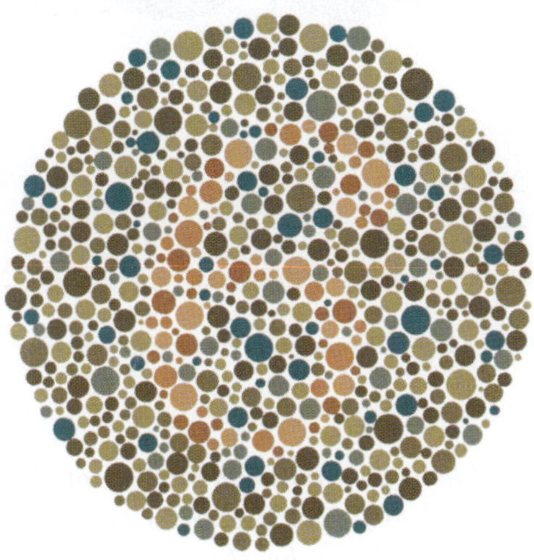

Figure 1-9a: Ischihara Plate 1 (normal patients should be able to read the number 6).

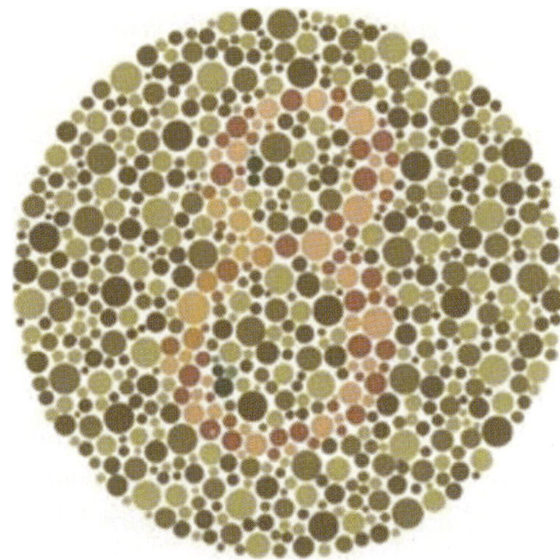

Figure 1-9b: *Ischihara Plate 2 (normal patients should be able to read the number 8, colour-blind patients may read this plate as 3).*

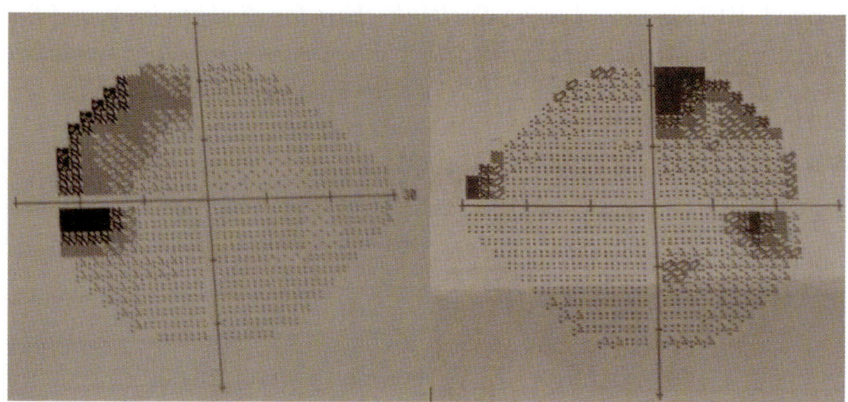

Figure 1-10: *Perimetery VF examination results.*

assessed at the bedside by confrontation method and by perimetery such as Goldman's (Figure 1-10). Fundoscopy is performed by direct oph-thalmoscopy at the bedside or by slit lamp examination in the eye department.

1-3-2iv *How to assess vision?*

VA: distant VA should be examined without and with corrective glasses and expressed as 6/6 (normal = the patient could see what a normal individual could see at 6 feet) or 20/20 (normal = the patient could see what a normal person could see at 20 metres). 6/12 means that a patient could see at 6 feet what a normal person could see at 12 feet and 10/20 means a patient could see at 10 metres what a normal individual could see at 20 metres. Near vision is assessed with and without reading glasses and is expressed as N5, N4 etc. where the N represents the size of font the patient could read.

CV: assessment of colour vision is important as many conditions affecting the retina and optic nerves could affect colour vision. Similarly patients with X-linked colour blindness would not be able to differentiate between green and red.

1-3-2v *How to assess VF with confrontation?*

To assess the patient's VF at the bedside, the confrontation method is used. The most common way of testing VF is to seat the patient on a chair and the doctor sits in front of the patient at an arm's length (50–60 cm away). I ask the patient to close one eye and look at the tip of my nose, I close my opposite eye, i.e. if the patient was asked to close his (her) left eye, I close my right eye and vice versa. I also focus on the patient's tip of the nose. I outstretch my left arm half way between the patient and myself and instruct the patient to keep looking at the tip of my nose while I bring my wiggling fingers from laterally to medially asking the patient to indicate when (s)he spots my moving fingers. I examine the four quadrants individually and compare the patient's VF with mine using my left hand to examine the temporal VF of the patient's right eye and compare it to my left temporal VF and I use my right hand to compare the patient's left nasal VF with my right nasal VF. I examine the other eye's VF in a similar fashion then examine both eyes at the same time to detect any visual inattention that can arise in parietal lobe lesions. You may use a pin with white head instead of fingers to test VF and if the pin head is small you could detect any significant scotomas and any enlarged blind spot. Using a red head pin helps the VF examination of central vision (Macular vision or colour vision). Remember that if the VA is poor VF examination would not be reliable.

1-3-2vi *How to perform fundoscopy?*

Direct fundoscopy requires the use of an ophthalmoscope. To perform direct ophthalmoscopy without dilating the pupils you need to seat the patient in a chair so that if possible you can access both sides, darken the room as much as possible, ask the patient to focus on a distant object and avoid looking into the light. These simple measures allow the pupil to dilate enough allowing direct ophthalmoscopy to be performed without eye drops. I carry out ophthalmoscopy in a systematic fashion as follows and use it to perform both ophthalmoscopy and examine the eyes themselves:

A normal fundus appearance to demonstrated in Figure 1-11.

1- I start with detecting the red reflex. From a 30–40 cm distance the pupil should appear red in an eye with clear media (cornea, lens and vitreous). If the pupil is black and the red reflex is absent then you cannot look at the retina. Absent red reflex could be due to: corneal opacity, exudates or pus in the anterior chamber, cataract, vitreous opacity or haemorrhage.

2- I then examine the anterior media starting with convex lens of 10d and examine the cornea, the anterior chamber, the iris, the lens and then the vitreous.

3- I then examine the optic disc systematically: disc margin (disc margins will be blurred in papilloedema and secondary optic atrophy), optic cup (this will be lost in papilloedema and enlarged in glaucoma), optic disc colour (this will be pale in optic atrophy), and optic disc swelling (this will be present in papilloedema and papillitis).

4- I then examine the retinal vessels: venous pulsations will be absent and the veins will be engorged in papilloedema. The arteries may show silver lining, nipping or atheroma in patients with chronic hypertension. Neovascularisation may be present in retinopathy.

5- I then examine the rest of the retina looking for:

   a. Haemorrhages in the subhyaloid layer (in subarachnoid haemorrhage), and splinter haemorrhages in hypertension.

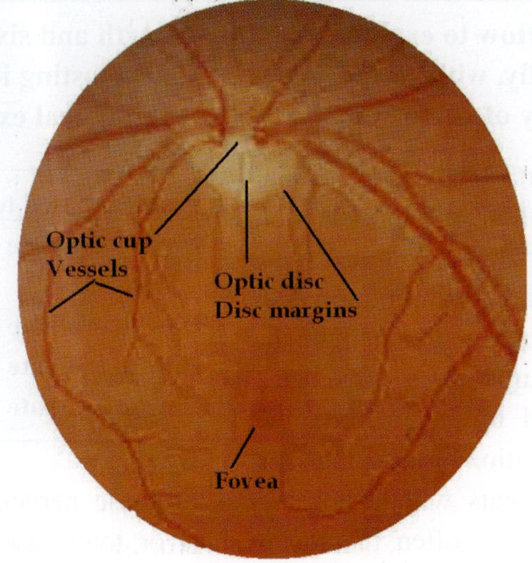

Figure 1-11: Photograph of a fundus demonstrating normal optic disc.

b. Exudates in hypertension and diabetes mellitus.
c. Other abnormalities such as nevus, pigmentation, pallor, or detachment.

Your personal notes:

....
....
....
....
....
....
....
....
....
....

Problem 1-4: How to examine the third, fourth and sixth cranial nerves efficiently, with confidence and make a lasting impression. (The smart way of performing neurological physical examination 3)

The third, fourth and sixth cranial nerves control eye movements. During undergraduate examinations, and postgraduate examinations in neurology, general medicine, ophthalmology and neurosurgery, candidates are often asked to demonstrate the physical examination of these muscles

> **Problem based tool box:**
> **How to examine eye**
>   **movements?**
> **How to evaluate diplopia?**
> **How to evaluate the pupils?**
> **How to evaluate ptosis?**

and nerves. Patients with abnormalities of these nerves are loved by examiners and they often feature as short or long cases during these assessments. Therefore mastering the physical examination of these nerves not only helps in the evaluation and diagnosis of patients but it is also helpful during these examinations.

III- The third cranial nerve (Oculomotor):
The third cranial nerve consists of somatic motor fibres and parasympathetic fibres. It innervates all the extra-ocular muscles except the lateral rectus and the superior oblique muscles. It supplies the superior, inferior and medial rectus muscles, and the inferior oblique muscle. It also supplies the majority of the elevator muscle of the superior eyelid. The third nerve parasympathetic fibres supply the constrictor muscles of the pupil and the ciliary muscle. Therefore complete third nerve palsy manifests with ipsilateral: ptosis, diplopia and dilated fixed pupil. The double vision is present in all directions of gaze. The two images are separated widely on looking laterally to the opposite side of third nerve palsy and the images come nearer to each other in lateral gaze to the same side as the palsy. The diplopia is not crossed, i.e. the right image belongs to the right eye and the images are side by side with slight tilt (Figure 1-12).

Where does the third nerve originate?
The third nerve originates in the midbrain (remember the formula 2C + 2MB = 4P + 4MO). It has two nuclei: the motor and the parasympathetic

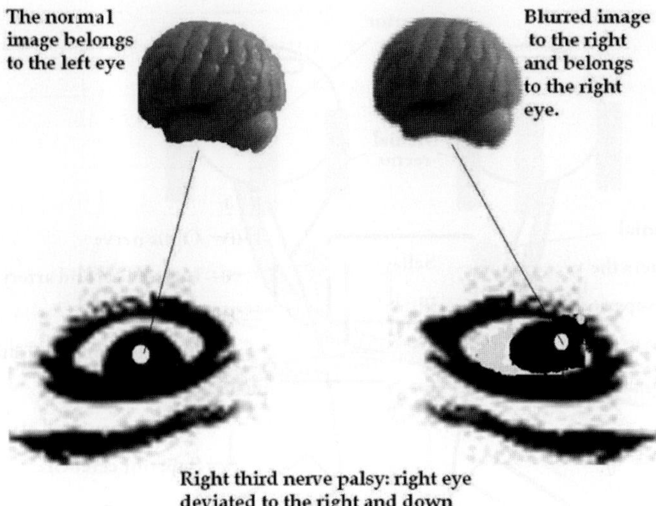

Figure 1-12: Uncrossed diplopia in third nerve palsy.

(Edinger Westphal) nuclei (Figure 1-13). The important anatomical locations where the third nerve is susceptible to compression that help localise the site of the lesion are summarised in Figure 1-13.

These sites include:

1- The superior orbital fissure: leading to complete ophthalmoplegia and ophthalmic trigeminal neuropathy as the third, fourth and sixth and the ophthalmic division of the trigeminal nerve (V1) enter the orbit via superior orbital fissure. Tumours either primary or secondary are primary causes of third nerve palsy at this location. In bigger and extensive tumours this syndrome can be associated with proptosis or compressive optic neuropathy.

2- The cavernous sinus (CS): the third nerve passes in the lateral wall of the CS together with the fourth nerve and ophthalmic (V1) and the maxillary (V2) divisions of the trigeminal nerve. So a CS syndrome leads to complete ophthalmoplegia associated with trigeminal nerve dysfunction in V1 and V2, and often proptosis due to obstruction of venous drainage of the orbit. The eye may be pulsatile and red in carotid-cavernous fistula (CCF).

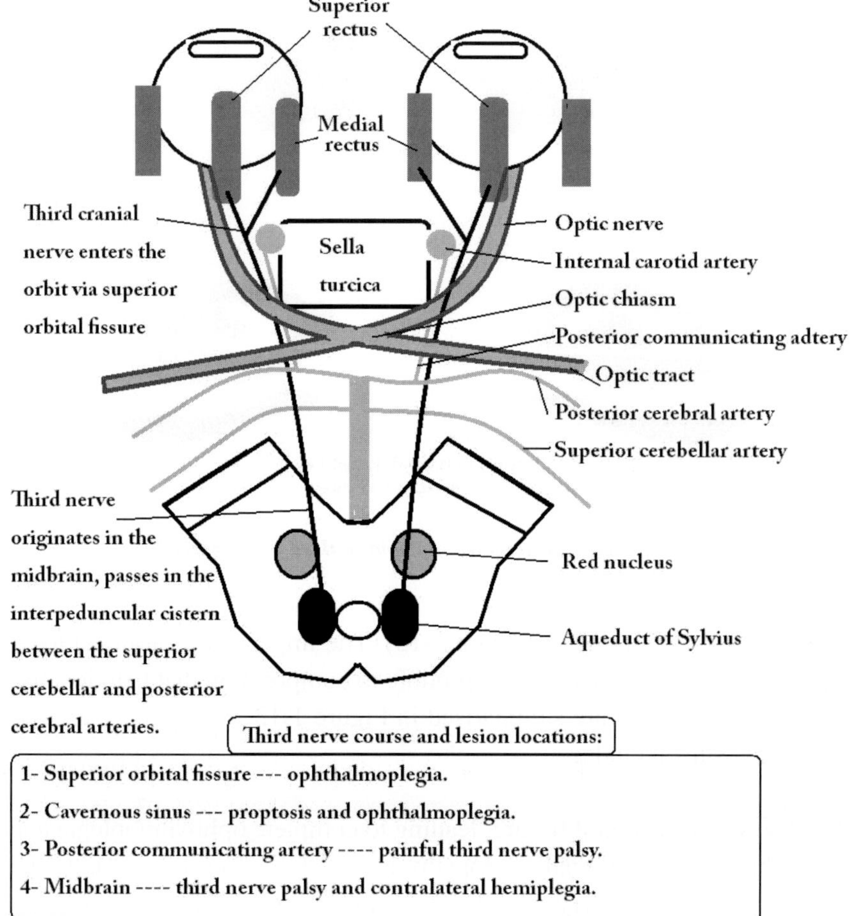

Figure 1-13: The course of the third nerve.

3-	The tentorial edge: the third nerve passes underneath the uncus of the temporal lobe near the tentorial edge and is often compressed by the herniated uncus during transtentorial herniation. Third nerve palsy is a true localising sign in raised ICP, meaning that any expanding lesion causing uncal herniation is located on the same side as the third nerve palsy. If the transtentorial herniation was severe it eventually pushes the contralateral cerebral peduncle against the contralateral tentorial edge leading to hemiparesis on the same side as the third nerve palsy (the hemiparesis is a false localising sign).

4- The posterior communicating artery (PComA) origin: the third nerve passes very close to the PComA origin from the internal carotid artery (ICA). Expanding PComA aneurysms are one of the commonest causes of painful third nerve palsy.

5- The interpeduncular cistern (IPC): the third nerve passes between the posterior cerebral artery (PCA) superiorly and the superior cerebellar artery (SCA) inferiorly in the IPC. An aneurysm of the SCA is a rare cause of third nerve palsy.

6- The midbrain: a lesion in the midbrain at the level of the third nerve nucleus leads to ipsilateral third nerve palsy and contralateral hemiparesis.

1-4-1 *How to examine the third nerve?*

i- Inspection may reveal ptosis, deviation of the eye laterally and downwards, and anisocorea (unequal pupils).

ii- Extra-ocular muscle movement examination (EOMME):

EOMME can be performed by manually opening the closed eye, asking the patient to focus on an object held at 30–40 cm in front of the patient, and asking if one or two images of the object are seen. If the patient can only see one image, ask the patient to let you know as soon as two images are seen. If the patient can see two images, ask the patient to describe the images. One image is usually clear and the other image less clear, in third nerve palsy the images are side by side. Ask the patient to describe when the images come together or further apart as you move the object in the directions of gaze. In third nerve palsy the images come closer together as you move the object laterally on the side of third nerve palsy and further apart as you move the object laterally on the contralateral side. I first move the object laterally to the far right then straight up and down while the right eye is abducted. Then I move the object horizontally to the far left and move the object up and down from that position. The value of this technique is the examination of each extra-ocular muscle individually (Figure 1-14).

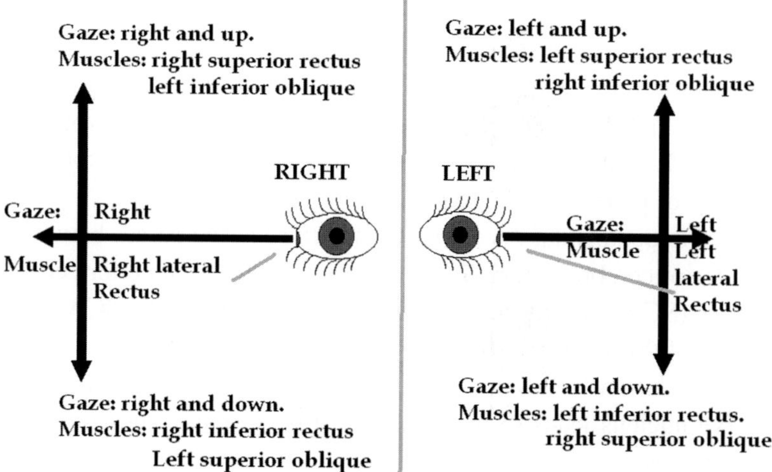

Figure 1-14: Schematic representation of extra-ocular muscle movements.

iii- Cover-uncover test:

When I discover that a patient has a squint or a strabismus (eye deviation with or without diplopia) I perform the Hirschberg test using a penlight to determine the type and degree of strabismus, the cross-over test to reveal latent as well as manifest strabismus and the cover-uncover test which reveals latent strabismus.

a) Hirschberg test: using a small penlight torch, direct the light to the eyes and ask the patient to look at it and observe the reflection of light in the eyes. Normal eyes with no strabismus show the reflection of the light in the centre of the pupils. Any deviation of more than one degree is considered abnormal.

b) Cross-over test: using the same light use an occluder to transfer from one eye to the other without interval and observe if the exposed eye moves. This will reveal any obvious or latent strabismus.

c) Cover-uncover test: in this test you cover and uncover the same eye sequentially and observe the eye as it moves in and out if strabismus was present (Figure 1-15).

These three tests are performed in that order.

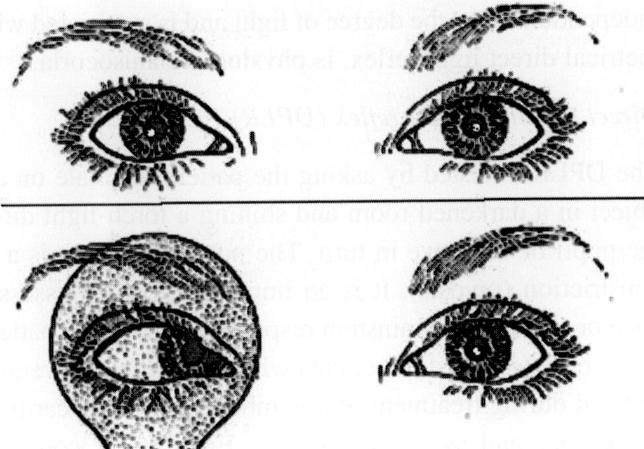

Figure 1-15: Demonstration of the cover-uncover test: top eye demonstrates that the light reflection of the right eye is lateral to mid pupil and once the eye is covered the eye deviates inwards (bottom set of eyes). Once the cover is removed the right eye moves out to return to previous position (top set of eyes).

iv- Examination of the pupils:

Examination of the pupils is essential in each patient. Normal pupils should be equal and reactive to light and accommodation (PERLA). Pupils must be studied by evaluating their size, shape, symmetry and activity (dilation and constriction).

1- *Evaluation of the size of the pupils:*

To evaluate size and symmetry of pupils, patients are asked to fixate on a faraway object to prevent the near reflex. The object must not be a light source to avoid the light reflex effect. Subsequently, the patient's face is illuminated from below with a weak light source, both pupils are simultaneously observed and their diameters are determined (in mm).

Normal pupils tend to be smaller in children, the elderly and subjects with dark iris. As a rule of thumb, anisocoria (unequal pupils) which change with changes of light conditions must be considered pathologic, while anisocoria which remains constant, independent from the degree of light and is associated with a symmetrical direct light reflex, is physiologic anisocoria.

2-   *Direct pupillary light reflex (DPLR):*

The DPLR is tested by asking the patient to fixate on a faraway object in a darkened room and shining a torch-light directly into the pupil of each eye in turn. The normal reaction is a pupillary constriction (myosis). It is an important test for assessing presence or absence of brainstem response in comatose patients and it is the only test used in patients who are artificially ventilated and sedated during treatment of a number of nervous, cardiovascular, respiratory and systemic diseases. Each reflex consists of five components: **stimulus, afferent, centre, efferent** and **effecter**. The stimulus in the DPLR is the light, the afferent is the ipsilateral optic nerve, the centre of the reflex is located in the tectum of midbrain at the level of the superior colliculus, the efferent is the ipsilateral third nerve and the effecter is the pupillary constrictor muscles (Figure 1-16). Normal pupils should constrict at the same speed and to the same extent unless there is a relative afferent pupillary defect (RAPD) due to visual impairment on the side of the sluggish pupil.

If neither pupil constricts to light the patient might be blind, has bilateral third nerve palsies, has damage of the midbrain or has paralysis of the constrictor muscles due instillation of mydriatic eye-drops.

3-   *Indirect pupillary light reflex or consensual light reflex (CPLR):*

To test the CPLR, light is shone in one eye and the pupil reaction of the other eye is observed. Normal pupils constrict when the light is shone in the other eye. The stimulus of this reflex is the light, the afferent is the ipsilateral optic nerve, the centre is the tectum of the midbrain, the efferent is the contralateral third nerve and effecter is the pupillary constrictors of the contralateral pupil (Figure 1-16).

If the reflex arc is intact, the DPLR must be equal to the CPLR (due to the double decussating pupillary fibres in the midbrain as well as the decussation of the nasal visual fibres in the

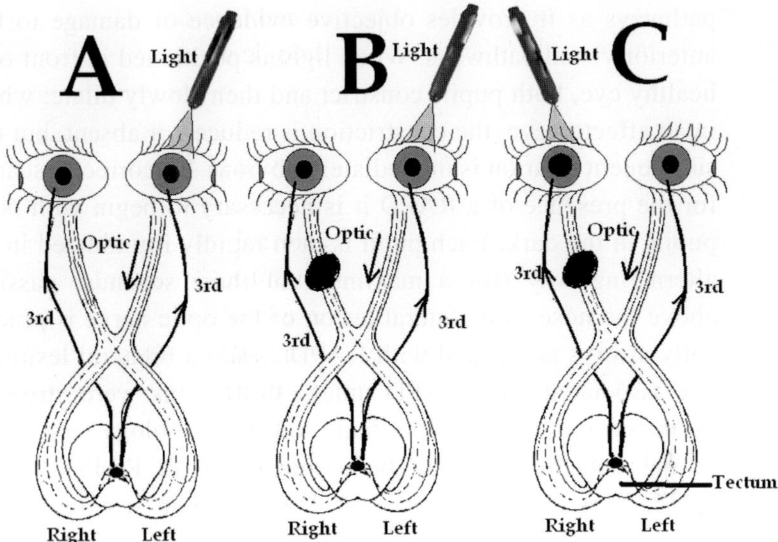

Figure 1-16: Diagram demonstrating the DPLR and CPLR arcs. A = Normal DPLR and CPLR in both eyes; B = normal CPLR in the right eye and normal DPLR in the left eye; C = normal CPLR in the left eye and absent DPLR in the right eye.

optic chiasm). The amplitude, latency and speed of pupillary constriction after a light stimulus are generally correlated to the visual acuity of the patient, except in cases in which the visual defects are secondary to a circumscribed foveal lesion or a bilateral cerebral lesion above the LGB (parietal, or occipital), in which pupillary activity is normal.

4- *Near pupillary reflex (NPR):*

The NPR is analysed by asking the patient to fixate on a faraway object and then to fixate on a near object positioned in front of the nose. Normal pupils constrict symmetrically and both eyes converge.

5- *Evaluation of relative afferent pupillary defect (RAPD):*

The presence of a relative afferent pupillary reflex (RAPD) is one of the most important signs in the assessment of visual pathways as it provides objective evidence of damage to the anterior visual pathways. When light is positioned in front of a healthy eye, both pupils constrict and then slowly dilate; while in an affected eye, the constriction is reduced or absent, but the subsequent dilation is immediately obvious. To correctly search for the presence of a RAPD it is necessary to begin with both pupils in the dark. Each pupil is then rapidly illuminated in an alternating way (for a maximum of three seconds) passing above the nose. A unilateral lesion of the optic nerve is practically always associated with RAPD, while a bilateral lesion is not associated with RAPD unless the lesions were strongly asymmetrical. On the other hand, retinal pathology (e.g. large retinal detachment) may be associated with RAPD. Slight RAPD may be present in some large macular lesions and in cases of amblyopia. It is generally not present in acute papilloedema, severe refractive defects, cataract, non-organic visual loss, and cerebral lesions.

Examination of the pupils is very helpful in diagnosis and management of patients (Table 1-2). Dissociation of light pupillary reflexes and NPR indicates the presence of midbrain pathology (Parinaud's syndrome, Argyll-Robertson's pupil) or the involvement of postganglionic parasympathetic fibres (Adie's tonic pupil).

Table 1-2: Pupillary signs and their interpretation

| Pupils' sizes | Pupillary reactions | | Conclusions |
	Right	Left	
Equal	Reactive	Reactive	Intact arc, normal
	Large fixed	Large fixed	Blindness, bilateral third palsies
	Small fixed	Small fixed	Pontine haemorrhage
Unequal	Large fixed	Reactive	Right third palsy
Unequal	Absent DPLR and present CLR	Reactive	Right optic neuropathy

v- Assessment of ptosis:

Droopy eyelids are common in the old age and may involve one or both eyelids. The drooping appearance may be due to: true *"eyelid ptosis"*, *"excess eyelid skin"*, *"brow ptosis"*, *"contralateral eyelid retraction"*, *"enophthalmos"*(sunken eye) or, a combination of the above. The treatments for these various problems are different and it is essential to distinguish which of the contributing factors are present in each patient so that an appropriate diagnosis and management plan can be provided.

IV- The fourth nerve (Trochlear):

The trochlear nerve arises from the midbrain (2C + 2MB = 4P + 4MO). It is the only cranial nerve that emerges from the back of the brain stem. It passes anterior around the ipsilateral cerebral peduncle into the anterior edge of the tentorium in the lateral wall of the CS before entering the orbit through the superior orbital fissure. Its slender shape, long intracranial course and posterior exit from the midbrain make it susceptible to injuries. It is also involved in superior orbital fissure and cavernous sinus syndromes. The fourth nerve supplies only the superior oblique muscle that depresses the eyeball. The causes of fourth nerve palsy can be broadly classified as congenital or acquired. Isolated congenital fourth nerve palsies may be heralded by head-tilting to the opposite side of the affected nerve in early childhood. In others, a congenital palsy may go unnoticed because of a compensatory mechanism allowing for alignment of the eyes when focusing on an object. Isolated acquired trochlear nerve palsies can be the result of numerous disorders. In most cases an underlying cause cannot be found (idiopathic palsy). Due to its long course within the cranium, the fourth nerve is susceptible to injury following head trauma. Depending on the site of nerve compression during trauma one or both nerves may be affected. Aneurysms at the superior cerebellar artery[4] or brain tumours may directly compress or result in an increase of ICP resulting in fourth nerve palsies. Disorders such as myasthenia gravis, diabetes, meningitis, microvascular disease (atherosclerotic vascular disease) or any cause of raised ICP may result in trochlear nerve palsy. In patients with compensated fourth nerve palsy, the removal of a cataract may restore clear vision to both eyes allowing the patient to become aware of their double vision. A child with a congenital palsy may be found doing a head-tilt by his or her parents or relatives. Children will very rarely complain of double vision. Adults with a new onset fourth nerve palsy will note two images, one on top of the other or angled in position when both eyes are open. Covering one eye, no matter which one is covered, will resolve the diplopia. The double vision will worsen when looking down or away from the affected side. If both nerves are affected (s)he may experience a horizontal diplopia (two images side by side) when looking downward. If a decompensated palsy is suspected, one should review old photographs to document a pre-existing head-tilt to support the diagnosis. Diagnosing fourth nerve palsy is for the most part a clinical one. Careful history taking and examination is the key to diagnosis. The Bielchowsky head-tilt test is one commonly used and reliable technique to diagnose isolated trochlear nerve palsies. Review of patient's old photographs can prove indispensable in diagnosing a decompensated palsy, obviating the need for additional testing.[4]

VI- Sixth cranial nerve examination (Abducens):

The abducens nerve arises from the pons (2C + 2MB = 4P + 4MO). It passes anterior into the CS before entering the orbit through the superior orbital fissure. Its long intracranial course makes it susceptible to injuries. It is also involved in superior orbital fissure and cavernous sinus syndromes. The sixth nerve supplies only the lateral rectus muscle that abducts the eyeball. It causes diplopia in the lateral gaze. The diplopia is crossed where the left image belongs to the right eye and vice versa (Figure 1-17). Sixth nerve palsy is considered a false localising sign in head injuries and raised ICP, however lesions at the tip of the petrous temporal bone may result in sixth nerve palsy (*Gradenigo's syndrome – Appendix I*).[5]

Examination of conjugate eye movements:

Conjugate eye movements are a very important part of the extra-ocular muscle assessment. These include examination of pursuit and saccade eye movements in addition to the aforementioned examination of third, fourth and sixth cranial nerves.

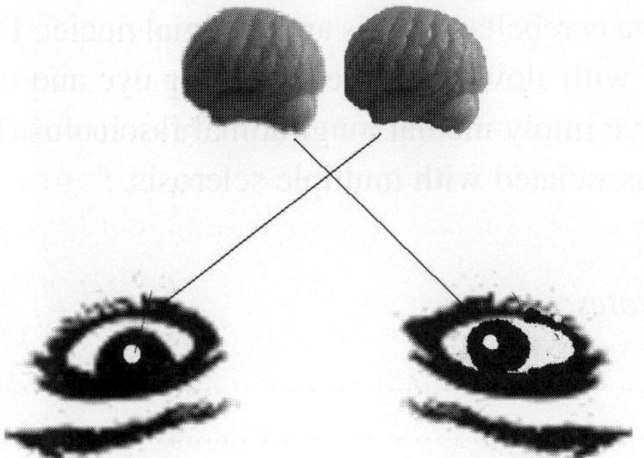

Figure 1-17: Sixth nerve palsy with crossed diplopia.

1- Smooth Pursuit eye movements:

The patient is asked to follow a finger as it is slowly moved to the left and to the right, and up and down. Make sure that the patient can see the finger clearly and do not exceed 60 degrees in total arc or 40 degrees per second. Normal eye tracking of a slowly moving discrete object generates a smooth eye movement that the examiner can easily see. Cerebellar or brain stem disease can cause saccadic eye tracking in which the patient repeatedly loses the target and then catches up with a small saccade. In most cases, abnormal pursuit is non-localising within the nervous system, although ipsilateral loss of pursuit can be ascribed to parietal lobe lesions.

2- Saccades eye movements:

The patient is asked to look back and forth between two outstretched fingers held about 12 inches apart in the horizontal and vertical plane. The latency of onset, speed, accuracy, and conjugate movement are observed. Saccadic eye movements are refixation movements that involve the frontal lobes (voluntary saccades), brain stem reticular formation (voluntary and involuntary saccades), and nuclei of third, fourth and sixth cranial nerves. Delayed saccades are seen in cortical and brainstem lesions, and slow saccades accompany brainstem disease. Inaccurate saccades (especially overshoots) are associated with lesions of the cerebellar vermis and fastigial nuclei. Dysconjugate eye movements with slowing of the adducting eye and overshoots of the abducting eye imply medial longitudinal fasciculus (MLF) pathology frequently associated with multiple sclerosis.

Your personal notes:

....

....

....

....

....

....

....

....

....

....

Problem 1-5:   How to examine the face (fifth and seventh cranial nerves) efficiently, with confidence and make a lasting impression. (The smart way of performing neurological physical examination 4)

The fifth cranial nerve (Trigeminal) is responsible for facial sensation and the seventh cranial nerve (Facial) is responsible for facial movements. During undergraduate examinations, and postgraduate examinations in neurology, general medicine, ophthalmology and neurosurgery candidates are often asked to demonstrate the

> **Problem based tool box:**
> **How to examine the face?**
> **How to examine the facial nerve?**
> **How to examine the fifth nerve?**

physical examination of the face. Patients with abnormalities of these nerves are loved by examiners and they often feature as short or long cases during these assessments. Therefore mastering this physical examination of these nerves not only helps in the evaluation and diagnosis of patients but is also helpful during these examinations.

V- The fifth cranial nerve (Trigeminal):

The fifth cranial nerve consists of somatic sensory and motor fibres. It innervates muscles of mastication (masseter, temporalis, medial and lateral pterygoids), tensor tympani, tensor veli palatini, mylohyoid and posterior belly of digastric muscle and is responsible for facial sensation. It consists of three divisions: ophthalmic (V1), maxillary (V2) and mandibular (V3).

1-5-1 *Where does the fifth nerve originate?*

The fifth nerve originates in the pons (remember the formula 2C + 2MB = 4P + 4MO). It has motor and sensory nuclei (Figure 1-18). The trigeminal sensory nucleus extends throughout the entire brainstem, from the midbrain to the medulla, and continues into the cervical cord, where it merges with dorsal horn cells of the spinal cord. The nucleus is divided anatomically into three parts. From caudal (Medulla) to rostral (Midbrain) they are the spinal trigeminal nucleus and tract (Descending Nucleus = DN),

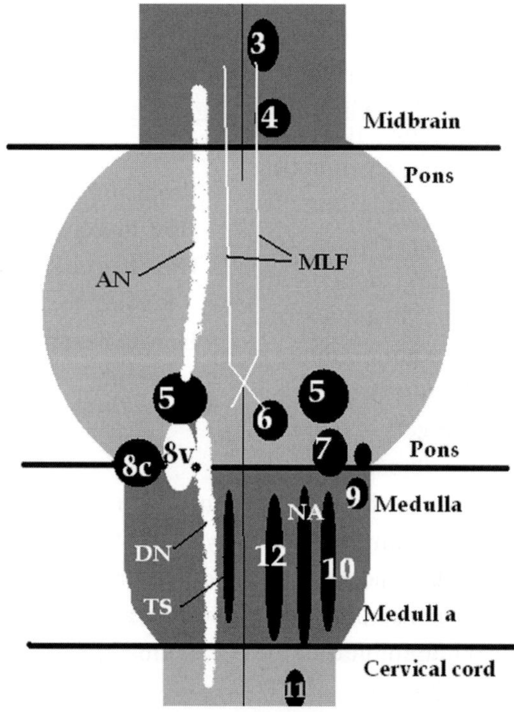

Figure 1-18: Cranial nerve nuclei in the brain stem: 3 = 3rd nerve nucleus, 4 = 4th nerve nucleus in midbrain, 5 = 5th nerve main nucleus with AN = ascending or mesencephalic 5th nerve nucleus and tract and DN = descending or spinal 5th nucleus and tract, 6 = sixth nerve, 8c = cochlear nucleus, 8v = vestibular nucleus, 9 = 9th nerve nucleus, 10 = 10th dorsal nucleus, 11 = accessory nucleus, 12 = hypoglossal nucleus, TS = tractus solitarius, NA = nucleus ambigious, and MLF = medial longitudinal fasciculus.

the main trigeminal nucleus,[5] and the mesencephalic trigeminal nucleus and tract (Ascending Nucleus = AN) (Figure 1-18).

The three parts of the trigeminal nucleus receive different types of sensory information. The spinal trigeminal (DN) nucleus receives pain/temperature fibres. The main trigeminal nucleus[5] receives touch/position fibres. The mesencephalic nucleus (AN) receives proprioception and mechanoreception fibres from the jaws and teeth. The spinal trigeminal nucleus contains a pain/temperature sensory map of the face and mouth. From the spinal trigeminal nucleus, secondary order neuron fibres cross the midline and ascend in the trigeminothalamic tract (TTT) to the contralateral thalamus. The TTT runs parallel to the spinothalamic tract (STT), which carries pain/temperature information from the rest of the body. Pain/temperature fibres are sent to thalamic nuclei. The central processing of pain/temperature information is markedly different from the central processing of touch/position information. Within the spinal trigeminal nucleus, information is represented in an onion skin fashion. The lowest levels of the nucleus (in the upper cervical cord and lower medulla) represent peripheral areas of the face (scalp, ears and chin). Higher levels (in the upper medulla) represent more central areas (nose, cheeks, lips). The highest levels (in the pons) represent the mouth, teeth, and pharyngeal cavity. The onion skin distribution is entirely different from the dermatome distribution of the peripheral branches of the fifth nerve. Lesions that destroy lower areas of the spinal trigeminal nucleus (but which spare higher areas) preserve pain/temperature sensation in the nose (V_1), upper lip (V_2) and mouth (V_3) while removing pain/temperature sensation from the forehead (V_1), cheeks (V_2) and chin (V_3). Analgesia in this distribution is "nonphysiologic" in the traditional sense, because it crosses over several dermatomes (Figure 1-19). Nevertheless, analgesia in exactly this distribution is found in humans after surgical sectioning of the spinal tract of the trigeminal nucleus. The spinal trigeminal nucleus sends pain/temperature information to the thalamus. It also sends information to the mesencephalon and the reticular formation of the brainstem. The

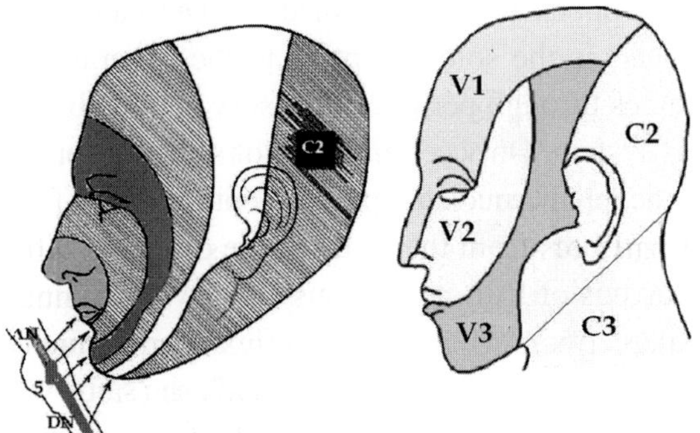

Figure 1-19: The onion ring map of facial sensation in the trigeminal nucleus in the brain stem and the V1, V2, V3 innervation of the face.

latter pathways are analogous to the spinomesencephalic and spinoreticular tracts of the spinal cord, which send pain/temperature information from the rest of the body to the same areas. The mesencephalon modulates painful input before it reaches the level of consciousness. The reticular formation is responsible for the automatic (unconscious) orientation of the body to painful stimuli. The main trigeminal nucleus represents touch/position sensation from the face. It is located in the pons, close to the entry site of the fifth nerve. Fibres carrying touch/position information from the face and mouth (via cranial nerves V, VII, IX, and X) are sent to the main trigeminal nucleus when they enter the brainstem. The main trigeminal nucleus contains a touch/position sensory map of the face and mouth, just as the spinal trigeminal nucleus contains a complete pain/temperature map. The main nucleus is analogous to the dorsal column nuclei (the gracile and cuneate nuclei) of the spinal cord, which contain a touch/position map of the rest of the body. From the main trigeminal nucleus, secondary fibres cross the midline and ascend in the trigeminal lemniscus to the contralateral thalamus. The trigeminal lemniscus runs parallel to the medial lemniscus, which carries touch/position information from the rest of the body to the thalamus. Some sensory information from the teeth and jaws is sent from the main trigeminal nucleus to the ipsilateral thalamus, via the small dorsal trigeminal tract. Thus touch/position information from the teeth and jaws is represented bilaterally in the thalamus (and hence in the cortex). The mesencephalic trigeminal nucleus (AN) is not really a "nucleus" it is a sensory ganglion (like the trigeminal ganglion) that happens to be imbedded in the brainstem. The mesencephalic "nucleus" is the sole exception to the general rule that sensory information passes through peripheral sensory ganglia before entering the central nervous system. Only certain types of sensory fibres have cell bodies in the mesencephalic nucleus: proprioception fibres from the jaw and mechanoreceptor fibres from the teeth. Some of these incoming fibres go to the motor nucleus of fifth nerve, thus entirely bypassing the pathways for conscious perception. The jaw jerk reflex is an example. Tapping the jaw elicits a reflex closure of the jaw, in exactly the same way that tapping the knee elicits a reflex kick of the leg. Other incoming fibres from the teeth and jaws go to the main nucleus of fifth nerve. This information is projected bilaterally to the thalamus. It is available for conscious perception. Activities like biting, chewing and swallowing require symmetrical, simultaneous coordination of both sides of the body. They are essentially automatic activities, to which we pay little conscious attention. They involve a sensory component (feedback about touch/position) that is processed at a largely unconscious level. The unusual anatomy of "mesencephalic fifth" has been found in all vertebrates, with the exception of lampreys and hagfishes. Lampreys and hagfishes are the only vertebrates without jaws. It is evident therefore, that information about biting, chewing and swallowing is singled out for special processing in the vertebrate brainstem, specifically in the mesencephalic nucleus.

1-5-2 *How to localise fifth nerve lesion?*

It is important to understand the common anatomical locations where the fifth nerve is susceptible to compression. Knowing these facts will help you localise the site of the lesion in clinical patient presentations.

1. The superior orbital fissure: leading to complete ophthalmoplegia and ophthalmic trigeminal (V1) neuropathy as the third, fourth, sixth and V1 enter the orbit via the superior orbital fissure. Primary or secondary tumours are the main causes of fifth nerve palsies at this location. In bigger and extensive tumours, this syndrome can be associated with proptosis or compressive optic neuropathy.
2. The cavernous sinus (CS): V1 and V2 pass in the lateral wall of the CS together with the third and fourth cranial nerves. So a CS syndrome leads to complete ophthalmoplegia associated with trigeminal nerve dysfunction in V1 and V2, and often proptosis due to obstruction of venous drainage of the orbit. The eye may be pulsatile and red in carotid-cavernous fistula (CCF).
3. Foramen ovale: where the sensory V3 enters and the motor V3 exits the skull base. Skull base tumours are the most common cause of V3 neuropathy at this location.
4. Meckel's cave: where the sensory trigeminal ganglion is located and the most common causes of lesions at this location are benign tumours in the form of meningioma or schwannoma leading to sensory impairment in all three divisions.

5. The cerebellopontiane angle (CPA): where the fifth nerve lies superior and can be affected in acoustic neuroma, CPA meningioma, epidermoid cyst and other tumours.
6. The root entry zone at the fifth nerve junction with the pons: compression at this location most often due to vascular compression leading to trigeminal neuralgia.
7. In the pons: leading to trigeminal neuropathy and contralateral hemiparesis, usually due to a cavernoma, arteriovenous malformation (AVM) or ischaemia.
8. In the medulla: causes loss of pain and temperature sensation in the face and the contralateral part of the body (*Wallenberg syndrome*).

1-5-3 How to examine the fifth nerve?

i- Test light touch in the three divisions of the trigeminal nerve using light cotton wisp. If the face is hairy avoid using stroke movements and use light touch only.
ii- Test for pain using sharp pin such as neurotip (Figure 1-20). The neurotip had two ends: blunt and sharp ends. Ask the patient to close his/her eyes and randomly test by the blunt and sharp ends of the neurotip. If the patient can identify the sharp end correctly each time then the patient had no impairment of pin prick (PP). Test all the divisions individually and systematically. If you find an area of impaired sensation, chart it by testing from abnormal to normal.
iii- Corneal reflex: the corneal reflex is an important reflex protects against corneal abrasions. The stimulus is light touch, the afferent is V1, the centre is in the pons, the efferent is facial nerve and the

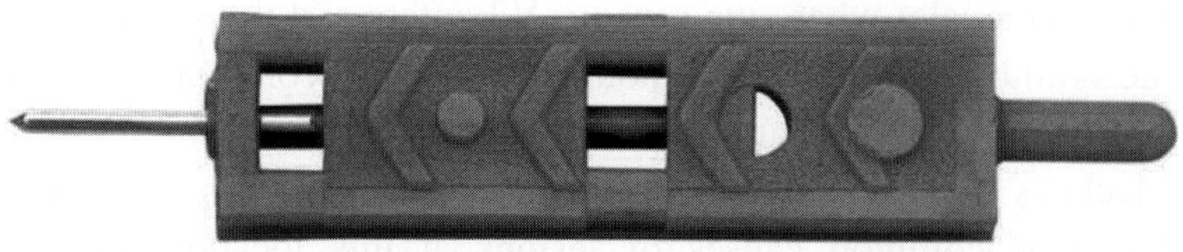

Figure 1-20: Neurotip used to test pin prick sensation (left end sharp and the right end is blunt).

effecter is the orbicularis oculi. Ask the patient to stare at a far object, use a wisp of sterile cotton, approach the eye from the lateral side to avoid the menace reflex (the menace reflex uses the optic nerve as afferent and is used to distinguish true blindness from functional visual symptoms), touch the cornea lightly, normal response leads to sudden closure of the eye.

iv- Test the strength of muscles of mastication by asking the patient to close the lower jaw tightly and feel the masseter and temporalis muscles, ask the patient to move the jaw from side to side against resistance to test the power of the pterygoids and to open the jaw against resistance to test the jaw openers.

VII- The seventh cranial nerve (Facial):

The seventh cranial nerve consists of somatic motor and gustatory fibres. It innervates muscles of facial expression, stapedius muscle and taste sensation from the anterior two thirds of the tongue. The taste sensation is carried by the chorda tympani that joins V3, passes in the middle ear, joins the facial in the facial canal in the temporal bone and finally as the nervus intermedius.

1-5-4 *Where does the seventh nerve originate?*

The seventh nerve originates in the pons (remember the formula 2C + 2MB = 4P + 4MO). It has motor and gustatory nuclei (Figure 1-21). The facial nucleus is located in the anterior part of the pons, its fibres pass posterior in the pons and loop around the sixth nerve nucleus before passing forward in the pons and exiting anterior towards the internal auditory meatus (IAM) through the CPA. In the IAM it joins the cochlear, and the superior and inferior vestibular nerves (Figure 1-21).

The relationship of the seventh and eighth nerves at the IAM is very important during surgery at this region. The seventh nerve occupies the anterior superior quadrant, the cochlear occupies the anterior inferior quadrant, the superior vestibular occupies the posterior superior quadrant and the inferior vestibular nerve occupies the posterior inferior quadrant (Figure 1-22).

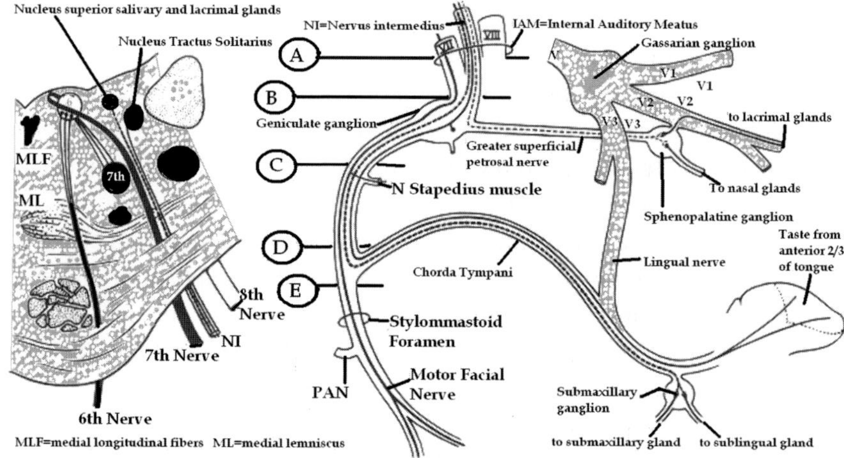

Figure 1-21: The course of the facial nerve and localisation of lesions (PAN =posterior auricular nerve, MLF = medial longitudinal fasciculus, ML = medial lemniscus, NI = nervus intermedius).

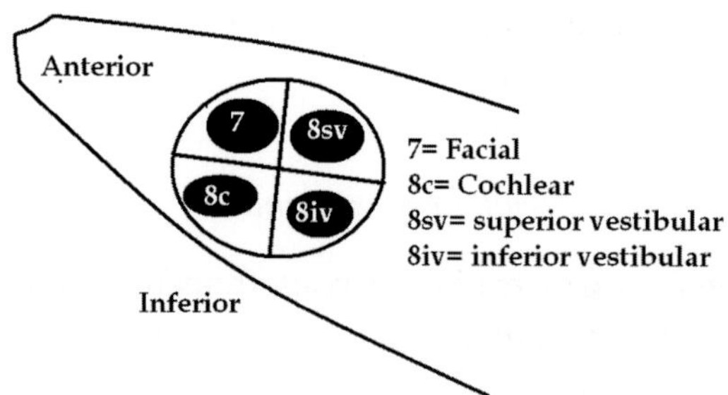

Figure 1-22: Schematic representation of the IAM and its contents.

The principal muscles supplied by the facial nerve are the frontalis, orbicularis oculi, buccinator, orbicularis oris, platysma, the posterior belly of the digastric muscle, and the stapedius muscle. In nuclear or infranuclear ("peripheral") lesions (lower motor neuron lesion = LMN), there is a partial to complete facial paralysis with smoothing of the brow, open eye, flat nasolabial fold, and drooping of the mouth ipsilateral to the lesion. Supranuclear ("central") lesions (upper motor neuron lesion = UMN) spares the eyebrow and eyelid musculature; there is flattening of the nasolabial fold and drooping of the mouth contralateral to the lesion. This distinction of LMN from UMN is very important as that will help localise the pathology. For example in a patient presenting with facial weakness that spares the upper half of the face (UMN) is more likely to be due to a lesion above the pons, and a patient presenting with a lesion involving all the face is likely to have a lesion in the pons outwards towards the face. The secretory and vasomotor fibres of the facial nerve go to the lachrymal gland, the mucous membranes of the nose and mouth, and the submandibular and sublingual salivary glands, and cutaneous sensory to the external auditory meatus and the region at the back of the ear. Abnormalities of taste include *ageusia* (lack of taste); *hypogeusia* (diminished taste acuity); and *dysgeusia* (unpleasant, obnoxious, or perverted taste).

1-5-5 *How to examine the seventh nerve?*

Careful and thoughtful observation is the key to discerning subtle signs of facial weakness. Note the blink, the nasolabial folds, and the corners of the mouth. Any asymmetry is the clue to unilateral facial weakness and is best perceived during conversation when the patient is unaware of being observed.

a. The blink reflex: The eyelid on the affected side closes just a trace later than the opposite eyelid.
b. The nasolabial folds: The weak one is flatter.
c. The mouth: The affected side droops and participates manifestly less in speaking.
d. Ask the patient to look up or wrinkle the forehead; inspect for asymmetry.
e. Ask the patient to close the eyes tightly. Look for incomplete closure or incomplete "burying" of the eyelashes on the affected side. Observe the nasolabial folds and mouth while the patient is concentrating on the eyes. As the orbicularis oculi contract tightly, there are milder associated contractions of muscles about the mouth and nose; these milder contractions are better suited to displaying slight weakness than when these muscles are tested directly.

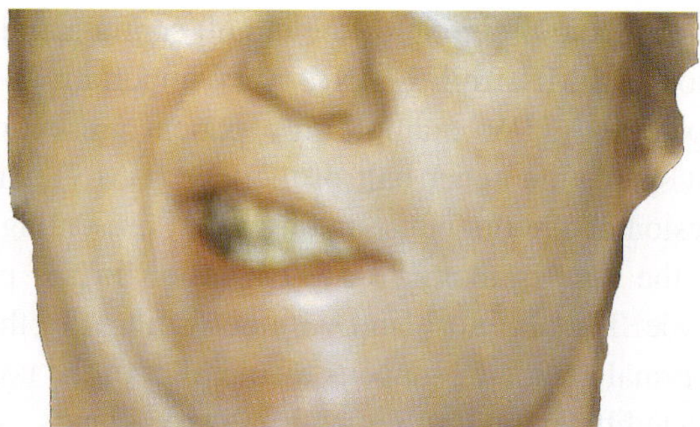

Figure 1-23: Photograph of right facial nerve palsy, demonstrating drooping of the side of the mouth.

f.   Ask the patient to smile or to show his/her teeth. Look for asymmetry about the mouth (Figure 1-23).

g.   The most subtle signs of mild facial weakness are the blink reflex and incomplete lid closure. Observe the blink reflex during conversation, or tap gently on the glabella with your index finger or reflex hammer in an attempt to bring out a mild asymmetry of blink.

h.   If you strongly suspect but are having difficulty confirming a mild facial weakness, ask the patient to lie flat on the examination couch with face up. Slide the patient's head off the examination couch so the head is below the body. This forces the eyelids to work against gravity. Now ask the patient to close both eyes and inspect for incomplete closure. Tap on the glabella and note asymmetry of the blink reflex.

i.   *Test for taste*: The four primary tastes are bitter, sweet, sour, and salty. Screen for disorders of sweet or salty taste with salt and sugar. With the patient's eyes closed and tongue protruded, take a tongue spatula and smear a small amount of salt or sugar on the lateral surface and side of the tongue. Instruct the patient to tell you the identity of the substance. Rinse the mouth thoroughly and repeat the test on the other side, using a different substance.

j.   Facial nerve reflexes:

   i. *Corneal reflex*: Stimulation of the cornea with a wisp of cotton produces reflex closure of both ipsilateral (strongest) and contralateral eyelids. The fifth nerve carries the afferent impulses and the facial nerve the efferent impulses.

ii. *Glabellar reflex*: Tapping the glabella leads to both eyes to close, with the contralateral response being weaker. The trigeminal nerve is the afferent side and the facial nerve the efferent side of the reflex. Light and sound can also produce the reflex, with the optic and acoustic nerves providing the afferent side. The response is weak or abolished in LMN facial weakness, present or exaggerated in UMN lesions, and exaggerated in Parkinsonism and cannot be voluntarily inhibited.

iii. *Palpebral-oculogyric reflex and Bell's phenomenon*: The eyeballs deviate upward when the eyes are closed, when awake and asleep. The afferent arc is proprioception carried through the seventh nerve to the medial longitudinal fasciculus (MLF). The third nerve to the superior rectus muscles forms the efferent side. In peripheral and nuclear lesions an exaggeration of this reflex is known as Bell's phenomenon.

iv. *Orbicularis oris reflex*: Percussion on the side of the nose or the upper lip causes ipsilateral elevation of the angle of the mouth and upper lip. The reflex arc is composed of the fifth and seventh nerves. Synonyms: nasomental, buccal, oral, or perioral reflex. This reflex disappears after about the first year of life, recurring with supranuclear facial nerve lesions and with extra-pyramidal diseases, such as Parkinsonism.

v. *Snout reflex*: Tapping the upper lip lightly causes bilateral contraction of the muscles around the mouth and base of the nose. The mouth resembles a snout. This is an exaggeration of the orbicularis oris reflex. It is present with bilateral supranuclear lesions and in diffuse cerebral diseases, such as various causes of dementia.

vi. *Suck reflex*: Sucking movements of lips, tongue, and mouth are brought about by lightly touching or tapping on the lips. At times merely bringing an object near the lips produces the reflex. Occurs in patients with diffuse cerebral lesions. The snout reflex occurs in similar circumstances.

vii. *Palmomental reflex*: A stimulus of the thenar area of the hand causes a reflex contraction ipsilaterally of the orbicularis oris and mentalis muscles. A number of normal individuals have this reflex, and also patients with diffuse cerebral disease. It is significant when other similar reflexes are also present.

1-5-6 *How to localise facial nerve lesions?*

1- UMN facial weakness alone or with upper limb weakness occurs in contralateral lesions of the motor cortex.

2- UMN facial weakness with hemiparesis occurs in contralateral lesions of internal capsule, or in midbrain.

3- LMN facial weakness with contralateral hemiparesis occurs in pontine lesions.

4- LMN facial weakness with sensori-neural deafness and vertigo occur in lesions of the CPA, or the IAM.

5- LMN facial weakness with conductive deafness and vertigo occur in lesions of the middle ear.

6- LMN facial weakness alone occurs in contralateral lesions in the facial canal, stylomastoid foramen and peripherally.

Your personal notes:

....

....

....

....

....

....

....

....

....

....

Problem 1-6: How to examine the eighth, ninth & tenth cranial nerves efficiently, with confidence and make a lasting impression. (The smart way of performing neurological physical examination 5)

The eighth cranial nerve (Vestibulo-Cochlear) is responsible for hearing and balance, the ninth cranial nerve (Glossopharyngeal) is responsible for swallowing and taste from posterior one third of the tongue, and the tenth cranial nerve (Vagus) is responsible for vocal cord movements and parasympathetic supply to the heart and gut. During undergraduate examinations, and postgraduate examinations in neurology, general medicine, ophthalmology and neurosurgery candidates

> **Problem based tool box:**
>
> **How to examine 8, 9 & 10 nerves?**
>
> **How to perform Weber's test?**
>
> **How to perform Rinné's test?**
>
> **How to perform the gag reflex?**
>
> **How to assess vestibular functions?**

are often asked to demonstrate the physical examination of the eighth cranial nerve. Patients with deafness are loved by examiners and they often feature as short or long cases during these assessments. Therefore mastering this physical examination of these nerves not only helps in the evaluation and diagnosis of patients but it is also helpful during these examinations.

VIII- The eighth cranial nerve (Vestibulo-Cochlear):

The eighth cranial nerve consists of three nerves: the cochlear and the superior and inferior vestibular nerves. The cochlear nerve is responsible for hearing and the vestibular nerves for balance.

1-6-1 *Where does the eighth nerve originate?*

The eighth nerve originates in the pons (remember the formula 2C + 2MB = 4P + 4MO). It has cochlear and vestibular nuclei (Figure 1-18). It emerges from the anterior lateral aspect of the pons and heads towards the IAM where it joins the facial nerve (Figure 1-22).

1-6-2 *How to examine the eighth nerve?*

Patients with eighth nerve problems complain of *deafness, tinnitus or vertigo*. The hearing level (HL) is quantified relative to "normal" hearing in decibels (dB), with higher dB indicating worse hearing. Hearing loss is often described as:

- Normal hearing: less than 25 dB in adults and 15 dB in children.
- Mild hearing loss: 25–40 dB.
- Moderate hearing loss: 41–65 dB.
- Severe hearing loss: 66–90 dB.
- Profound hearing loss: 90 dB or above.
- 100 dB hearing loss is nearly equivalent to complete deafness for that particular frequency. A score of 0 is normal. It is possible to have scores less than 0, which indicates better than average hearing.

Testing of hearing at the bedside:
These tests may be used for initial assessment, but formal audiometry is preferable. It is essential to mask the other ear by putting a finger in the other ear and rubbing the tragus at the same time. Alternatively, continuous rubbing of a piece of paper between thumb and index finger near the masked ear to produce a consistent broadband sound would be sufficient. However, to test for loud noises, you need to use a Barany noise box. Tuning forks are often used to test hearing at chosen frequencies, but whisper, rubbed fingers and a ticking watch can be used.

1- Whispered voice test:

   This is a useful screening test but may not be sensitive in children. The examiner stands at an arm's length (0.6 metres) behind the seated patient (to prevent lip reading) and whispers a combination of numbers and letters (for example, "6-E-4"), and then asks the patient to repeat the sequence. The examiner should quietly exhale before whispering to ensure as quiet a voice as possible. If the patient responds incorrectly, the test is repeated using a different number/letter combination. The patient is considered to have passed the screening test if they repeat at least three out of a possible six numbers or letters

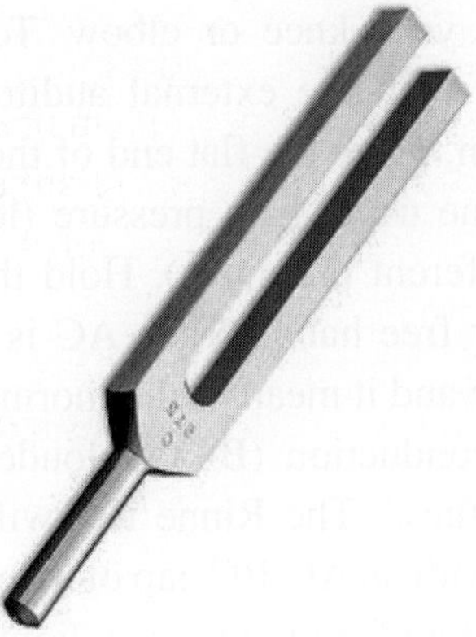

Figure 1-24: A 512 Hz tuning fork to test hearing.

correctly. Each ear is tested in turn, starting with the ear with better hearing. During testing the non-test ear is masked by gently occluding the auditory canal with a finger and rubbing the tragus in a circular motion. The other ear is assessed similarly with a different combination of numbers and letters.

2- Tuning fork bedside tests:

You need a high frequency tuning fork to perform the following tests. Use 512 Hz or 256 Hz tuning fork for these tests (Figure 1-24).

i- Compare the patient's air conduction (AC) with yours:

Strike the fork (TF) against your elbow or knee, hold the TF in line with the patient's external auditory meatus (EAM) till the patient does not hear any more sound, immediately place the TF in line with your own EAM. If you can detect the sound the patients AC is worse than yours (patient is deafer than you). Repeat the process on the other side. Remember to mask the opposite ear.

ii- Rinne's test:

Use tuning fork of 512 Hz, but those of 256 Hz may be better. A heavy tuning fork is better as a light one produces a sound that fades away too quickly. Produce a sound level of 90 dB by striking the TF against your knee or elbow. To test AC, hold the TF directly in line with the external auditory canal. When testing bone conduction, place the flat end of the stem of the TF against the mastoid bone using firm pressure (loudness varies by up to 15 dB with different pressures). Hold the patient's head steady with your other free hand. When AC is louder than BC, this is Rinne's positive and it means either normal or sensorineural deafness. If bone conduction (BC) is louder than AC, it indicates conductive deafness. The Rinne test will reliably detect a conduction defect with an AC-BC gap of at least 30–40 dB. However, it is not a substitute for pure tone audiometry.

iii- Weber's test:

A 512 Hz TF is placed in the midline of the patient's forehead. If the sound is louder on one side than the other, the patient may have either an ipsilateral (the ear hears the sound loudest) conductive hearing loss or a contralateral sensorineural hearing loss.

iv- Speech discrimination test (SDT):

SDT helps determine how well a person hears and understands speech. Spondee or spondaic words are the speech stimuli used to obtain the speech reception threshold (SRT). A spondee is defined as a two-syllable word spoken with equal stress. The SRT is the softest intensity level at which a patient can correctly repeat 50% of the words. Word recognition scoring is a common clinical approach to evaluate a person's ability to hear and understand speech. Lists of 20 to 50 words are presented to the patient at supra-threshold levels, usually 30 dB above threshold. The list is phonetically balanced, which means it has speech sounds that occur as often as they would in everyday conversation. Out of this list, a percentage is calculated based on correctly repeated words. Word recognition scores of 90% or higher are considered normal while scores below this level indicate a problem with word recognition. Patients with conductive hearing loss usually show excellent word recognition. Patients with cochlear lesions have poorer discrimination. Patients with retrocochlear lesions usually have even poorer discrimination scores which sometimes may be exacerbated by the phenomenon of "rollover". Rollover is thought to occur as a result of changes in code intensity due to loss of monotonic stimulation and may be indicative of retro-cochlear pathology.

1-6-3 *How to test vestibular functions (balance)?*

Problems with the vestibular system cause central vertigo. This sensation may be described by patients in a variety of ways: spinning, tilting, pushed to one side, light headedness, clumsiness, or even blacking out. If blackout was documented, a peripheral cause of the dizziness is rarely if ever at fault. Vertigo of vestibular origin is characterised by worsening on sudden movements of the head and change in posture.

1- Observe for spontaneous nystagmus:

Ask the patient to fixate on a stationary target in the neutral gaze position with best corrected vision (glasses or contact lenses in place). Observe for nystagmus. If nystagmus is observed, note its amplitude, direction, and effect of target fixation. Lesions of the labyrinth and eighth vestibular (8v) produce intense, direction-fixed, horizontal-rotary nystagmus that is enhanced under Fresnel lenses. (These lenses were invented by French physicist Augustin-Jean Fresnel. Originally developed for lighthouses, the design enables the construction of lenses of large aperture and short focal length without the weight and volume of material required in conventional lens design. Fresnel lens therefore, is thinner, passing more light and allowing lighthouses to be visible over much longer distances. In nystagmus, these lenses are used to make the image less clear and enhance nystagmus.) The nystagmus also intensifies when gazing in the direction of the fast phase (Alexander's law). This pattern can be seen in lesions causing irritation (beating toward the affected ear) and destruction (beating toward the unaffected ear) of the labyrinth, 8v, or (rarely) the 8v-nuclei. In contrast, lesions of the brain stem, cerebellum, and cerebrum cause less intense, direction-changing horizontal, vertical, torsional, or pendular nystagmus that is diminished under Fresnel lenses. Examples include periodic alternating nystagmus (PAN), congenital nystagmus, and lesions of the vermis.

2- Look for gaze nystagmus:

The patient is asked to look at a target placed 20 to 30 degrees to the left or right off centre for 20 seconds. Gaze-evoked nystagmus is observed and change in nystagmus direction, type, or intensity of spontaneous nystagmus. The ability to maintain eccentric gaze is under control of the brainstem and the vermis (flocculonodular lobes). When these mechanisms fail to hold the eyes in the eccentric position, the eyes drift toward the midline (exponentially decreasing velocity), followed by refixation saccades toward the target. Such gaze-evoked nystagmus is central in origin and always beats in the direction of intended gaze. In contrast, enhancement of peripheral spontaneous nystagmus (linear slow component velocity) occurs without direction change when gazing in the direction of the fast phase. Causes of gaze-evoked nystagmus include a drug effect (sedatives, anti-epileptics), alcohol, brain tumours, and cerebellar degenerative syndromes.

3- Fixation Suppression Test:

The patient is asked to fixate on his/her own index finger held out in front at an arm's length. The examination chair is rotated up to 2 Hz while the patient stares at his/her finger. The examiner observes for a decrease in the visual-vestibular nystagmus that was evoked during rotation without ocular fixation. The modulation of nystagmus invoked by rotation is a central nervous system phenomenon heavily dependent on the cerebellar flocculus. Failure of fixation suppression in the presence of adequate visual acuity implies floccular dysfunction. This test is similar in nature to the fixation suppression performed after caloric stimulation during electro-oculography.

4- Head Thrust Test (Head Impulse Test):

The patient is asked to fixate on a target on the wall in front of them while the examiner moves the patient's head rapidly to each side. The examiner looks for any movement of the pupil during the head thrust and a refixation saccade back to the target. Either direct observation of pupillary movement or the use of an ophthalmoscope is employed to document eye movement. This test was introduced by Halmagyi and Curthoys (1988). The head impulse test was described as a reliable sign of reduced vestibular function in the plane of rotation for the ear ipsilateral to the head thrust. The observation of eye movement during the manoeuvre is a sign of decreased neural input from the ipsilateral ear to the vestibulo-ocular reflex (VOR) because the contralateral ear is in inhibitory "saturation" and cannot supply enough neural activity to stabilise gaze. In such instances, the eye travels with the head during the high-velocity movement, and a refixation saccade is necessary to fixate the target. Bilateral refixation movements are seen frequently in cases of ototoxicity.

5- Postheadshake Nystagmus:

The patient's head is tilted forward 30 degrees and the examiner shakes the patient's head in the horizontal plane at 2 Hz for 20 seconds and observes for postheadshake nystagmus and notes the direction and any reversal of nystagmus. Fresnel lenses are used to avoid fixation and make the nystagmus more obvious. The manoeuvre may be repeated in the vertical direction. Postheadshake nystagmus is considered a pathologic sign of imbalance in the vestibular inputs in the plane of rotation. In nystagmus caused by peripheral causes the nystagmus is directed toward the stronger ear with small reversal phase sometimes observed. Signs of central aetiology include prolonged nystagmus, vertical nystagmus following horizontal headshake ("cross coupling"), and dysconjugate nystagmus.

6- Vestibular Caloric Test (VCT):

The VCT is a test of the vestibulo-ocular reflex (VOR) that involves irrigating cold or warm water or air into the external auditory canal. It is commonly used by audiologists and other trained professionals to validate a diagnosis of asymmetric function in the peripheral vestibular system. Caloric test is usually a subtest of the electronystagmography (ENG) battery of tests. It is one of several tests which can be used to test for brainstem death (BSD). Cold (not more than seven degrees less than normal, 30°C) or warm (not more than seven degrees above normal, 44°C) water or air is irrigated into the external auditory canal, usually using a syringe. In patients with an intact cerebrum: if the water is cold relative to body temperature (30°C), the eyes turn toward the ipsilateral ear, with horizontal nystagmus (quick horizontal eye movements) to the contralateral ear. If the water is warm (44°C) the eyes turn toward the contralateral ear, with horizontal nystagmus to the ipsilateral ear. Absent reactive eye movement suggests vestibular weakness of the horizontal semicircular canal of the side being stimulated. In comatose patients with cerebral damage, the fast phase of nystagmus will be absent as this is controlled by the cerebrum. As a result, using cold water irrigation will result in deviation of the eyes toward the ear being irrigated. If both phases are absent, this suggests the patient's brainstem reflexes are also damaged and carries a very poor prognosis. The acronym COWS is used to remember: "Cold water = fast phase of nystagmus to the side Opposite from the cold water filled ear, Warm water = fast phase of nystagmus to the Same side as the warm water filled the ear".

IX- The ninth cranial nerve (Glossopharyngeal):
The ninth cranial nerve supplies the stylopharyngeal muscle and carries sensation from the back of the tongue and the larynx, is responsible for taste sensation from the posterior third of the tongue, and supplies the parotid gland.

1-6-4 Where does the ninth nerve originate?

The ninth nerve originates in the medulla oblongata (remember the formula $2C + 2MB = 4P + 4MO$). Its sensory fibres end up in the spinal tract of the trigeminal nerve. The ninth nerve can be regarded as a purely sensory nerve.

1-6-5 How to examine the ninth cranial nerve?

The ninth nerve can only be evaluated as such. The main tests used are:

1- Pharyngeal sensation:

Touch the back of the throat gently with an orange stick on either side of the midline and ask the patient to compare both sides. If in doubt you can use a long pin to test for pain.

2- The gag reflex (GR):

The GR is a reflex contraction of the back of the throat, evoked by touching the back of throat. The GR helps prevent choking. The afferent of the reflex is the ninth nerve, which inputs to the nucleus solitarius (Figure 1-18), and the efferent is the vagus nerve from the nucleus ambiguus. Absence of the gag reflex can be a symptom of a number of damages to the ninth nerve, the tenth nerve, or brainstem. However, studies indicated that up to one-third of healthy people do not have a GR. The GR sometimes is triggered intentionally to induce vomiting, by those who suffer from bulimia nervosa.

X- The tenth cranial nerve (Vagus):

The vagus nerve is the only nerve that starts in the brainstem and extends, through the jugular foramen, down below the head, to the neck, chest and abdomen, where it contributes to the innervations of the viscera. Besides output to the various organs in the body, the tenth nerve conveys sensory information about the state of the body's organs to the central nervous system. The left tenth nerve is mainly sensory and the right is mainly motor, however 80–90% of the fibres are sensory.

1-6-6 *Where does the tenth nerve originate?*

The tenth nerve originates in the medulla oblongata (remember the formula 2C + 2MB = 4P + 4MO). It passes through the jugular foramen together with the internal jugular-sigmoid sinus junction, the ninth and 11th cranial nerves, and then passes in the carotid sheath where they are joined by the internal carotid artery (Figure 1-25).

In the superior mediastinum, the tenth nerve gives out its recurrent laryngeal nerve (RLN). The RLN supplies the laryngeal muscles that move the vocal cords. The left RLN loops around the arch of the aorta while the right RLN loops around the subclavian artery. Therefore the left RLN is less likely to be stretched during anterior cervical surgery (longer and medially located), e.g. during approach to cervical discs where the larynx and pharynx are retracted to the right during left-sided approach and to the left during right-sided approach. Hence hoarseness is more common after

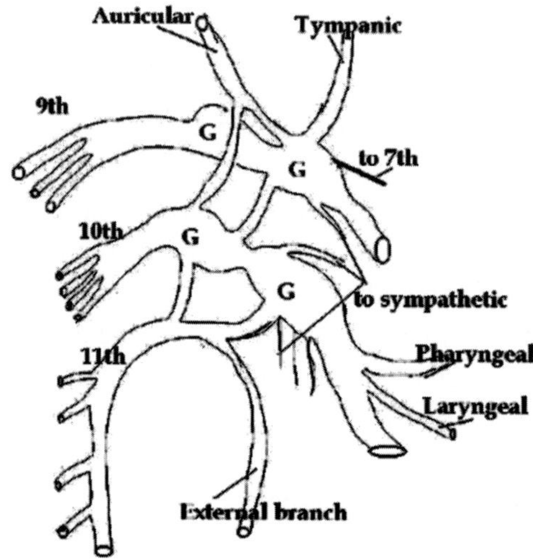

Figure 1-25: Diagram of the ninth and tenth cranial nerves (G = ganglion).

right-sided approaches. Damage to the vagus causes dysphonia or hoarseness, while stimulation of the vagus nerve produces bradycardia. Because
the right vagus is mainly motor, stimulation of the right vagus produces
bradycardia and diarrhoea, while stimulation of the left which is purely sensory does not have these side effects and is used to treat epilepsy and
depression. The vagus nerve supplies motor parasympathetic fibres to all
the organs from the neck down to the second segment of the transverse
colon, except the suprarenal (adrenal) glands. The vagus also controls a few
skeletal muscles, namely: the cricothyroid, the levator veli palatini, salpin-
gopharyngeus, palatoglossus, palatopharyngeus, and the superior, middle
and inferior pharyngeal constrictor muscles of the larynx (for speech). This
means that the vagus nerve is responsible for such varied tasks as heart rate,
gastrointestinal peristalsis, sweating, and quite a few muscle movements in
the mouth, including speech (via the RLN) and keeping the larynx open for
breathing. It also receives some sensation from the outer ear, via the auricular branch (Alderman's nerve) and part of the meninges. The right tenth
nerve innervates the sinoatrial node. The vagus nerve has three nuclei associated with cardiovascular control: the dorsal motor nucleus, the nucleus
ambiguus and the solitary nucleus. The parasympathetic output to the heart

comes mainly from neurons in the nucleus ambiguus and to a lesser extent from the dorsal motor nucleus. The solitary nucleus receives sensory input about the state of the cardiovascular system, being an integration hub for the baroreflex. Anticholinergics such as atropine and scopolamine are called vagolytic because they inhibit the action of the vagus on the heart, gastrointestinal tract and other organs. Anticholinergics increase heart rate and are used to treat bradycardia and asystole. Vagus nerve stimulation (VNS) therapy using a pacemaker-like device implanted in the chest is a treatment used since 1997 to control seizures in epilepsy patients and has recently been approved for treating drug-resistant cases of clinical depression. VNS may also be achieved by one of the vagus manoeuvres: holding the breath for a few seconds, dipping the face in cold water, coughing, or tensing the stomach muscles as if to bear down to have a bowel movement (valsalva manoeuvre). Patients with supraventricular tachycardia (STV), atrial fibrillation (AF), and other illnesses may be trained to perform vagus manoeuvres (or find one or more on their own). Vagus nerve blocking vagotomy (cutting of the vagus nerve) is a now-obsolete therapy that was performed for peptic ulcer. Vagotomy is currently being researched as a less invasive alternative weight loss procedure to gastric bypass surgery. Excessive activation of the vagus nerve during emotional stress can cause vasovagal syncope because of a sudden drop in blood pressure and heart rate. Vasovagal syncope affects young children and women more often. It can also lead to temporary loss of bladder control under moments of extreme fear. Vagus damage leads to loss of the GR and deviation of the uvula away from the side of lesion, and there is failure of palate elevation.

1-6-7 *How to examine the tenth cranial nerve?*

1- Inspection of the uvula:

The uvula should be midline in normal patients and deviated to the other side of vagus lesion. Ask the patient to say "Aah" and watch the uvula movements.

2- Gag reflex (GR):

The gag reflex was discussed under the ninth cranial nerve.

Your personal notes:

....
....
....
....
....
....
....
....
....
....

Problem 1-7:   How to examine the 11th and 12th cranial nerves efficiently, with confidence and make a lasting impression. (The smart way of performing neurological physical examination 6)

The 11th cranial nerve (accessory) is responsible for innervating the sternocleidomastoid (SCM) and the trapezium muscles and the 12th cranial nerve (hypoglossal) is responsible for tongue.

> **Problem based tool box:**
> **How to examine the tongue?**
> **How to examine the 11th nerve?**
> **How to examine the 12th nerve?**
> **How to localise lesions of 11th and 12th cranial nerves?**

During undergraduate examinations, and postgraduate examinations in neurology, general medicine, ophthalmology and neurosurgery candidates are often asked to demonstrate the physical examination of these two nerves. Patients with tongue paralysis or torticollis are loved by examiners and they often feature as short or long cases during these assessments. Therefore mastering this physical examination of these nerves not only helps in the evaluation and diagnosis of patients but it is also helpful during these examinations.

XI- The eleventh cranial nerve (Accessory):

Anatomically, the 11th nerve consists of two components: cranial part that eventually joins the tenth nerve and spinal part that supplies the SCM and trapezium muscles. The 11th nerve supplies also the palatoglossus muscle of the tongue, the only muscle of the tongue not supplied by the 12th nerve. The cranial component however is now considered part of the vagus and not part of the accessory nerve proper. Therefore in practice when you are asked to examine the 11th nerve, concentrate on examining the spinal component.

1-7-1 *Where does the 11th nerve originate?*

The 11th nerve originates in the medulla (remember the formula 2C + 2MB = 4P + 4MO). However, what we consider in practice as the 11th nerve arises from the cervical spinal cord, it ascends up through the foramen magnum and out through the jugular foramen joining the vagus and glossopharyngeal nerves (Figure 1-26).

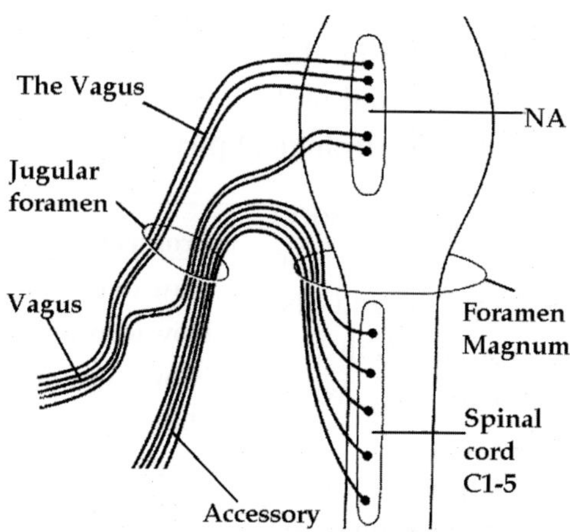

Figure 1-26: The 11th cranial nerve (NA = nucleus ambiguus).

1-7-2 *How to examine the 11th nerve?*

Patients with 11th nerve problems complain of *torticollis or drooping of the shoulder.* The sternocleidomastoid (SCM) muscle tilts and rotates the head, so torticollis is either caused by spasm ipsilateral to the torticollis or weakness of the contralateral SCM. The trapezium muscle has several actions on the scapula, including shoulder elevation and adduction. Range of motion and strength testing of the neck and shoulders can be measured during a neurological examination to assess function of the spinal accessory nerve. Limited range of motion or poor muscle strength is suggestive of damage to the 11th nerve. Damage of the 11th nerve can be caused by injury to the spinal accessory nerve most commonly iatrogenic during head and neck surgery.

- Inspect the SCM and trapezium muscles looking for wasting, fasciculation or deformity of the neck.
- To assess the SCM power, ask the patient to turn the head to one side against resistance.
- To assess the strength of trapezium muscle, ask the patient to shrug the shoulders against resistance.

XII- The twelfth nerve (Hypoglossal):

The 12th cranial nerve supplies all the tongue muscles apart from the palatoglossus which is supplied by the 11th cranial nerve as mentioned before.

1-7-3 *Where does the 12th nerve originate?*

The 12th nerve arises from the hypoglossal nucleus in the medulla oblongata (remember the formula 2C + 2MB = 4P + 4MO) and emerges in the pre-olivary sulcus separating the *olive* and the *pyramid*. It then passes through the hypoglossal canal. On emerging from the hypoglossal canal, it gives off a small meningeal branch and picks up a branch from the anterior ramus of C1. It spirals behind the vagus nerve and passes between the internal carotid artery and internal jugular vein lying on the carotid sheath. After passing deep to the posterior belly of the digastric muscle, it passes to the submandibular region to enter the tongue. It supplies motor fibres to all of the muscles of the tongue, except the palatoglossus muscle which is innervated by the 11th nerve, which runs in part with the vagus nerve.

1-7-4 *How to examine the 12th cranial nerve?*

To test the function of the 12th nerve, the patient is asked to stick out their tongue. If there was loss of function on one side (unilateral paralysis) the

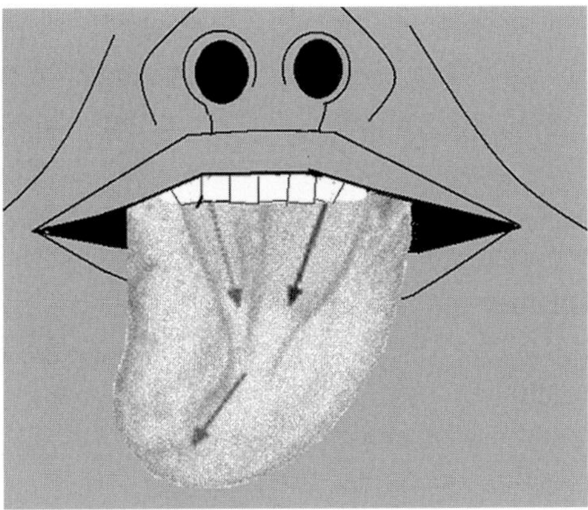

Figure 1-27: Photograph of a right paralysed hypoglossal.

tongue will appear atrophic on the paralysed side and may have some fasciculations. The tongue points towards the affected side (Figure 1-27).

The strength of the tongue can be tested by getting the patient to poke the inside of his/her cheek, and feeling how strongly the patient can push a hand pushed against the patient's cheek.

Problem 1-8:   How to examine the motor system efficiently, with confidence and make a lasting impression. (The smart way of performing neurological physical examination 7)

Examination of the motor system is very important in all patients, particularly in the upper and lower limbs. Symptoms related to dysfunction of the motor system include the following:

> **Problem based tool box:**
> **How to examine the motor system?**
> **How to assess muscle tone and power?**
> **What is the MRC grades?**
> **How to demonstrate deep reflexes?**
> **How to localise a lesion along the motor system pathways?**

- Weakness.
- Stiffness of the limbs.
- Slowness.
- Tremor or shaking.
- Abnormal movements.
- Poor hand grip.
- Leg gives way.
- Falls.

To examine the motor system you need to assess the following components:

1- Muscle shape and mass.
2- Abnormal movements.
3- Muscle tone.
4- Muscle power.
5- Reflexes.

Always observe first (muscle mass and shape), inspect second (individual muscles for abnormal movements), palpate third (muscle tenderness, tone and power), and use specials bedside tests last (reflexes).

- Observe: Carefully observe the patient to detect any twitches, tremors, dyskinesia, other involuntary movements, or any unusual paucity of movements. Note the patient's posture and gait.
- Inspect: Next closely inspect several individual muscles for muscle wasting, hypertrophy or fasciculation. Fasciculations are best

observed in the small muscles of the hand, shoulder girdle muscles, and the thigh muscles.

- Palpate: Palpate for muscle tenderness if you suspect myositis.

1-8-1 *How to assess muscle tone?*

- Muscle tone: To assess the muscle tone, ask the patient to relax, flex and extend the patient's fingers, wrist, and elbow, flex and extend patient's ankle and knee. Normally there is a small, continuous resistance to passive movement. Observe for decreased (flaccid) or increased (rigid/spastic) muscle tone. Abnormal muscle tone can be described as:

1- Hypotonia:

Hypotonia means decreased muscle tone. It can either be congenital or acquired. Congenital hypotonia is called benign congenital hypotonia and is usually detected during infancy. An infant with hypotonia exhibits a floppy quality (rag doll) feeling when (s)he is held. Infants with this problem lag behind in acquiring certain fine and gross motor developmental milestones that enable a baby to hold his/her head up when placed prone, balance themselves or sit upright and remain seated without falling over. Since the muscles that support the bone joints are so soft, there is a tendency for hip, jaw and neck dislocations in these infants and their joints can be hyperextended. Some children with hypotonia may have trouble feeding if they are unable to suck or chew for long periods. A child with hypotonia may also have problems with speech or exhibit shallow breathing. Acquired hypotonia may occur in muscular dystrophy.

2- Flaccidity (flaccid tone):

Flaccidity also means reduced or absent muscle tone. This is often indicative of LMN lesions in the anterior horn cells, e.g. in motor neuron disease (MND) or poliomyelitis, peripheral nerve such as in peripheral nerve injuries, radiculopathy or peripheral nerve compression. In acute spinal cord injury (spinal shock) the muscle tone can be flaccid despite the lesion being UMN in nature.

3- Hypertonia:

Hypertonia means increased muscle tone. This can be spastic, rigid or myotonic in nature:

a- Spasticity:

Spasticity is characterised by a velocity-dependent increase in tonic stretch reflexes with exaggerated tendon jerks, resulting from hyper-excitability of the stretch reflex and is one of UMN signs. A key sign of spasticity is velocity dependent increase in resistance to passive stretch of muscles. Spasticity is a disorder of the central nervous system (CNS) in which certain muscles continually receive a message to tighten up and contract. The nerves leading to those muscles are unable to regulate themselves, permanently and continually over-firing commands to tighten and contract the muscles. This causes stiffness or tightness of the muscles and may interfere with gait, movement, and speech. Spasticity is seen in spastic diplegia, spastic cerebral palsy, multiple sclerosis, MND, and UMN lesions of the pyramidal system (Figure 1-28).

The identification of the location of the lesion causing the weakness can be made by the identifying the type and distribution of weakness and any associated cranial nerve palsies or sensory level (Table 1-3).

1-8-2 *How to localise a motor lesion along motor pathways?*

b- Muscle Rigidity:

Muscle rigidity describes an increase in muscle tone, leading to a resistance to passive movement throughout the range of motion. In contrast, spasticity is rate-dependent and only elicited upon a high speed movements and when the resistance overcomes the spasticity the muscle gives way is called clasp knife. There are different types of rigidity:

i) Cogwheel rigidity (jerky resistance) seen in extrapyramidal disorders such as Parkinsonism.

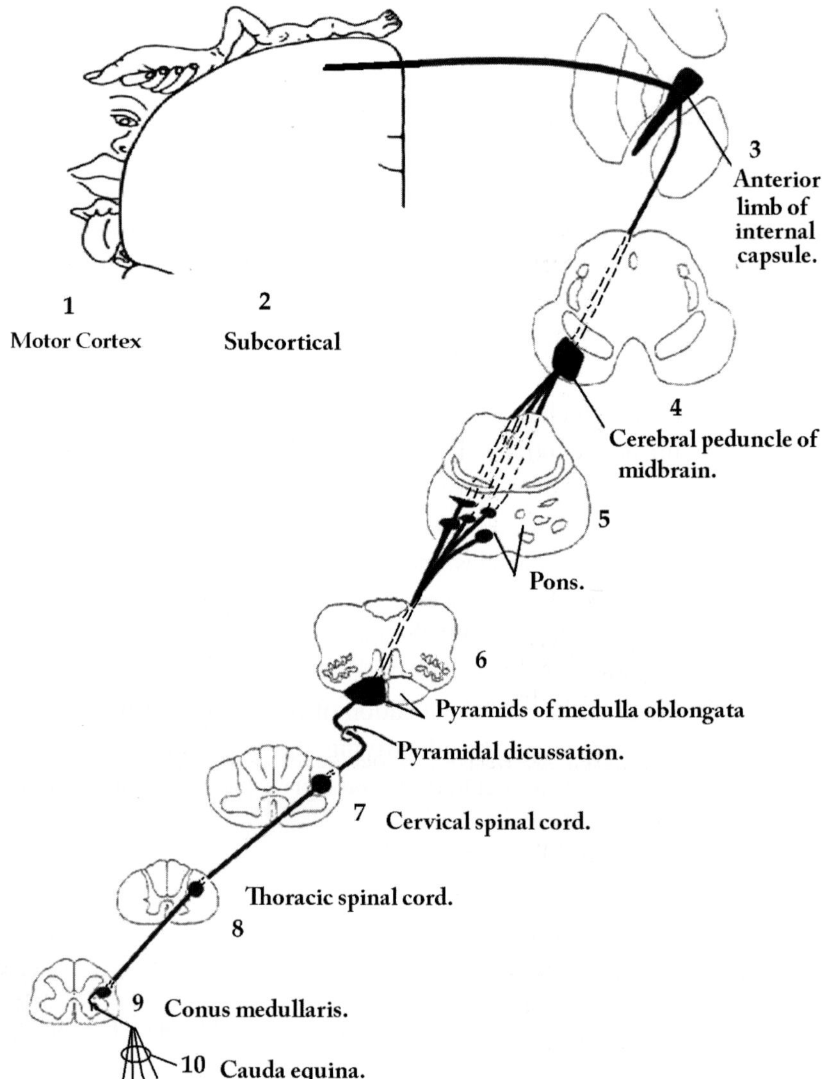

Figure 1-28: Schematic representation of the motor pathways (pyramidal system).

Table 1-3: Localisation of lesions causing motor weakness: correlate these lesions with diagram in Figure 1-28 above

Lesion location	Weakness		Associated nerve palsy	Associated sensory level
	Type	Distribution		
1- Motor cortex	UMN	One limb	None	None
2- Subcortical	UMN	Hemiparesis	None	None
3- Int. capsule	UMN	Hemiparesis	UMN- Facial	None
4- Midbrain	UMN	Hemiparesis	LMN- Third	None
5- Pons	UMN	Hemiparesis	LMN- Facial	None
6- Medulla	UMN	Hemiparesis	LMN- 12th	None
7- Cervical cord	UMN	Tetraparesis	None	At C3 to C8
8- Thoracic cord	UMN	Paraparesis	None	At T1 to T12
9- Conus	Mixed	Paraparesis	None	At L1 to L5
10- Cauda equina	LMN	Paraparesis	None	At L1 to S1

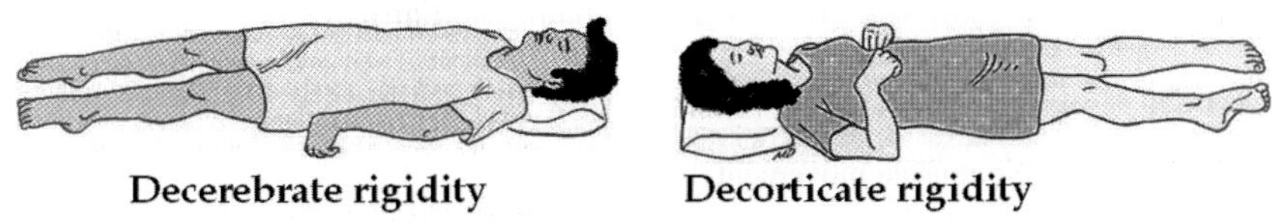

Figure 1-29: Decerebrate and decorticate rigidities.

ii) Lead-pipe rigidity (continuous rigidity). These various forms of rigidity can be seen in different forms of movement disorders such as Parkinson's.

iii) Decerebrate rigidity: this is spasticity in extensor muscles described in animals with brain stem transaction (Figure 1-29).

iv) Decorticate rigidity: this spasticity in the flexor muscles described in patients with diffuse axonal injury (DAI) (Figure 1-29).

1-8-3 *How to assess muscle power?*

- Muscle power:

Test muscle strength by having the patient move against your resistance. Make sure that you test across one joint at a time by holding the limb by

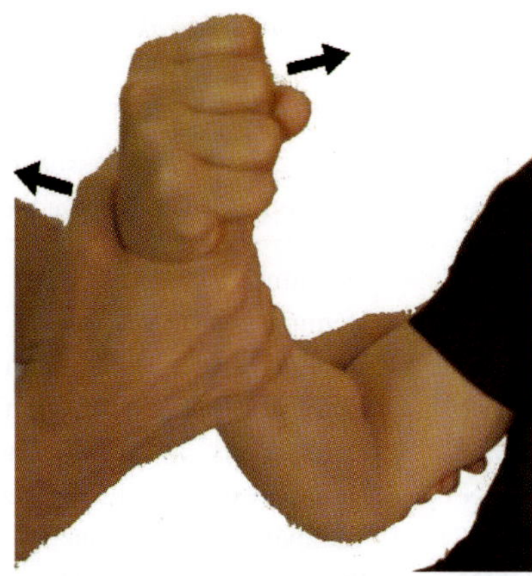

Figure 1-30: Diagram demonstrating how to examine muscle strength in the upper and lower limbs.

Table 1-4: MRC scale for grading muscle power

Grade	Description
0	No muscle movement
1	Visible muscle movement, flicker, but no movement at the joint
2	Movement at the joint, but not against gravity
3	Movement against gravity, but not against added resistance
4	Movement against resistance, but less than normal
5	Normal strength

the other hand, e.g. testing the power across the elbow joint ask the patient to flex the elbow, hold the upper arm by one hand and the forearm by the other hand and ask patient to flex against your resistance then extend against resistance (Figure 1-30). Always compare one side to the other and grade muscle strength on MRC (Medical Research Council) scale from 0 to 5 (Table 1-4).

Test the following muscle groups:

1- Finger abduction (C8, T1, ulnar nerve): ask the patient to spread their fingers apart and keep them apart against your resistance. Use your two index fingers to exert the resistance (Figure 1-31).

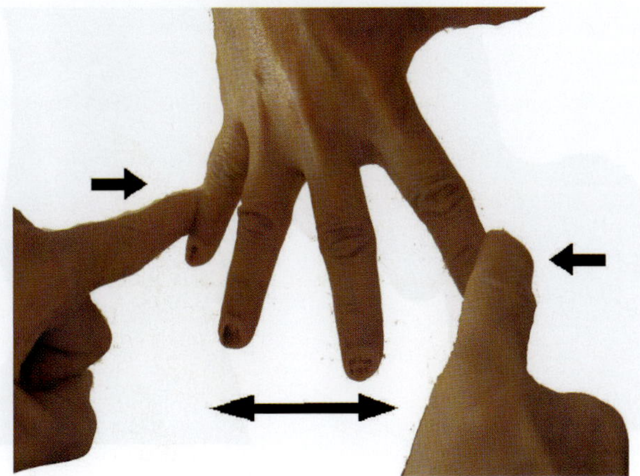

Figure 1-31: Finger abduction.

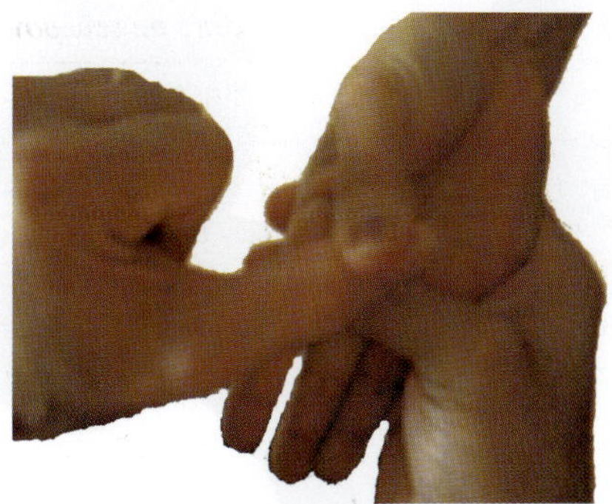

Figure 1-32: Thumb opposition.

2- Opposition of the thumb (C8, T1, median nerve): ask the patient to bring his/her thumb towards the little finger against resistance or ask the patient to oppose the thumb and index together and prevent you opening the formed ring (Figure 1-32).

3- Hand grip: ask the patient to squeeze two of your fingers as hard as possible (C7, C8, T1) (Figure 1-33).

4- Extension at the wrist (C6, C7, C8, radial nerve): ask the patient to make a fist and exert pressure to overcome it (Figure 1-34).

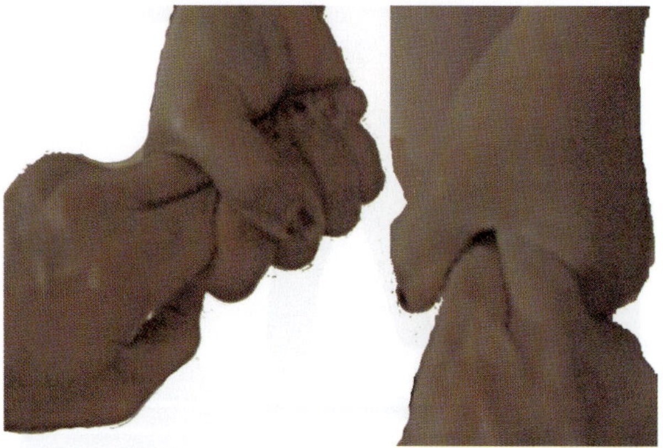

Figure 1-33: Assessment of hand grip.

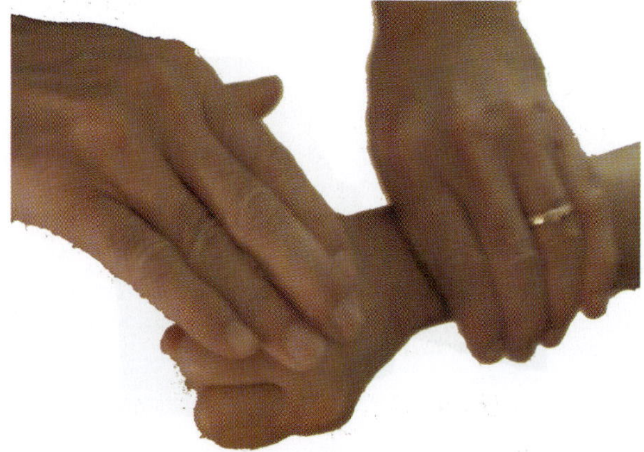

Figure 1-34: Wrist extension.

5- Flexion at the elbow (C5, C6, biceps): ask patient to flex the elbow against resistance (Figure 1-30).

6- Extension at the elbow (C6, C7, C8, triceps): ask the patient to extend the elbow against your resistance (Figure 1-35).

7- Shoulder abduction (mainly C5, deltoid): ask patient to abduct the shoulders to 90 degrees with the elbow flexed but hands apart, exert pressure down to abduct the shoulders asking patient to resist your pressure (Figure 1-36).

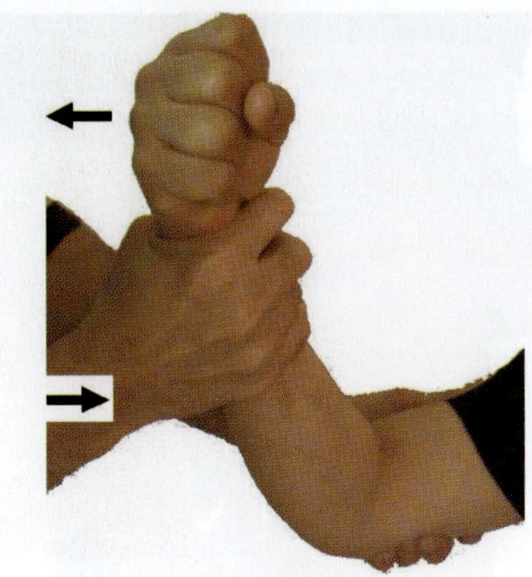

Figure 1-35: Elbow extension.

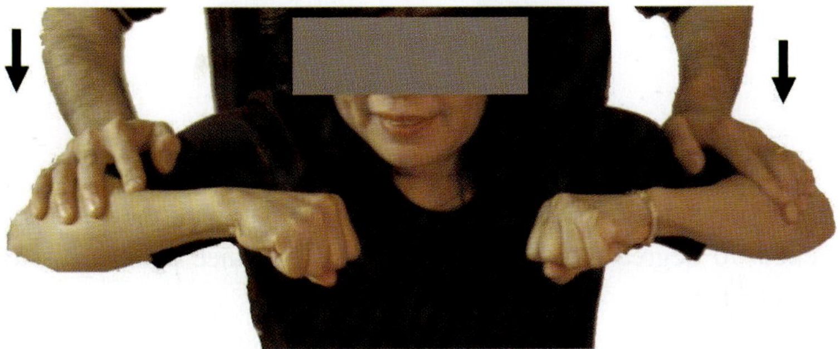

Figure 1-36: Shoulder abduction.

8- Flexion at the hip (L2, L3, L4, iliopsoas): ask the patient to elevate the knee against resistance (Figure 1-37).

9- Adduction at the hips (L2, L3, L4, adductors): ask the patient to flex the hip and knee by 90 degrees and bring the knee to the opposite side against resistance.

10- Abduction at the hips (L4, L5, S1, gluteus medius and minimus): from the same position above ask patient to move the knee outwards against resistance.

11- Extension at the hips (S1, gluteus maximus): ask patient to resist your attempt to elevate the thigh.

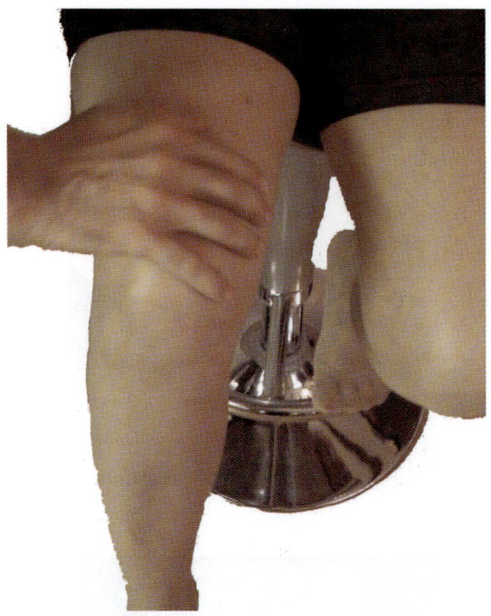

Figure 1-37: Illustration of hip flexion.

12- Extension at the knee (L2, L3, L4, quadriceps): with the knee and hip flexed 90 degrees ask patient to extend the knee against resistance (Figure 1-38).

13- Flexion at the knee (L4, L5, S1, S2, hamstrings): from the same previous position ask patient to flex the knee against resistance (Figure 1-39).

14- Dorsiflexion at the ankle (L4, L5): ask patient to dorsiflex the foot against resistance (Figure 1-40).

15- Plantar flexion (S1): ask patient to push against your hand as if pushing an accelerator of a vehicle (Figure 1-41).

16- Extensor hallucis longus (L5): ask patient to dorsiflex the big toe against resistance (Figure 1-42).

17- Pronator drift: Ask the patient to out-stretch both upper limbs straight forward for 20–30 seconds with palms up, and eyes closed. Instruct the patient to keep the arms still while you tap them briskly downward. The patient will not be able to maintain extension and supination and drifts into pronation with UMN disease.

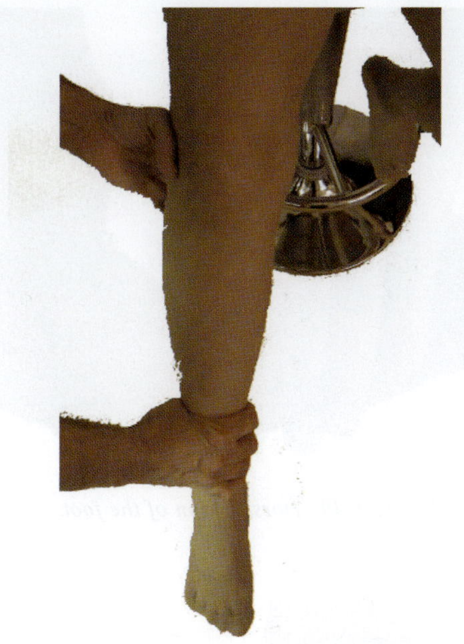

Figure 1-38: Knee extension.

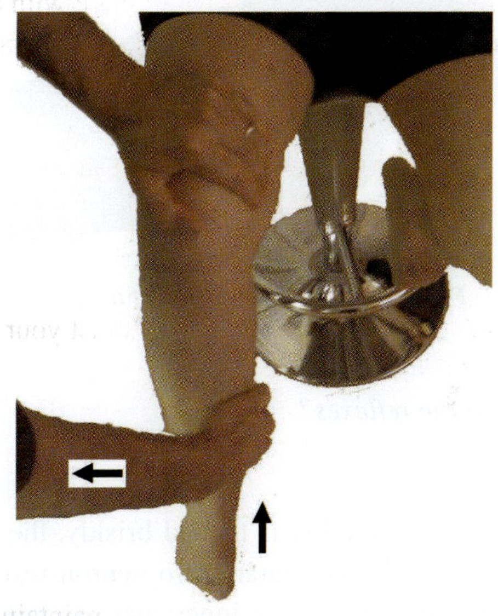

Figure 1-39: Knee flexion.

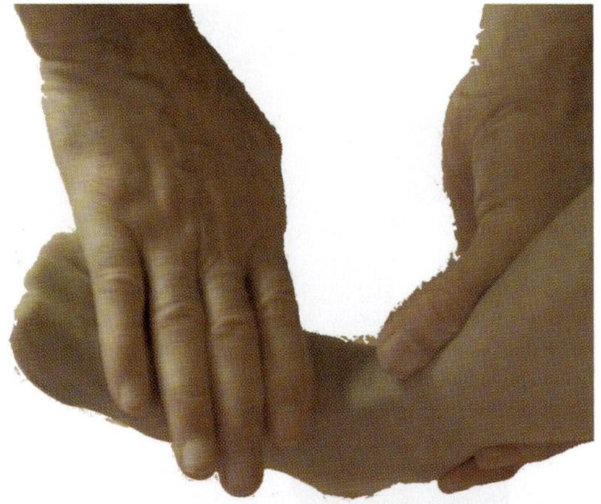

Figure 1-40: Dorsiflexion of the foot.

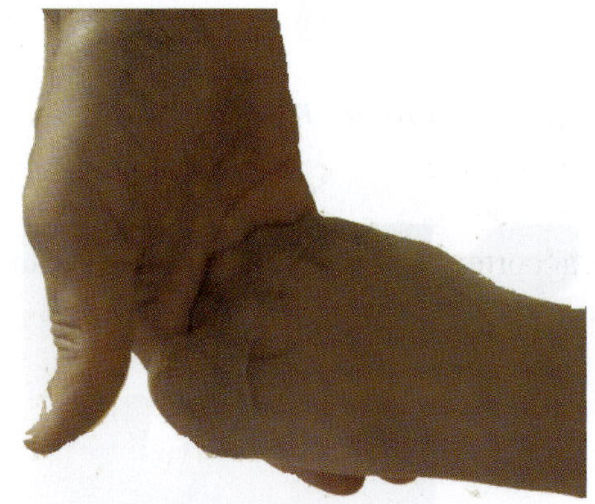

Figure 1-41: Plantar flexion of the foot.

1-8-4 *How to elicit the reflexes?*

• **Reflexes:**

Normally when a muscle tendon is tapped briskly, the muscle immediately contracts. This is an involuntary two-neuron reflex arc involving the spinal or brainstem segment that innervates the muscle. The afferent neuron whose cell body lies in a dorsal root ganglion or sensory ganglion

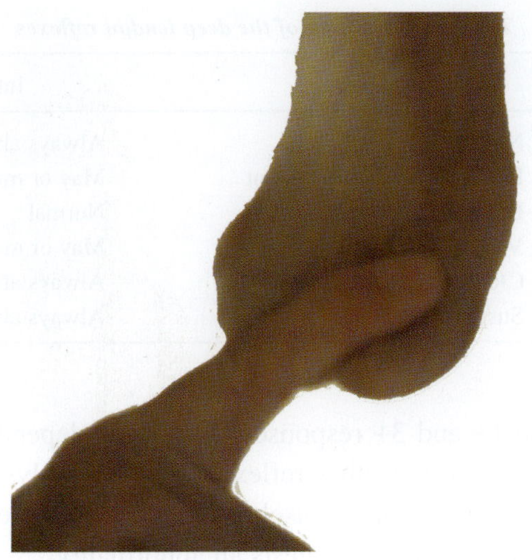

Figure 1-42: Extensor hallucis longus examination.

of the cranial nerves, innervates the muscle or Golgi tendon organ associated with the muscle;[6] the efferent neuron is an alpha motor-neuron in the anterior horn of the spinal cord or the motor nucleus of a cranial nerve. The cerebral cortex and a number of brainstem nuclei exert influence over the sensory input of the muscle spindles by means of the gamma motor-neurons that are located in the anterior horn of the spinal cord; these neurons supply a set of muscle fibres that control the length of the muscle spindle itself. The reflexes could be either normal, hypo- or hyperreflexia:

Hyporeflexia: is an absent or diminished response to tapping. It usually indicates a disease that involves one or more of the components of the two-neuron reflex arc itself.

Hyperreflexia: refers to hyperactive or repeating (clonic) reflexes. These usually indicate an interruption of corticospinal and other descending pathways that influence the reflex arc due to a UMN lesion, that is, a lesion above the level of the reflex pathways.

By convention the deep tendon reflexes are graded as in Table 1-5.

Table 1-5: Grading of the deep tendon reflexes

Grade	Description	Interpretation
0	No response	Always abnormal
1+	Present with reinforcement	May or may not be abnormal
2+	Brisk	Normal
3+	Very brisk	May or may not be abnormal
4+	Clonic (repeating) response	Always abnormal
5+	Sustained clonus	Always abnormal

Whether the 1+ and 3+ responses are normal depends on what they were previously, what the other reflexes are, and analysis of associated findings such as muscle tone, muscle strength, or other evidence of disease. Asymmetry of reflexes suggests an abnormality.

Methods: In a screening examination you will usually find it more convenient to integrate the reflex examination into the rest of the examination of that part of the body, e.g. do the upper extremity reflexes when examining the rest of the upper extremity. When an abnormality of the reflexes is suspected or discovered, the reflexes should be examined as a group with careful attention paid to the method of the examination. Valid test results are best obtained in a fully relaxed patient and not thinking about what you are doing. After a general explanation, mingle the specific instructions with questions or comments designed to distract the patient to talk at some length about some unrelated topic. If you cannot get any response with a specific reflex, have the patient strongly contract a muscle not being tested, e.g.

- In the upper extremity ask the patient to clench their teeth tightly or have the patient make a fist with one hand while the opposite extremity is being tested.
- If the reflex being tested is in the lower limbs, have the patient perform the Jendrassik manoeuvre, to reinforce the reflex. The patient's fingers of each hand are hooked together so each arm can forcefully pull against the other. The split second before you are ready to tap the tendon, say pull.[7,8]

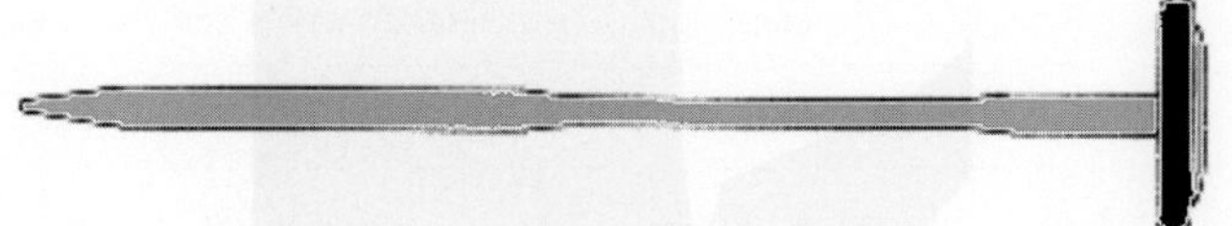

Figure 1-43: The reflex hammer.

The best position to perform these reflexes is for the patient to be sitting on the side of the bed or examination couch. Use a reflex hammer (Figure 1-43). Hold the hammer so that movement occurs at the wrist joint of your hand not at your elbow. Use a brisk but not painful tap. Use your wrist, not your arm, for the action. In an extremity a useful manoeuvre is to elicit the reflex from several different positions, rapidly shifting the limb and performing the test.

Use varying force and note any variance in the response. Note the following features of the reflex response: the amount of hammer force necessary to obtain contraction, the velocity of contraction, the strength and duration of the muscle contraction, the duration of relaxation phase, and the response of other muscles nearby. When a reflex is hyperactive, that muscle often will respond to the testing of a nearby muscle. A good example is reflex activity of a hyperactive biceps or finger reflex when the brachioradialis tendon is tapped. This is termed overflowing of a reflex. After obtaining the reflex on one side, always go immediately to the opposite side for the same reflex so that you can compare them. These are the reflexes tested normally:

Jaw Jerk (JJ): Place the tip of your index finger on a relaxed jaw, one that is about one-third open. Tap briskly on your index finger and note the speed as the mandible is flexed.

Pectoralis Jerk (PJ): The chest is exposed, feel the pectoris major muscle tendon, ask patient to relax, place index and middle fingers over the tendon and tap it with the reflex hammer. Observe the muscle contraction.

Deltoid Jerk (DJ): Feel the tendon of the deltoid about 1/3 the lateral aspect of the upper arm, put two fingers over the tendon, tap gently with reflex hammer, and watch the deltoid muscle for any contraction.

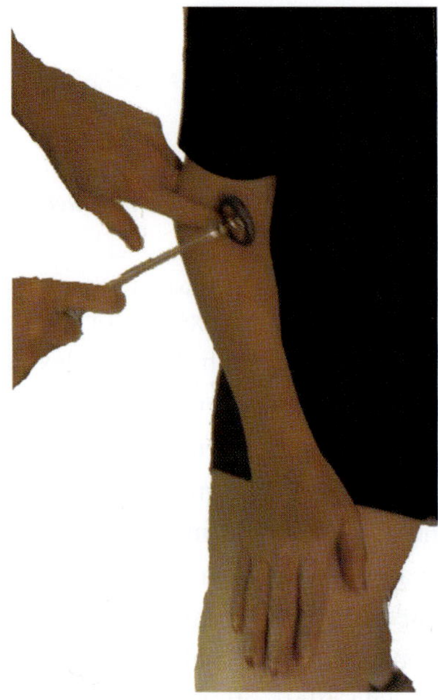

Figure 1-44: Demonstration of the biceps jerk.

Biceps Jerk (BJ): The forearm should be supported, either resting on the patient's thighs or resting on the forearm of the examiner. The arm is midway between flexion and extension. Place your thumb or index firmly over the biceps tendon, with your fingers curling around the elbow, and tap briskly (Figure 1-44). The forearm will flex at the elbow.

Triceps Jerk (TJ): Support the patient's forearm by cradling it with yours or by placing it on the thigh, with the arm midway between flexion and extension. Identify the triceps tendon at its insertion on the olecranon process, and tap just above the insertion (Figure 1-45). There is extension of the forearm.

Brachioradialis (Supinator) Jerk (SJ): The patient's arm should be supported. Identify the brachioradialis tendon at the wrist. It inserts at the base of the styloid process of the radius, usually about 1 cm lateral to the radial artery. If in doubt, ask the patient to hold the arm as if in a sling (flexed at

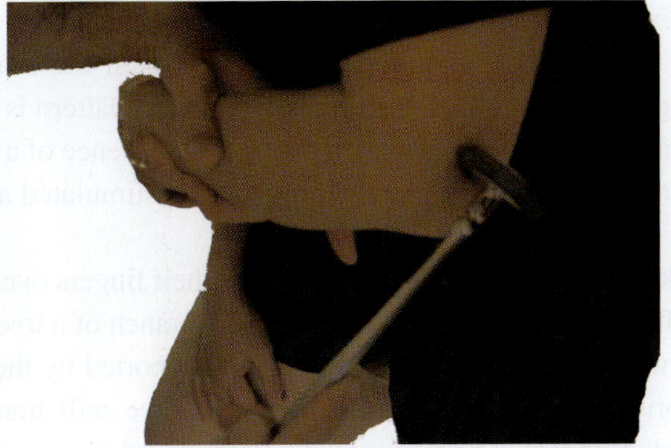

Figure 1-45: Triceps jerk.

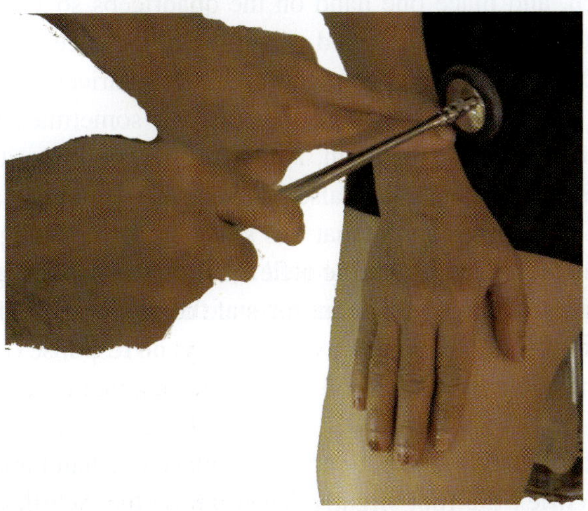

Figure 1-46: Demonstration of the brachioradialis jerk.

the elbow and halfway between pronation and supination) and then flex the forearm at the elbow against resistance from you. The brachioradialis and its tendon will then stand out. Place the thumb of the hand supporting the patient's elbow on the biceps tendon while tapping the brachioradialis tendon with the other hand (Figure 1-46). Observe three potential reflexes as you tap. Brachioradialis reflex: flexion and supination of the forearm.

Biceps reflex: flexion of the forearm. You will feel the biceps tendon contract if the biceps reflex is stimulated by the tap on the brachioradialis tendon. Finger jerk: flexion of the fingers. The usual pattern is for only the brachioradialis reflex to be stimulated. But in the presence of a hyperactive biceps or finger jerk reflex, these reflexes may be stimulated also.

Finger Jerk (FJ): Have the patient gently curl their fingers over your index finger, much as a bird curls its claws around the branch of a tree. Then raise your hand, with the patient's hand now being supported by the curled fingers. Tap briskly on your fingers so that the force will transmit to the patient's curled fingers. The response is a flexion of the patient's fingers.

Patellar (Knee) Jerk (KJ): Let the knees swing free by the side of the bed or couch, and place one hand on the quadriceps so you can feel its contraction. If the patient is in bed, slightly flex the knee by placing your forearm under both knees by contraction of the quadriceps with extension of the leg. If the reflex is hyperactive there is sometimes concomitant adduction of the ipsilateral thigh. Adduction of the opposite thigh and extension of the opposite leg also can occur simultaneously if those reflexes are hyperactive. Note that this so-called crossed thigh adduction or leg extension tells you that the reflexes in the opposite leg are hyperactive. They tell you nothing about the state of the reflex in the leg being tested. Use the Jendrassik manoeuvre if there is no response (Figure 1-47). The KJ is mediated by the L3 and L4 nerve roots, mainly L4.

Ankle Jerk (AJ): With the patient sitting, place one hand underneath the sole and dorsiflex the foot slightly. Then tap on the Achilles tendon just above its insertion on the calcaneus. If the patient is in bed, flex the knee and invert or evert the foot somewhat, cradling the foot and lower leg in your arm. Then tap on the tendon. If no response is obtained, have the patient face a chair and kneel on it with the knees resting against the back of the chair, the elbows on the top of the back, and the feet projecting over the seat. First dorsiflex the foot slightly and tap on the tendon.[9] Use the Jendrassik manoeuvre if this does not work. This position is well suited to observing the relaxation phase of the reflex in patients with suspected thyroid disease (Figure 1-48).

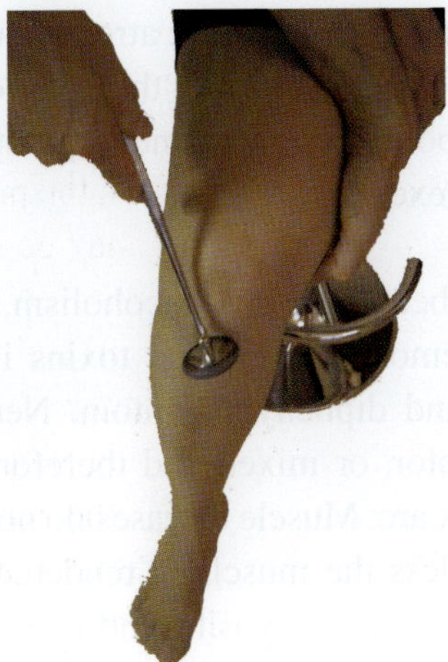

Figure 1-47: The knee jerk.

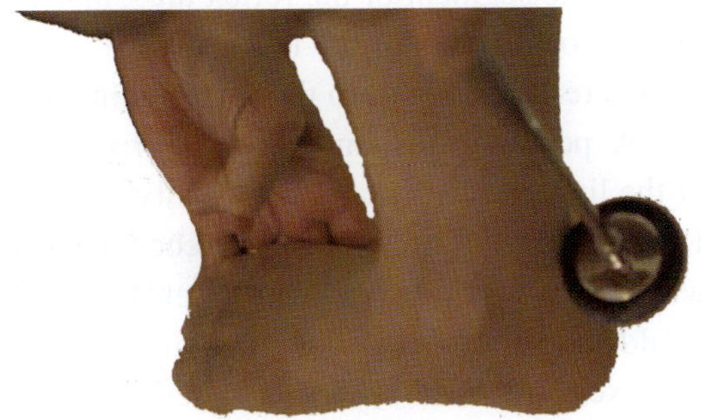

Figure 1-48: Ankle jerk.

1-8-5 *How to interpret reflex findings?*

Clinical significance: Absent stretch reflexes indicate a lesion in the reflex arc itself. Associated symptoms and signs make localisation possible in most cases:

- Absent reflexes and sensory loss in the distribution of the nerve supplying the reflex means that the lesion involves the afferent arc of the reflex; either the nerve or the dorsal horn.

- Absent reflex with paralysis, muscle atrophy, and fasciculation means the lesion involves the efferent arc; the anterior horn cells (AHC) or efferent nerve, or both. Peripheral neuropathy is the most common cause of absent reflexes.

The causes include diabetes mellitus, alcoholism, amyloidosis, uraemia; vitamin deficiencies, remote cancer; and toxins including lead, arsenic, isoniazid, vincristine, and diphenylhydantoin. Neuropathies can be predominantly sensory, motor, or mixed and therefore can affect any or all components of the reflex arc. Muscle diseases do not produce a disturbance of the stretch reflex unless the muscle is rendered too weak to contract. This occasionally occurs in polymyositis and muscular dystrophy.

- Hyperactive stretch reflexes are seen when there is interruption of the cortical supply to the LMN, an UMN lesion. The interruption can be anywhere above the segment of the reflex arc. Analysis of associated findings enables localisation of the lesion.
- Pendular stretch reflexes: insult to the cerebellum may lead to pendular reflexes. A pendular response is not brisk but involves less damping of the limb movement than is usually observed when a deep tendon reflex is elicited. Patients with cerebellar lesions may have a KJ that swings forwards and backwards several times. A normal or brisk KJ would have little more than one swing forward and one back. Pendular reflexes are best observed when the patient's legs are allowed to hang and swing freely off the end of an examination couch.

The deep tendon reflexes are useful localising signs to determine the site of the lesion (Table 1-6).

Other reflexes:
A number of other reflexes are examined at the same time as examining the tendon jerks. These include:

Cremasteric reflex (CR): Elicited in males by stroking the medial side of the thigh and observing elevation of the ipsilateral testicle. CR is absent in L1 and L2 lesions.

Table 1-6: Deep tendon reflexes and localisation

Abbreviation	Name of reflex	Level/site
JJ	Jaw jerk	Trigeminal nerve
PJ	Pectoralis jerk	C4
DJ	Deltoid jerk	C5
BJ	Biceps jerk	Mainly C6
SJ	Supinator jerk	Mainly C6
TJ	Triceps jerk	Mainly C7
FJ	Finger jerk	C8 and T1
KJ	Knee jerk	L3 and L4
AJ	Ankle jerk	S1

Posterior tibial reflex (PTR): Elicited by taping the tibialis posterior tendon, just behind the lateral malleolus. The reflex is absent in L5 nerve lesion.

Plantar reflex (PR): The plantar response is an important reflex to master and understand its significance. Stroking the lateral aspect of the sole of each foot with the end of a reflex hammer or a key will produce flexion of the toes. Extension of the big toe with fanning of the other toes is abnormal (a positive Babinski). The afferent reflex arc is S1 nerve root (Figure 1-49). An absent PR means LMN of the S1 nerve root or anterior horn cell of S1. Babinski positive means there was an UMN lesion. However Babinski positive will also be observed in drowsy individuals, comatose patients and in infants.

The abdominal reflex: Use a blunt object such as a key or tongue depressor spatula. Stroke the abdomen lightly on each side in an inward and downward direction above (T8, T9, T10) and below the umbilicus (T10, T11, T12). Note the contraction of the abdominal muscles and deviation of the umbilicus towards the stimulus (Figure 1-50).

Anal wink (AW): Elicited by striking the skin around the anus and observing the anus reaction. The afferent arc is innervated by S3-5.

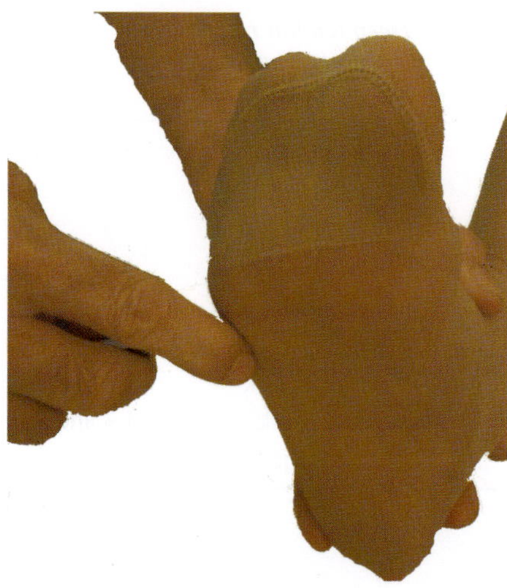

Figure 1-49: Eliciting the plantar response.

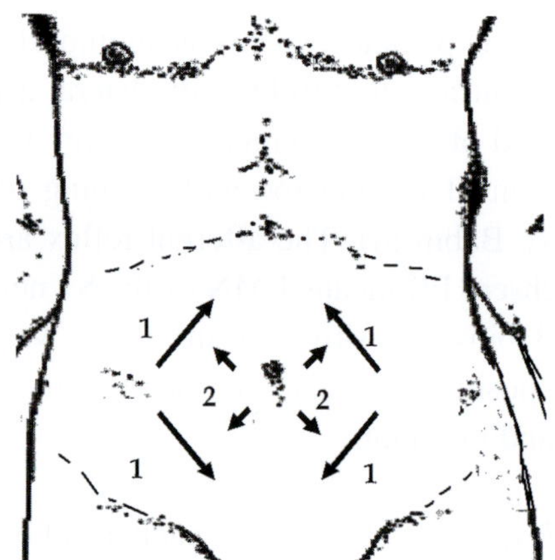

Figure 1-50: Diagram of the abdominal reflex. Number 1 denotes the direction of the abdominal stroke. Number 2 denotes the normal direction of movements of the umbilicus in a normal reflex arc.

Your personal notes:

....
....
....
....
....
....
....
....
....
....

Problem 1-9:   How to examine the sensory system, coordination and gait efficiently and make a lasting impression. (The smart way of performing neurological physical examination 8)

Examination of the sensory system is very important in all patients, particularly in the upper and lower limbs. Symptoms related to dysfunction of the sensory system include the following:

- Numbness.
- Pins and needles.
- Sensory impairment.
- Lack of sensation.
- Pain.
- Abnormal sensation.

<u>Problem based tool box:</u>
Where do different sensation carried?
How to assess the spinothalamic pathways?
How to assess the posterior columns?
How to assess cortical sensation?
How to assess coordination and cerebellar signs?

To examine the sensory system you need to consider the following facts:

1- Pain and temperature are transmitted via the spino-thalamic tracts (STT) that crosses to the opposite side within two to six segments of the spinal cord anteriorly (Figure 1-51).

2- Proprioception, vibration and light touch are transmitted via the posterior column (PC) that crosses to the opposite side in the medulla oblongata (Figure 1-51).

3- Stereognosis (SG), one-point localisation (OPL) and two-point discrimination (TPD) require intact STT and PC and intact sensory cortex (area 312 in the post-central gyrus).

4- You need to compare sides, and up and down to detect abnormal sensation and once you detect an area of altered sensation map it out by moving from abnormal to normal to establish dermatomal sensory loss or sensory level.

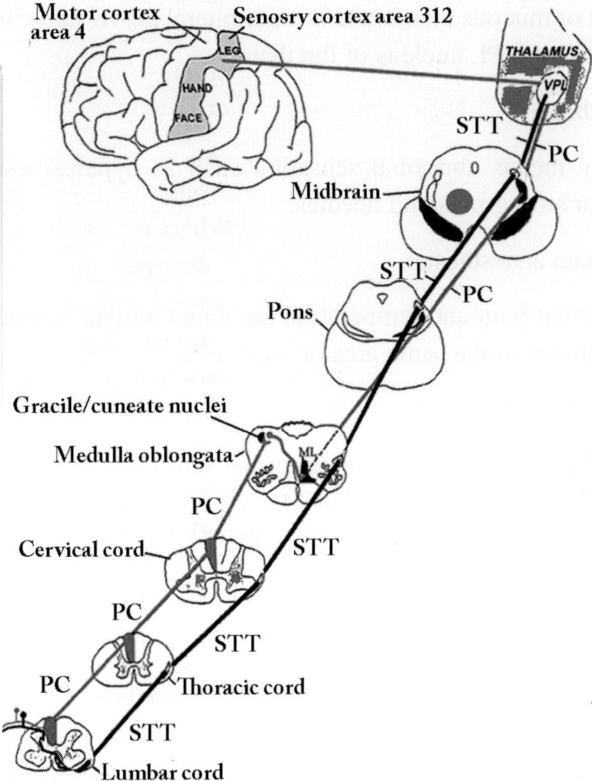

Figure 1-51: The sensory pathways. VPL = Ventro-posterio-lateral thalamic nucleus.

5- Always examine pain, temperature, touch, proprioception and vibration sense before examining cortical sensation (SG, OPL and TPD).

Abnormal sensory findings or focal sensory neurological deficits include:

1- Anaesthesia or hypoesthesia:

Complete lack of sensation (anaesthesia) or impaired sensation (hypoesthesia) occurs when pain, temperature and touch are interrupted in the area of skin or mucous membrane in a peripheral nerve, nerve trunk, nerve root, the STT or VPL nucleus of the thalamus.

2- Paraesthesia:

Paraesthesia means abnormal sensation such as hyperesthesia, burning sensation, or strong pins and needles.

3- Dissociate anaesthesia:

This means that pain and temperature are intact on one side and proprioception is absent in the same area or vice versa.

4- Sensory level:

This denotes the level of lack or abnormal sensation. For example if we say patient X had a sensory level at T10, we mean that patient X is unable to feel the sensation below the level of T10 (the umbilicus).

1-9-1 How to localise a lesion along the sensory pathway?

To test and identify the correct sensory level you need to know the sensory landmarks on the body (Table 1-7 and Figure 1-52).

1-9-2 How to examine the spinothalamic sensory pathways?

1-9-2i Examination of light touch:

Use a wisp of cotton to test for light touch; do not stroke the skin if the skin is hairy as that would not be testing light touch. Gently touch the skin with the patient's eyes open in normal area first so that the patient understands what is being tested. Then examine touch in systematic fashion with the patient's eyes closed. Map any abnormal area by moving from abnormal to normal.

1-9-2ii Examination for pain and temperature:

Because pain and temperature are transmitted in the STT, testing pain often is sufficient in most clinical scenarios. To test pain sensation, use a

Table 1-7: *Localisation of sensory dermatomes and sensory levels*

Dermatome/Level	Description of the area
C2	The occipital region of the scalp.
C3	The lateral aspect of the neck.
C4	The shoulder area.
C5	The lateral area of the upper arm around the deltoid.
C6	The thumb and extends above the wrist in the forearm.
C7	The middle finger and extends above the wrist.
C8	The little finger and extends above the wrist in the forearm.
T1	The arm pit.
T4	The nipple area.
T6	The xiphoid level.
T10	The umbilicus.
T12	The symphysis pubis.
L2	Lateral thigh.
L3	Around the front of the knee.
L4	Medial calf/ medial malleolus.
L5	The big toe.
S1	Lateral border of the foot.
S3–5	Saddle area.

neurotip (Figure 1-20). Use similar technique to that used to test trigeminal sensation. Use the sharp end and the blunt end in normal area first so the patient understands what you are testing and ask the patient to distinguish the two sensations. With the patient's eyes closed test the skin in a systematic fashion using random sharp and blunt pricks and ask the patient to identify the sensation by uttering the word "sharp" if (s)he thinks that the sharp end was used and the word "blunt" if (s)he thinks that the blunt end was used. Map from abnormal to normal. Testing temperature is often omitted if pain sensation was normal. However, you can use a tuning fork (TF) heated or cooled by water and ask the patient to identify "hot" or "cold". Test the following areas: shoulders (C4), (T1) and outer (C5) aspects of the arms, thumbs (C6), middle fingers (C7) and little fingers (C8), front of both thighs (L2), front of the knees (L3), medial (L4) and lateral (L5) aspect of both calves and lateral border of the feet (S1).

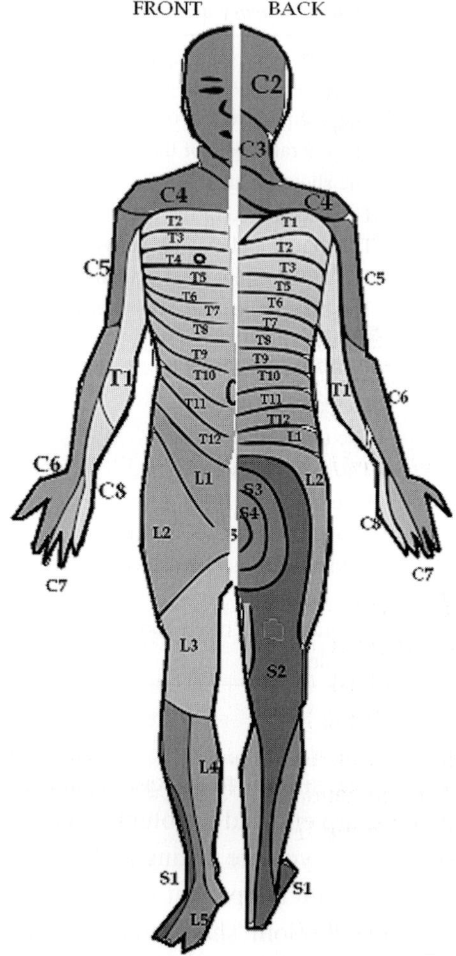

Figure 1-52: Sensory dermatomes and sensory levels.

1-9-3 *How to assess integrity of posterior columns?*

1-9-3i *Examination of joint position and joint movements:*

To examine for joint position and joint movement (JPM) hold the distal phalanx of the big toe between your thumb and index, holding the sides of the toe rather than superior-inferior surface to avoid the use of other sensation such as pressure. Move the phalanx up or down, show the

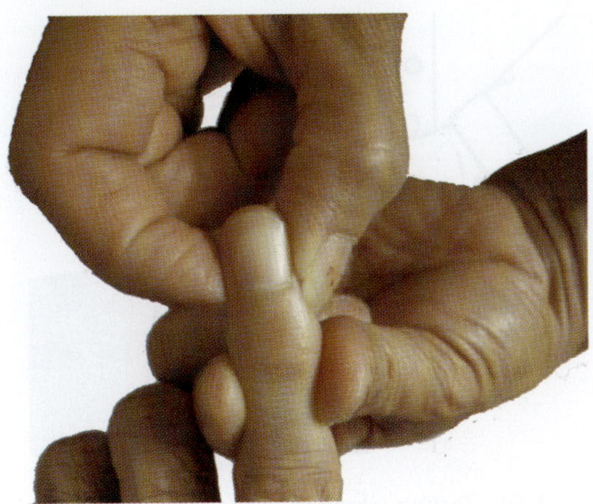

Figure 1-53: *Joint position and joint movement technique at the distal interphalangeal joint of the index finger.*

patient these movements to explain what is up and what is down with the eyes open, ask the patient to close his/her eyes and move the phalanx up and down at random and ask the patient to report if the movement was up or down (Figure 1-53). If the IPM sensation is absent at the big toe repeat the test at the ankle joint, then the knee if the JPM was absent at the ankle. Similarly test JPM in the hand starting distally and moving proximally till you find a joint at which the JPM is intact.

1-9-3ii *Vibration sense examination:*

You require a tuning fork (TF) of 128 Hz. Show the patient what you are testing by striking the TF and placing its vibrating base at a bony prominence that you are sure is normal, e.g. mastoid or sternum. Repeat the test with the TF not vibrating so there is no doubt about what you are looking for. Once you are satisfied that the patient knows what you are testing, place the vibrating TF stem with the patient's eyes closed on the distal interphalangeal joint in the index finger and big toe in each limb, if vibration sense absent proceed proximally to the wrists and malleoli, if absent proceed to elbow and patellae, if absent proceed to clavicles, greater trochanters and spinous processes (Figure 1-54).

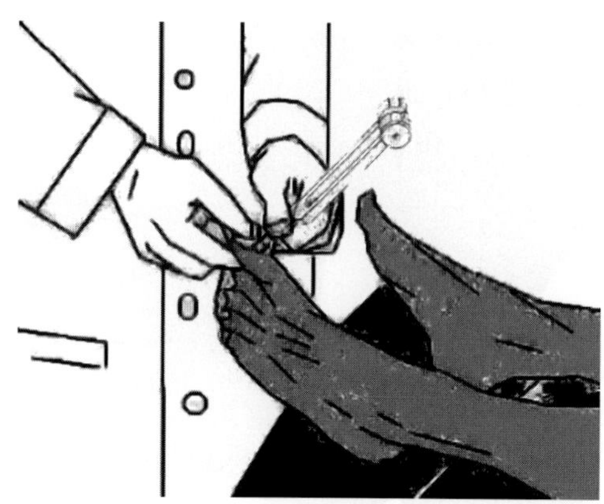

Figure 1-54: Testing vibration in the interphalangeal joint.

1-9-4 *How to examine cortical sensation?*

Proceed to examine these if the aforementioned sensations were normal and you suspect a parietal lobe problem.

1-9-4i *Stereognosis:*

To check stereognosis place a familiar object in the patient's hand (coin, paper clip, pencil, etc.). Ask the patient to identify the object.

1-9-4ii *One-point localisation:*

With the patient's eyes closed touch the skin with a pen to make a mark, give the pen to the patient in the untested hand and ask him (her) to make a similar mark where (s)he thought (s)he felt you had made your mark. Measure the distance between the two marks. On the distal phalanx should be few millimetres; on the trunk should be about 10 mm (Figure 1-55).

1-9-4iii *Two-point discrimination:*

Use an opened paper clip or a specific calliper that has two points to touch the patient's finger pads in two places simultaneously. Randomly alternate the test by touch with one or two points, ask the patient to identify "one"

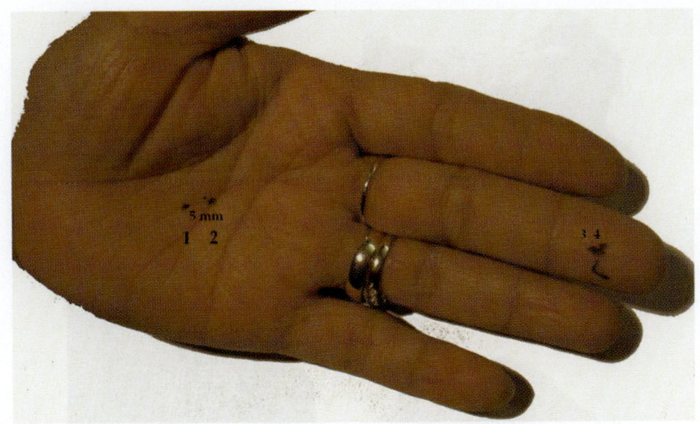

Figure 1-55: One point localisation on the palm compared to the tip index.

or "two". Find the minimal distance at which the patient can discriminate. On the tip of the fingers it should be very few millimetres, while on the palm could be 5–6 mm.

1-9-4iv *Graphesthesia:*

With the blunt end of a pen or pencil, draw a large number (2, 5, 6, 9 etc.) in the patient's palm. Ask the patient to identify the number.

1-9-5 *How to assess coordination?*

Coordination is dependent on the integrity of proprioception, visual cues, vestibular system and the cerebellum. The following tests are often used to assess coordination.

1-9-5i *Finger nose test:*

Ask the patient to touch your finger then the tip of his/her nose repetitively and observe over shooting (Figure 1-56).

1-9-5ii *Heel-shin test:*

Ask the patient to slide the heel of one leg over the front of the shin of the other (Figure 1-57).

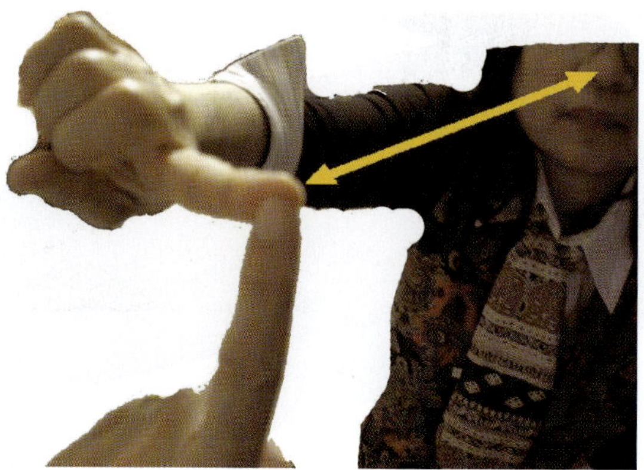

Figure 1.56: Finger nose test, patient tries to touch examiner's finger than his/her nose repetitively while the examiner changes the position of his finger.

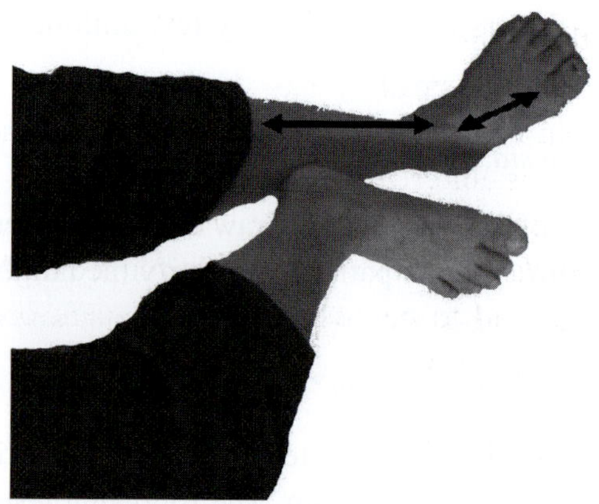

Figure 1-57: The heel-shin test.

1-9-5iii *Disdiadokinesis:*

Ask the patient to stretch their hands supine in front and then to rapidly move in pronation/supination movements. Alternatively ask the patient to mimic playing the piano with the fingers, or ask the patient to tap the distal thumb with the tip of the index finger as fast as possible, or ask the patient to strike one hand on the thigh, raise the hand, turn it over, and then

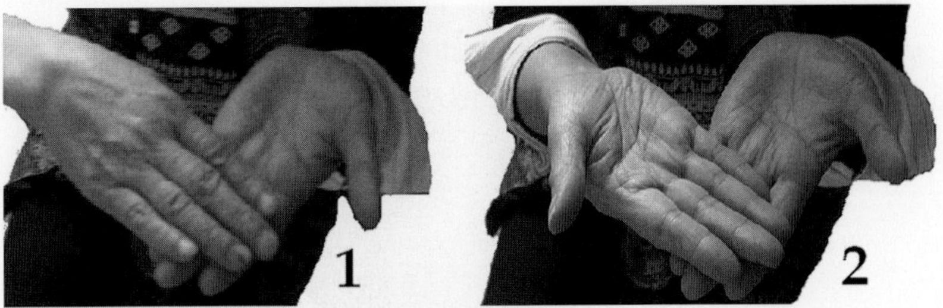

Figure 1-58: *Alternative tapping of the palm and dorsum of the right hand.*

strike it back down as fast as possible, or ask the patient to tap your hand with the ball of each foot as fast as possible. Observe the speed and symmetry of movements (Figure 1-58).

1-9-5iv *Romberg test:*

Please be aware that if this test is positive, i.e. patient is dependent almost entirely on their vision to steady themselves in space and have no proprioception the patient may fall to the ground, so be prepared to catch the patient if they are unstable. To perform the test, ask the patient to stand with the feet together (Figure 1-59). Ask the patient to close his/her eyes for five to ten seconds without support, while you are ready to support the patient. The test is said to be positive if the patient becomes unstable (indicating a vestibular or proprioception problem).

1-9-5v *How to assess gait?*

Ask the patient to walk across the room, turn and come back, observe posture, hand swing and steadiness. Then ask the patient to walk heel-to-toe (Figure 1-60) in a straight line (tandem gait) and observe any unsteadiness. Ask the patient to walk on their toes in a straight line and then on their heels in a straight line. Finally ask the patient to hop in place on each foot and do a shallow knee bend rise from a sitting position.

1-9-5vi *How to assess inattention?*

Some patients may have inattention for sensory information from one side of the body often seen in parietal lobe lesions. To look for inattention you

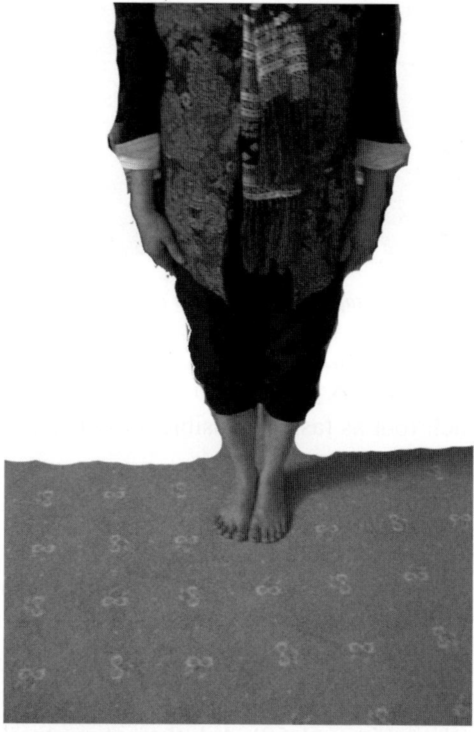

Figure 1-59: To perform Romberg test ask patient to stand with the feet together, stand behind the patient to support her/him.

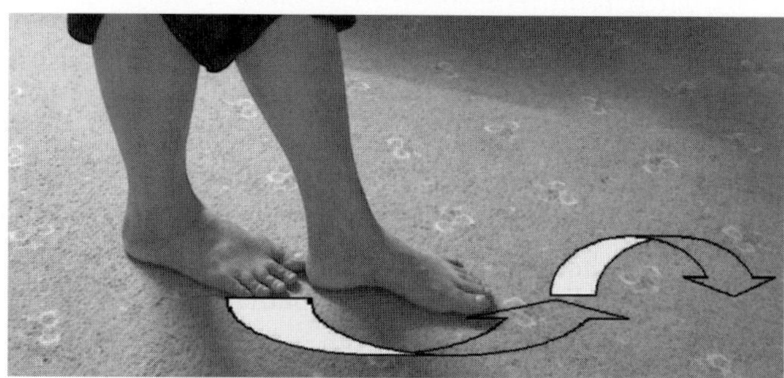

Figure 1-60: Tandem gait.

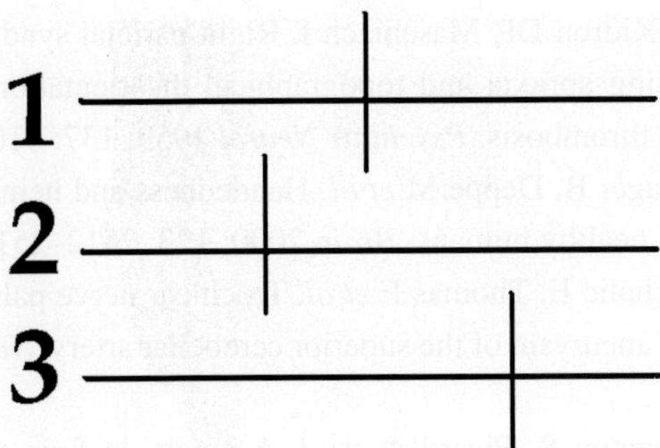

Figure 1-61: Line bisection and inattention: 1 normal midline bisection, 2 in right hemi neglect, and 3 in left hemi neglect.

have to present the patient with simultaneous stimulation of the left and right sides of the body as follows:

- *Visual inattention:* If the visual fields were tested individually and both were normal, look for inattention by presenting visual cues simultaneously in the two visual fields. Ask the patient to focus on a distant object, use both hands and present moving index fingers in the temporal field of each eye simultaneously and ask the patient to point to the moving finger. Inattention is present when the patient always points to one side only when both fingers were moving.

- *Sensory inattention:* With the patient's eyes closed, ask the patient to say "right" when the right palm is touched and "left" when the left palm is touched. Sensory inattention is present when the patient identifies only one side when both palms were touched at the same time.

- *Line bisection test:* Draw a line on a paper and ask the patient to draw a line across the middle of the line. Patient with inattention will bisect the line to one side (Figure 1-61).

References

1. Mayer E, Martory MD, Pegna AJ *et al.* A pure case of Gerstmann syndrome with a subangular lesion. *Brain* 1999; 122: 1107–1120.

2. Bornstein B, Kidron DP, Maschiach I. Right parietal syndrome spatial inattention, dressing apraxia and topographical disorientation, following right carotid artery thrombosis. *Psychiatr Neurol* 1959; 137: 310–324.

3. Knecht S, Drager B, Deppe M *et al.* Handedness and hemispheric language dominance in healthy humans. *Brain* 2000; 123: 2512–2518.

4. Collins T, Mehalic E, Thomas F *et al.* Trochlear nerve palsy as the sole initial sign of an aneurysm of the superior cerebellar artery. *Neurosurgery* 1992; 30: 258–261.

5. Bléry M, Chagnon S, Picard A *et al.* A report on four cases, including a Gradenigo-Lannois syndrome. *J Radiol* 1980; 61: 677–681.

6. Garnit R. The functional role of the muscle spindles: facts and hypotheses. *Brain* 1975; 98: 531–556.

7. Delwaide PJ, Toulouse P. The Jendrassik manoeuvre: quantitative analysis of reflex reinforcement by remote voluntary muscle contraction. *Adv Neurol* 1983; 39: 661–669.

8. Gassel MM, Diamantopoulos E. The Jendrassik manoeuvre. *Neurology* 1964; 14: 555–560, 640–642.

9. Impallomeni M, Kenny RA, Flynn MD *et al.* The elderly and their ankle jerks. *Lancet* 1984; 1: 670–672.

Your personal notes:

....

....

....

....

....

....

....

....

....

....

Chapter 2: Neurological Investigations

Problem 2-1:   Computerised tomographic scan (CT): How to interpret CT-based images?

Computerised tomographic scan (CT) is a method used to generate three-dimensional image of an object, e.g. the brain from a series of two-dimensional X-ray images taken around a single rotational axis (Figure 2-1).

Problem based tool box:

CT pros and cons

Hyperdense lesions

Isodense lesions

Hypodense lesions

Ring lesions

Each image is a computer-generated image of a volume of an object or organ based on X-ray absorption (electron density). By convention the right side of the body is projected on the left side of the image as if you are looking into a mirror. Each CT image (slice) is 1.25 to 10 mm thick and related to an axis on the scout view (Figure 2-2).

2-1-1: *How can I read a plain CT image of the brain?*

The easy way to read an image is to view the image systematically starting from one location, e.g. one corner and scan the whole image square by square and note any abnormalities. To spot abnormalities you need to be familiar with the normal anatomy of the organ under investigation. Normal CT brain image demonstrates the following anatomy (Figure 2-3):

1- Brain tissue as a shade of grey (1).
2- CSF in the ventricles as shade of dark (2) hypodense compared to brain which means it is darker than brain.
3- Bone (skull) as a shade of white (3) hyperdense = whiter than brain.

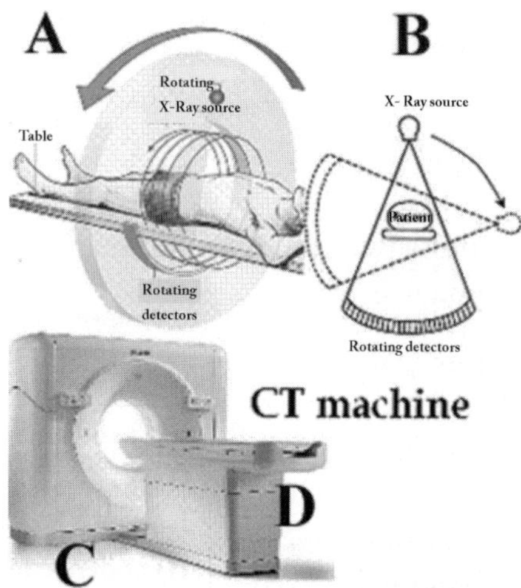

Figure 2-1: Diagram of CT scanner. A = The axis of rotation of X-ray source and detectors, B = schematic representation of X-ray tube and detectors rotation, C = image of the CT scanner gantry housing the X-ray tubes and detectors, and D = motorised table to feed the patient into the scanner gantry.

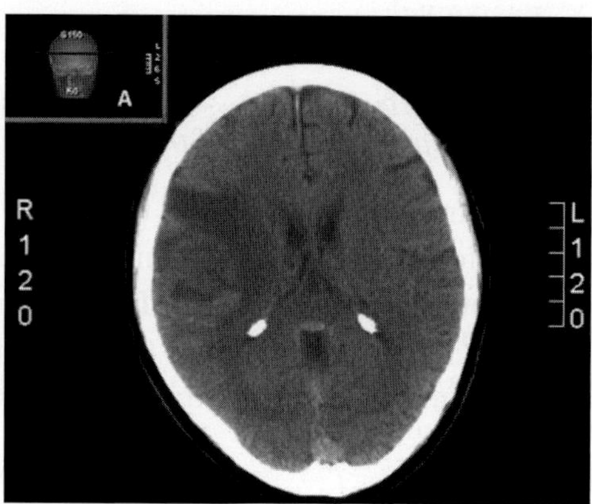

Figure 2-2: CT scan slice of the head 1.5 mm thick, the exact location of the image is shown on the scout view (A).

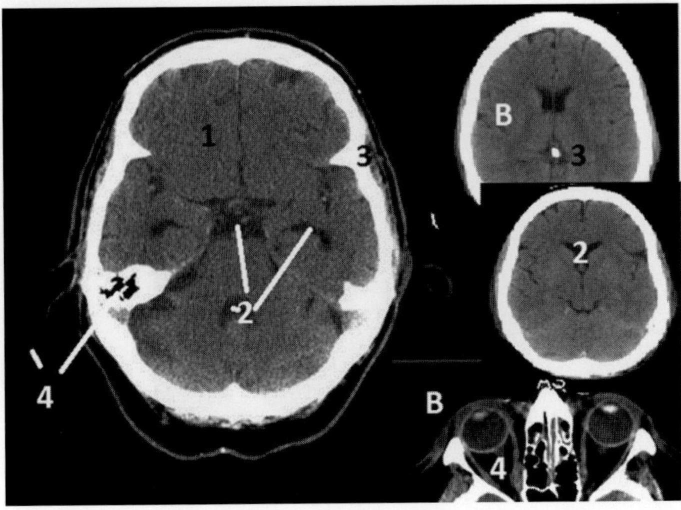

Figure 2-3: Normal CT brain showing skull bone (3-A), pineal calcification (3-B), air (4), and fat in the orbit (4-B).

4- Air, e.g. in the mastoid air cells, paranasal sinuses and around the head will appear as very dark (4), hypodense.
5- Fat, e.g. in the orbits will also appear as dark (5), hypodense.
6- Calcification, e.g. in the choroid plexus or pineal body will appear as white (6), hyperdense.

In summary normal CT scan appearance of CSF, fat and air is hypodense (dark) and bone and calcification appearance on CT is hyperdense (white). These descriptions are valid when the image-window level is set for soft tissue (brain) as the images can be manipulated using windowing features, e.g. brain, bone, spine, etc. (Figure 2-4). Each density can be assigned a Hounsfield number. Sir G Hounsfield invented the CT scan in 1967 and it was publicly announced in 1972. Although CT scan images are obtained in the axial plane, the data can be reconstructed in multiple orthogonal planes (Figure 2-5).

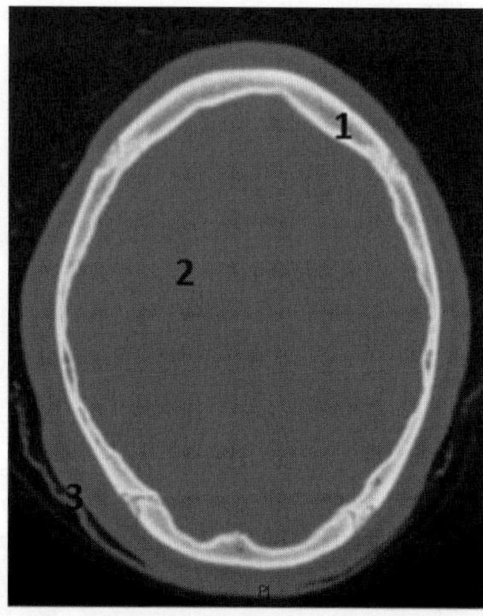

Figure 2-4: Axial CT head using bone window demonstrating the skull inner and outer tables (hyperdense) and the scalp slightly hyperdense.

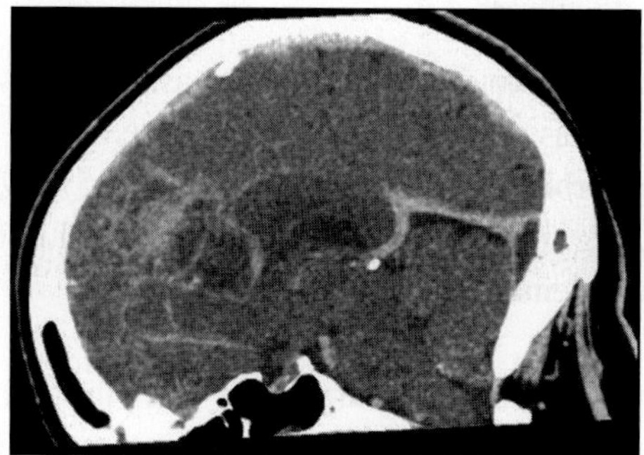

Figure 2-5: CT scan reconstructions in sagittal plane.

2-1-2 *What are the uses of CT scan?*

CT scan of the head is used to evaluate the following conditions:

- Head trauma:

In head trauma CT is proved to be a very valuable tool. It can detect skull fractures, fluid levels in paranasal sinuses, diffuse axonal injury, brain

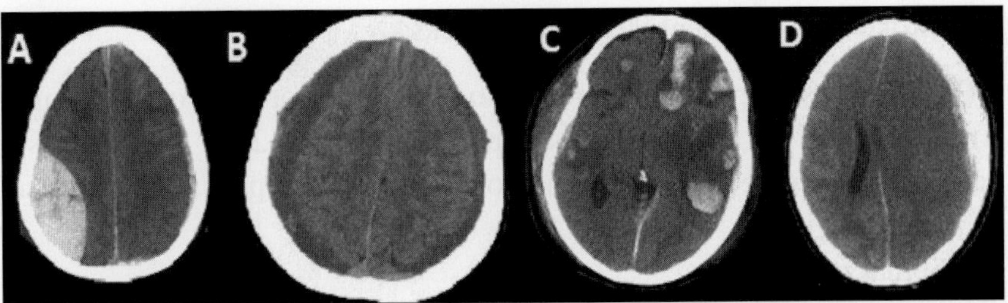

Figure 2-6: CT images in head injuries: A = right hyperdense bilenticular mass (extradural haematoma), B = right hypodense sickle-shaped collection (chronic subdural haematoma), C = multiple hyperdense lesions spread in the two cerebral hemispheres (contusions), and D = left sickle-shaped hyperdense collection (acute subdural haematoma) associated with swelling of the left cerebral hemisphere and midline shift.

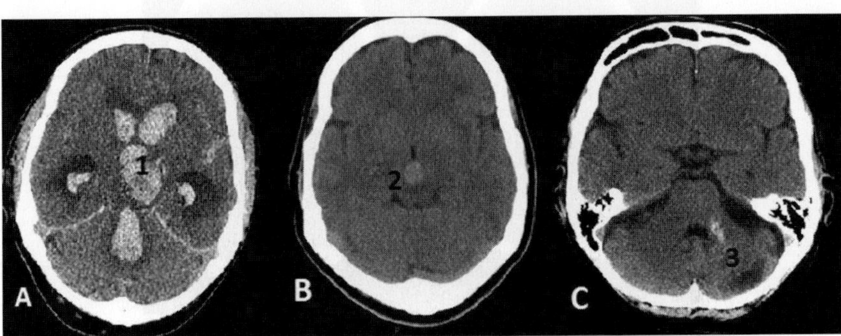

Figure 2-7: Plain CT scan images of spontaneous intracranial haemorrhage: A = intraventricular bleed (1), B = hyperdense basilar tip aneurysm (2), and C = calcification in the cerebellum due to AVM (3).

swelling, intracranial air, extradural haematoma (Figure 2-6A), subdural haematoma (Figures 2-6B and 2-6D), and cerebral contusion (Figure 2-6C).

- Spontaneous intracranial haemorrhage:

Acute blood in the cranial cavity appears hyperdense on CT. CT is proved to be very valuable in the diagnosis of subarachnoid haemorrhage (SAH) confirming the diagnosis and sometimes demonstrating an underlying aneurysm or AVM (Figure 2-7).

- Strokes and transient ischaemic attacks:

CT scan is used in patients suspected to have stroke or cerebral ischaemia. An established stroke appears as hypodense (Figure 2-8). If there was a haemorrhage in the infarct, the haemorrhage would appear as hyperdense.

- Spinal trauma:

CT is proved to be very valuable in assessing patients with spinal trauma particularly the cervical spine when an area is obscured by the shoulders, e.g. the cervico-thoracic junction. It is also very valuable in reconstructing the spine to evaluate its stability (Figure 2-9).

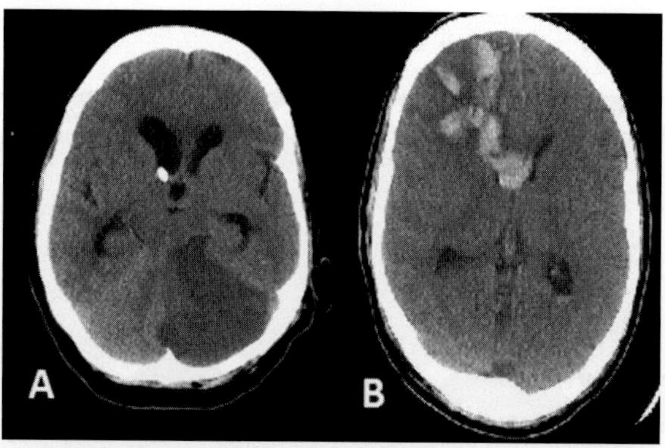

Figure 2-8: Plain CT scan images of cerebellar stroke (A), B = haemorrhage in the right frontal lobe with some blood layering in the left occipital horn.

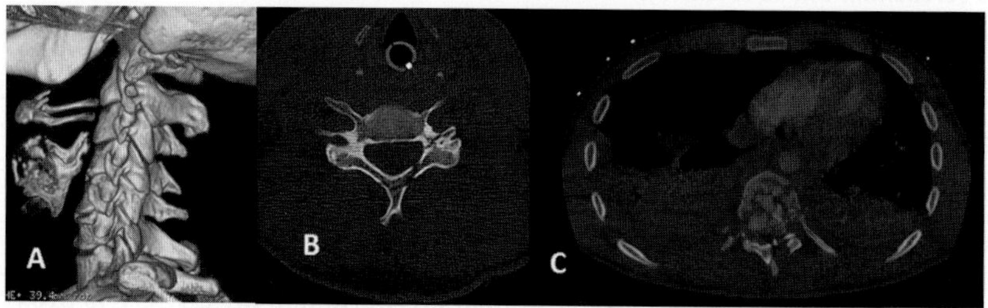

Figure 2-9: CT scan images of the spine: A = 3D reconstruction of cervical spine, B = axial image of C7 with fracture in the left lamina, and C = burst fracture of thoracic vertebra with bilateral haemothorax.

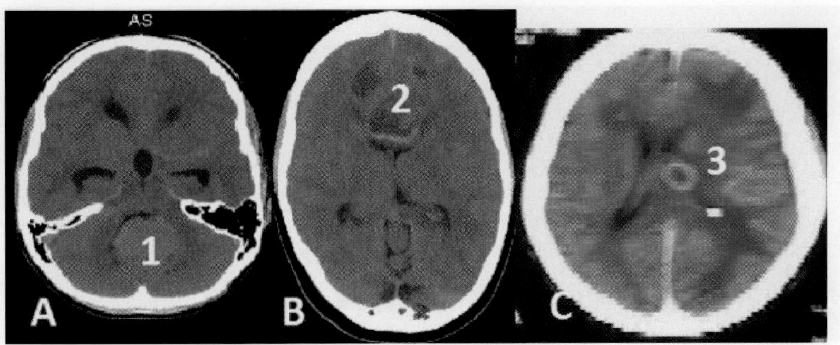

Figure 2-10: CT scan images of patients with raised ICP: A = posterior cranial fossa tumour (1) with hydrocephalus, B = butterfly glioma (2), and C = multiple abscesses, one in the left thalamus (3).

- Suspected raised intracranial pressure (ICP):

Patients suspected to have raised ICP such as those presenting with headache, nausea and vomiting, patients with papilloedema, patients with focal neurological deficits, patients with seizures and patients with reduced consciousness or comatose (Figure 2-10).

- Stereotactic targeting:

CT can be used in conjunction with stereotactic frames or frameless image guided technology to biopsy lesions in the brain, insert electric leads in the brain, insert catheters, chemicals or cells, and localise lesions during surgery (Figure 2-11).

- Surgical planning:

Neurosurgery is image dependent and almost no neurosurgical procedure is carried out without neuro-image guidance. From 1990s most neurosurgical procedures are carried out using image guided systems that are able to track the surgical field and display the corresponding location on an image space created on the computer workstation.

- Assessment of paranasal sinuses, temporal bone, skull bone and facial bones and their lesions.

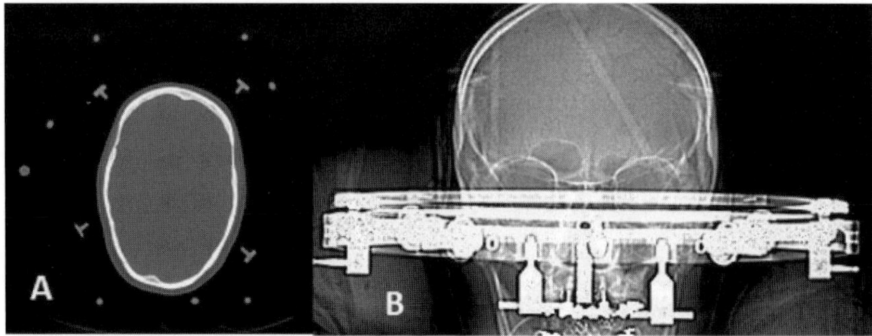

Figure 2-11: Plain CT scan images planning for stereotactic biopsy: A = axial slice with nine fiducials and B = scout view showing the stereotactic frame ring.

- Radiotherapy planning.
- Staging of malignancies by performing CT scan of chest, abdomen and pelvis.

IV contrast is used after plain CT to highlight breakdown in the blood brain barrier (BBB). Some lesions enhance well (homogenous enhancement), others have mixed enhancement and others do not enhance at all.

2-1-3 *What enhancement patterns are seen on CT?*

1- Homogenous enhancement is seen in Figure 2-12:

    a. Meningiomas.
    b. Vestibular schwannomas.

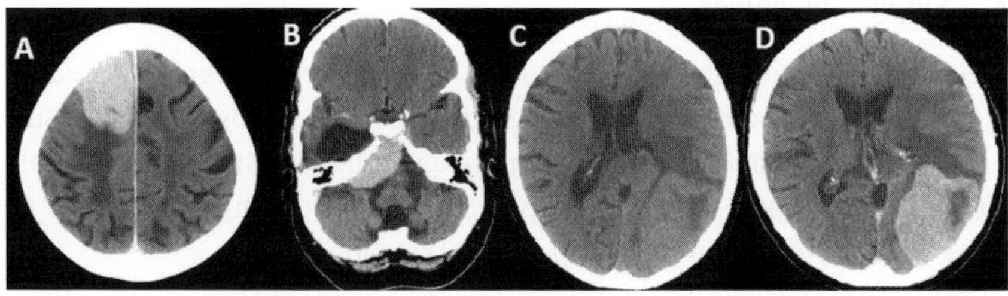

Figure 2-12: Examples of homogenous enhancing lesion: A, B, C, and D meningiomas; C before contrast and D after contrast injection.

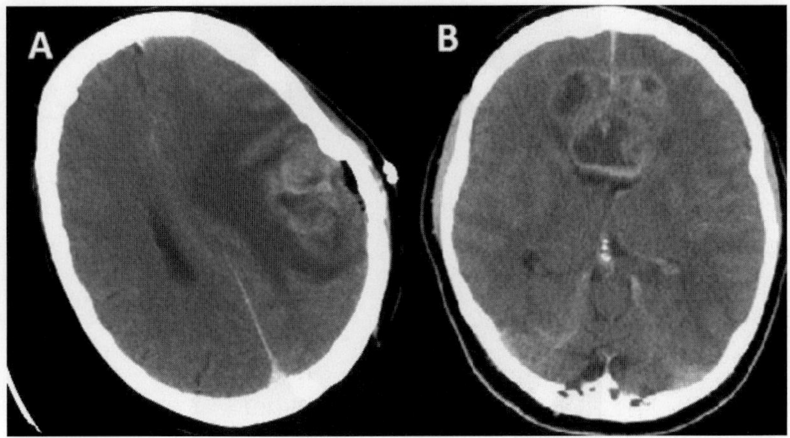

Figure 2-13: Examples of non-uniform mixed enhancing lesions: A metastasis and B glioblastoma multiforme (GBM).

    c.   Haemangioblastoma nodules.
    d.   Pilocytic astrocytoma.
    e.   Haemangiopericytoma.
    f.   Ependymoma.

2- Mixed enhancement is seen in Figure 2-13:

    a.   High grade gliomas.
    b.   Metastases.
    c.   Medulloblastoma.
    d.   Pituitary adenomas.
    e.   Craniopharyngiomas.
    f.   Inflammatory lesions.

3- Peripheral enhancement is seen in Figure 2-14:

    a.   Abscess (ring enhancing lesion).
    b.   Cystic metastasis.
    c.   Cystic high grade glioma.
    d.   Luxury perfusion in acute infarct (2% after two days).
    e.   Cystic astrocytoma.
    f.   Inflammatory cyst.

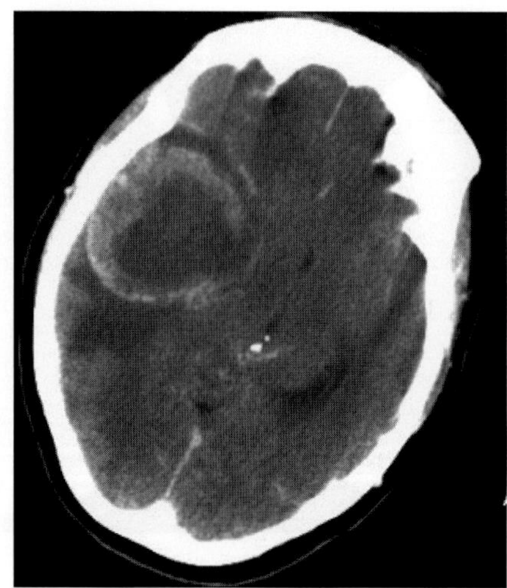

Figure 2-14: Examples of ring enhancing lesion (metastasis).

4- No enhancement is seen:

  a.   Infarction.
  b.   Arachnoid cyst.
  c.   Cholesterol cyst.
  d.   Lipoma.
  e.   Grade I astrocytoma.
  f.   Epidermoid cyst.

2-1-4 *What are the advantages of CT?*

CT has higher resolution and ability to image inside the skull. It can demonstrate bone very well, e.g. skull lesions, bony involvement and bone density. It can also demonstrate haemorrhages. Modern CT scanners have the added advantage of 3D reconstruction.

2-1-5 *What are the disadvantages of CT?*

One of the disadvantages of CT is the fact that it utilises ionising radiation and is considerate moderate to high risk investigation. Although CT

Table 2-1: Comparison of radiation dose of CT and other X-rays

Investigation	mSv (Effective dose)	Millirem
Chest X-ray	0.1	10
Head CT	1.5	150
Chest CT	5.8	580
Abdominal CT	5.3	530
Chest, abdomen and pelvis CT	9.9	990

represents about 7% of all radiological investigations using X-rays it is responsible for 47% of total collective radiation dose.[1] Due to the rise in using CT, the total medical radiation had increased despite that it had reduced in other areas (Table 2-1).

Another disadvantage of CT is reaction to contrast materials. Allergic reaction can occur and contrast material can lead to kidney failure, particularly in those who had pre-existing renal insufficiency or diabetes mellitus.

Problem 2-2:   Magnetic resonance imaging (MRI): How to interpret MRI-based images?

MRI scanning is a method used to visualise an organ, e.g. the brain using a powerful magnet to align the nuclei (hydrogen atoms) in the tissues. The aligned atoms are then systematically excited by radiofrequency fields to temporarily alter their alignment. When the hydrogen atoms re-align themselves, they emit

Problem based tool box:	
MRI pros and cons	
T1-weighted	**FLAIR**
T2-weighted	**MPRage**
CISS	**Diffusion**
Gadolinium	**DTI**

signal used to generate MRI images (Figure 2-15). This signal can be manipulated by additional magnetic fields to build up different image types.

MRI is very useful in neurological (brain and spine), musculoskeletal, cardiovascular, and oncological (cancer) imaging. The first human MRI scan was in 1977.

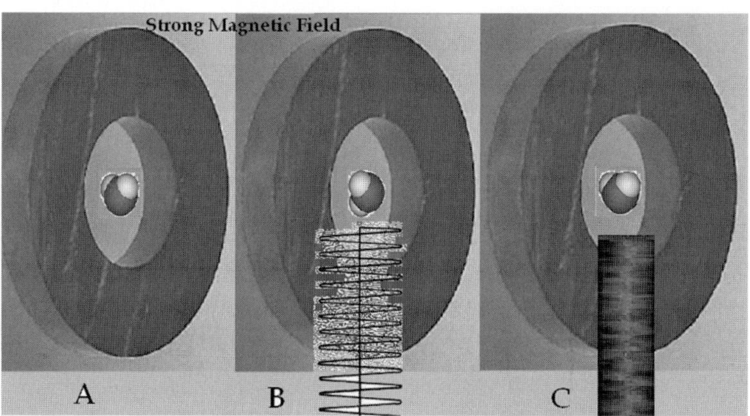

Figure 2-15: Mechanism of MRI: A = atoms are aligned within a strong magnet, B = radiofrequency field deflects the aligned atoms, and C = once the radiofrequency field is switched off, the atoms re-align themselves in the magnet and emit the signal.

2-2-1 *How can I read an MRI image of the brain?*

The easy way to read an image is to view the image systematically starting from one location, e.g. one corner and scan the whole image square by square and note any abnormalities. To spot abnormalities you need to be familiar with the normal anatomy of the organ under investigation under different MRI sequences.

2-2-2 *What are the different MRI sequences?*

1- T1-weighted MRI:

T1-weighted MRI sequences are obtained by using short TR and TE. Repetition time (TR) is the time interval between radiofrequency pulses and TE is time to echo. To obtain T1-weighted a TR of about 500 ms and TE of about 30 ms are used. Lesions with short T1 are bright and those with long T1 are dark. Bright T1-signal include: fat in lipomas and dermoids, subacute haemorrhage (metHb), high protein content (colloid cyst), and melanin (metastatic melanoma). Paramagnetic materials have short T1 and are bright, e.g. gadolinium (Figure 2-16). Long T1 is dark, e.g. bone, calcification, CSF and air (Figure 2-16).

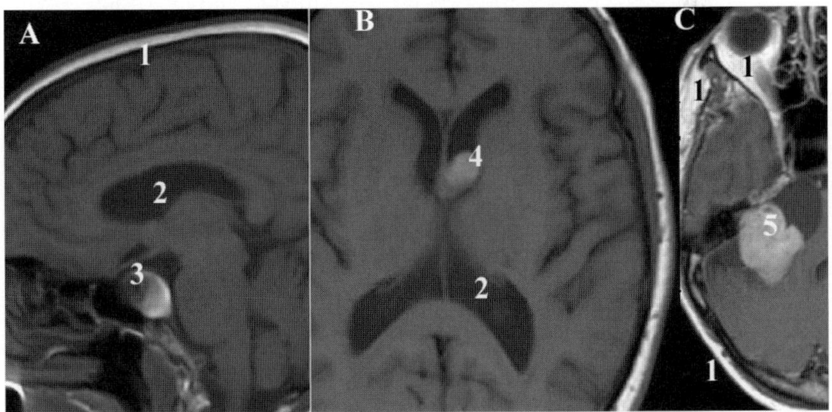

Figure 2-16: T1-MRI 1 = fat, 2 = CSF, 3 = Rathke cyst, 4 = colloid cyst, and 5 = gadolinium-enhanced vestibular schwannoma.

2- T2-weighted MRI:

T2-weighted MRI sequences are obtained by using long TR and TE. To obtain T2-weighted a TR of about 2000 ms and TE of about 100 ms are used. Lesions with short T2 are bright and those with long T2 are dark. Bright T2-signal include: fat in lipomas and dermoids, acute haemorrhage (deoxyHb), haemosidrin, physiological iron, and mucinous material. CSF is also bright on T2 (Figure 2-17). Long T2 is dark, e.g. bone, calcification, flowing blood (flow void in arteries and AVMs) and air (Figure 2-17).

The easy way to recognise T1 and T2 is to look at the ventricles, if the ventricles are bright then it is almost certainly T2-weighted and if they are dark it is most likely T1-weighted.

3- MPRage sequence:

Magnetisation Prepared Rapid Gradient Echo is a fast 3D gradient echo pulse sequence using a magnetisation preparation pulse like TurboFLASH. Only one segment or partition of a 3D data record is obtained per inversion preparation pulse. After the acquisition, for all rows a delay time (TD) is used to prevent saturation effects. MPRage is designed for rapid acquisition with T1-weighted dominance. Fast gradient echoes are characterised by their rapid sampling

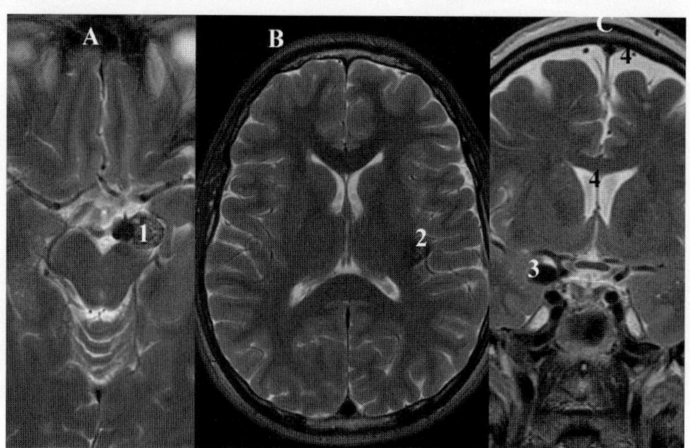

Figure 2-17: T2-weighted images 1 and 3 = flow void, 2 = haemosidrin, and 4 = CSF.

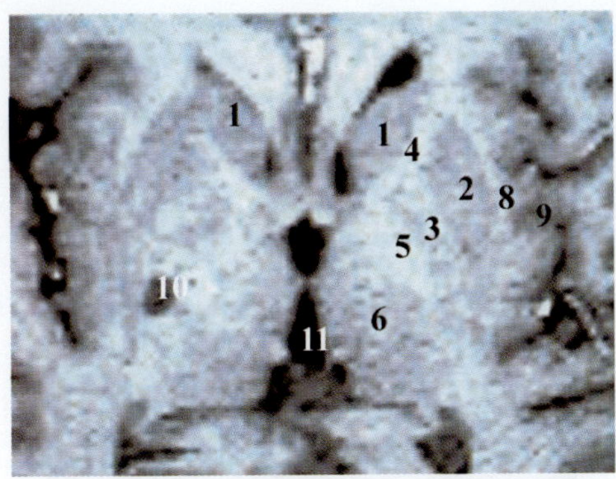

Figure 2-18: MPRage, 1 = caudate nucleus, 2 = putamen, 3 = globus pallidum, 4 = anterior limb of internal capsule (IC), 5 = posterior limb of IC, 6 = thalamus, 8 = external capsule, 9 = insular cortex, 10 = lesion in the pallidum, and 11 = third ventricle.

time, high signal intensity and image contrast while approaching steady state (the echo is collected during the time when tissues are experiencing T1 relaxation). The rapid speed of the acquisition makes it an excellent alternative to breath-hold abdominal imaging, neuro, dynamic bolus, MR angiography and cardiac imaging. MPRage is very useful in delineating the basal ganglia and other internal brain structures because of better contrast between the grey and white matters (Figure 2-18).

4- FLAIR sequence:

Fluid attenuated inversion recovery (FLAIR) produces strongly T_2-weighted image and suppressed CSF signal. This is accomplished by 180° inversion pulse. A relatively long TI is used to allow the longitudinal magnetisation of CSF to return to the null point before SE imaging. Thus, the CSF signal is completely suppressed for cortical or periventricular areas, and lesions with typical T_2 prolongation in the brain that are adjacent to spinal fluid become much more conspicuous compared with conventional T_2 imaging (Figure 2-19). FLAIR sequence is very useful in acute multiple sclerosis and acute infarction. FLAIR removes CSF partial volume artifact that obscures these lesions on T2-weighted images.[2]

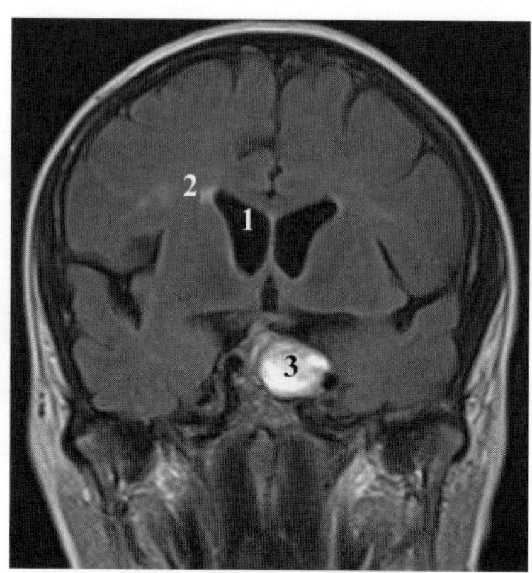

Figure 2-19: FLAIR images demonstrating periventricular high signal lesions in the right hemisphere (2) and very dark signal of suppressed CSF (1). It also demonstrates high signal in clotted aneurysm (3).

5- CISS sequence:

Constructive Interference Steady State (CISS) is a stimulated T2 echo, where two true fast spin echo sequences are acquired with differing RF pulses and then combined for strong T2-weighted high resolution 3D images. These spinecho sequences are normally affected by dark phase dispersion bands, which are caused by patient induced local field inhomogeneities and made prominent by the relatively long TR used. The different excitation pulse regimes offset these bands in the two sequences. Combining these images result in a picture free of banding. The image combination is performed auto-matically after data collection, adding some more time to the reconstruction process. The advantage of the 3D CISS sequence is its combination of high signal levels and extremely high spatial resolution. CISS is used to image the inner ear, cranial nerves and cerebellum, e.g. in small acoustic or vascular compression in trigeminal neuralgia (Figures 2-20 and 2-21).

6- Diffusion sequences:

Various pulse sequences are modified to enhance signal loss resulting from water molecules that show significant diffusion versus those with more

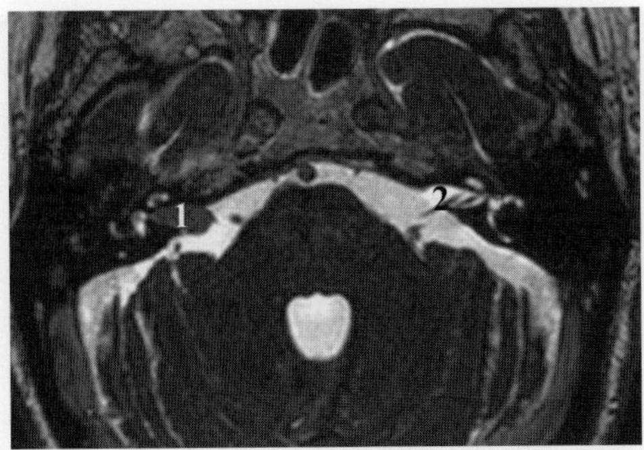

Figure 2-20: CISS image demonstrating small right vestibular schwannoma (1) and clear VII/VIII nerves and cochlea (2) on the left.

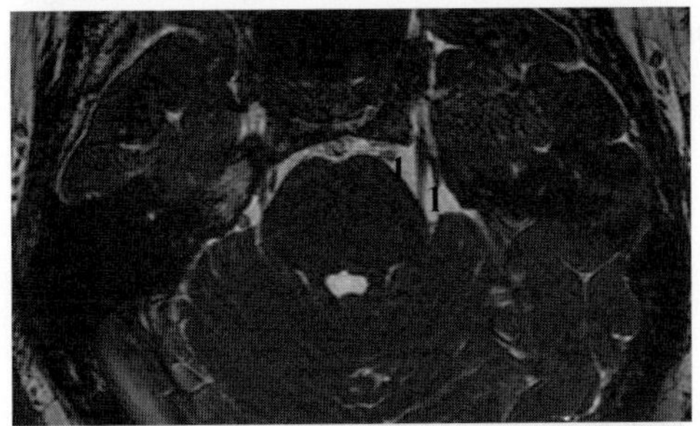

Figure 2-21: CISS image demonstrating trigeminal nerves (1). Note the vascular compression on the right and clear nerve on the left (1).

restricted diffusion. Certain pathologies show restriction of diffusion, such as cytotoxic oedema and demyelination. With a diffusion-weighted pulse sequence, these abnormalities can be made more obvious (Figure 2-22).

Depending on the particular gradient/gradients used, anisotropic diffusion can be detected, as occurs normally in white matter tracts. This can be used in fibre tracking: diffusion tensor imaging (DTI) (Figure 2-23).

7- STIR sequences:

STIR (short TI inversion recovery) sequence can be used for fat suppression, where a relatively short inversion time is used to null the fat signal while maintaining water and soft tissue signal. This sequence is useful to

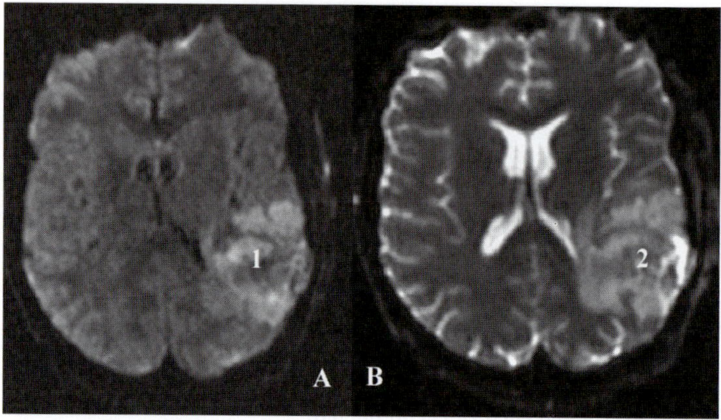

Figure 2-22: Diffusion MRI image demonstrating restricted diffusion of water molecules in an acute infarction (1).

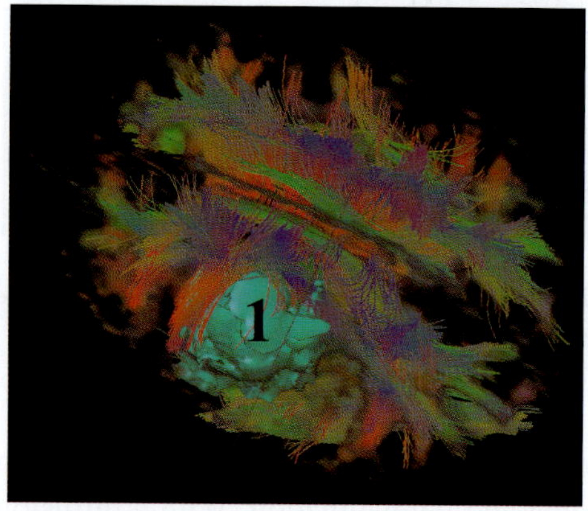

Figure 2-23: DTI image of fibre tracking around a brain tumour (1) identifying a surgical corridor through which the tumour was removed without affecting the white matter tracts.

distinguish lipomas from other types of tumours or to suppress fat surrounding a lesion making it more obvious. One drawback of this sequence is the partial loss of proton signal during the TI time. Also the TR time must be longer than that of a spin echo sequence for recovery of longitudinal magnetisation.

2-2-3 *What are the uses of MRI?*

MRI scan of the head is used to evaluate the following conditions:

- Head trauma:

CT scan is the main neuroimaging modality in head injuries. However, MRI can provide the same or even better information in head injuries, but significant numbers of patients with head injuries requiring brain imaging are ventilated at the time of the scan making MRI less desirable. When CT is not available MRI is often used (Figure 2-24).

- Spontaneous intracranial haemorrhage:

Acute blood in the cranial cavity appears high signal on MRI. Although CT is the main brain imaging used in spontaneous intracerebral haematoma and SAH, MRI proved very valuable in the diagnosis of delayed subarachnoid haemorrhage, aneurysms and AVMs (Figure 2-25).

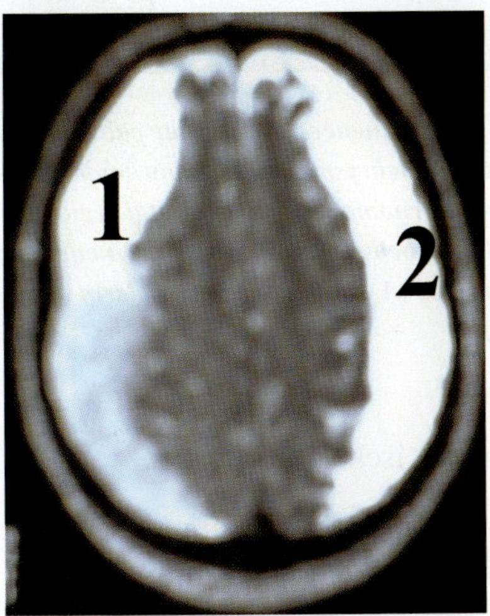

Figure 2-24: MRT T2-weighted image in a patient with bilateral chronic subdural haematomas (1 and 2) who had MRI because the CT was out of commission for service. Note the layering of the blood on the right side (1) indicating that there was fresher bleed on that side.

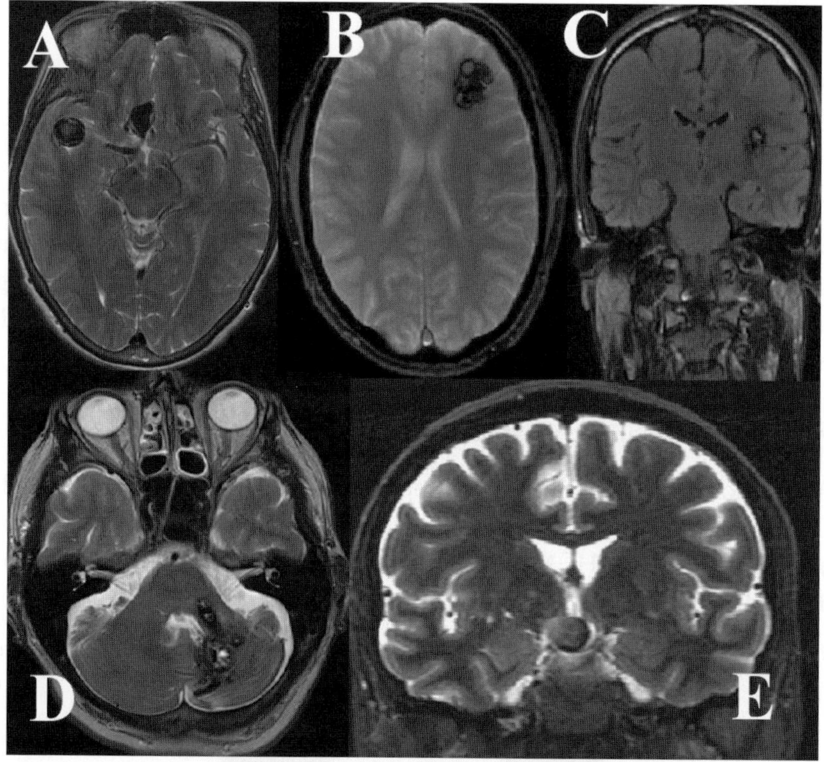

Figure 2-25: Different MRI sequences in vascular causes of spontaneous intracranial haemorrhage: A = multiple aneurysms one in right middle cerebral artery and one in anterior com artery, B = cavernoma in the left frontal region, C = cavernoma in the left insula, D = AVM in left cerebellum, and E = giant aneurysm in tip of basilar artery. Dark signals denote flow void (A and D) or haemosiderin (B, C, and E) due to previous haemorrhage (B and C).

- Strokes and transient ischaemic attacks:

MRI is a better imaging modality and more sensitive in acute ischaemia particularly using diffusion images (Figure 2-22).

- Spinal conditions:

MRI scan is the investigation of choice in the spine and virtually replaced CT and myelography. MRI is excellent in demonstrating bony,

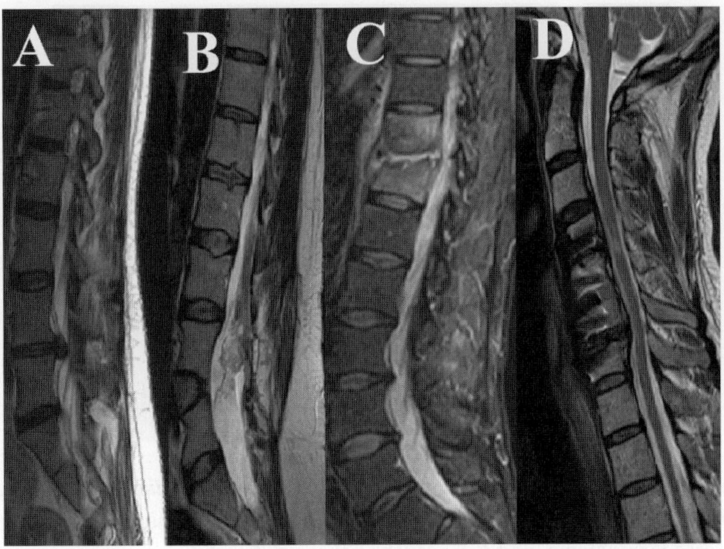

Figure 2-26: MRI images of the spine: A = T2-weighted demonstrating L4/5 disc prolapse, B = T2 demonstrating L4 hemivertebra and epidermoid, C = STIR image of T11/12 discitis, and D = T2 demonstrating screw plate fixation of C3 to C7 and intradural gliosis.

disc, dural, extradural, intradural or intramedullary lesions in the spine (Figure 2-26).

- Suspected raised intracranial pressure (ICP):

Patients suspected to have raised ICP such as those presenting with headache, nausea and vomiting, patients with papilloedema, patients with focal neurological deficits, and patients with seizures are best investigated by MRI (Figure 2-27).

- Stereotactic targeting:

MRI is used in conjunction with stereotactic frames or frameless image guided technology to biopsy lesions in the brain, insert electric leads in the brain, insert catheters, chemicals or cells, and localise lesions during surgery (Figure 2-28).

                                   Chapter 2

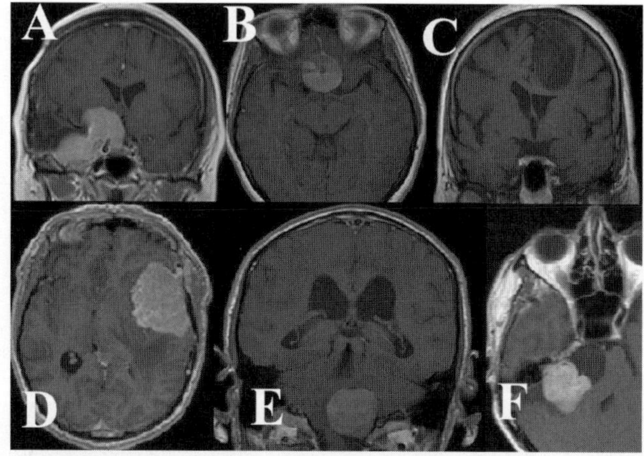

Figure 2-27: MRI images of patients with raised ICP: A = medial wing meningioma, B =olfactory groove meningioma, C =astrocytomas, D =haemaniopericytoma, E =posterior fossa meningioma, and F =acoustic neuroma.

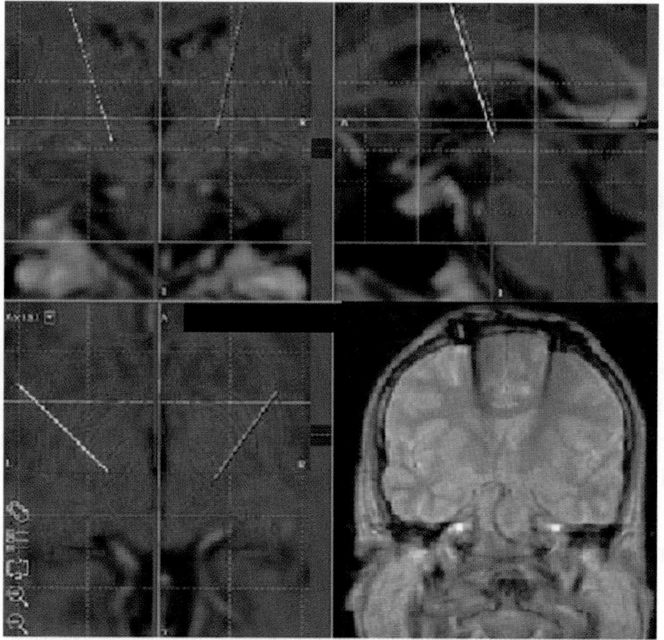

Figure 2-28: Screen shot of bilateral deep brain stimulation (DBS) plan with stereotactic atlas overlies an MRI and post-operative MRI showing the DBS electrode artifacts.

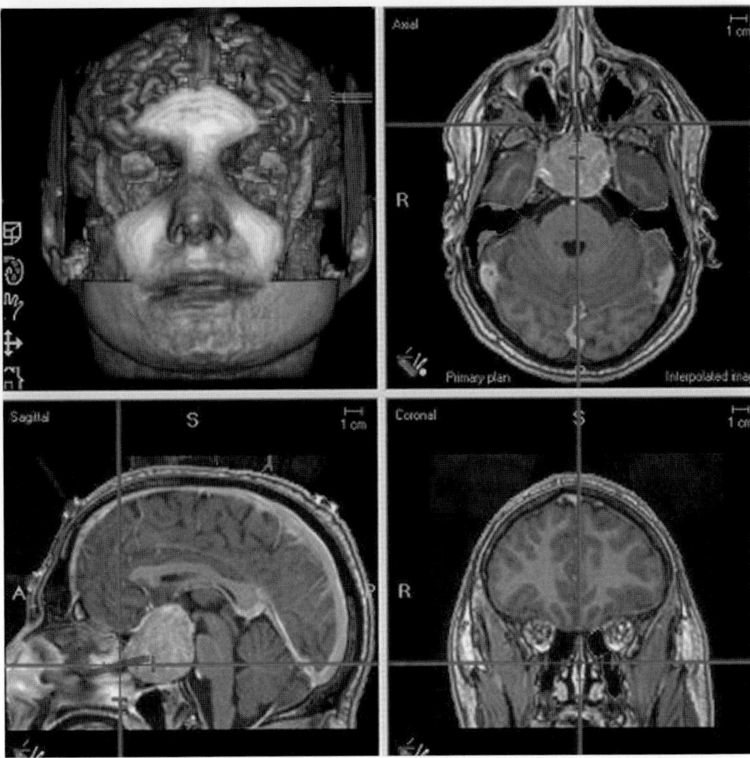

Figure 2-29: Screen shot of pre-operative surgical plan for transsphenoidal pituitary surgery.

- Surgical planning:

MRI scan is the main planning modality of brain operations using image guided systems, e.g. tumour surgery (Figure 2-29), gamma knife or cyber-knife stereotactic radiosurgery.

2-2-4 *What lesions enhance on MRI scan?*

IV contrast is used after plain T1-weighted imaging using gadolinium to highlight breakdown in the BBB. Some lesions enhance well (homogenous enhancement), others have mixed enhancement and others do not enhance at all.

1- Homogenous enhancement is seen in:

    a.   Meningiomas.
    b.   Vestibular schwannomas.
    c.   Haemangioblastoma nodules.
    d.   Pilocytic astrocytoma.
    e.   Haemangiopericytoma.
    f.   Ependymoma.

2- Mixed enhancement is seen in:

    a.   High grade gliomas.
    b.   Metastases.
    c.   Medulloblastoma.
    d.   Pituitary adenomas.
    e.   Craniopharyngiomas.
    f.   Inflammatory lesions.

3- Peripheral enhancement is seen in:

    a.   Abscess (ring enhancing lesion).
    b.   Cystic metastases.
    c.   Cystic high grade gliomas.
    d.   Luxury perfusion in acute infarcts (2% in two days).
    e.   Cystic astrocytoma.
    f.   Inflammatory cysts.

4- No enhancement is seen in:

    a.   Infarction.
    b.   Arachnoid cyst.
    c.   Cholesterol cyst.
    d.   Lipoma.
    e.   Grade I astrocytoma.
    f.   Epidermoid cyst.

2-2-5 *What are the advantages of MRI?*

In summary MRI has several advantages: excellent tissue contrast and resolution, multiplaner imaging capability, no-ionising radiation and ability to detect motion of water molecules.

2-2-6 *What are the disadvantages of MRI?*

The main disadvantage of MRI imaging is its inability to overcome metal and motion artifacts that can limit its use. It cannot be used in patients who have pacemaker, neurostimulator or a pump, metal clips on intracranial vessels or metal fragments in the eyes. Some patients also find the MRI set-up too claustrophobic and are unable to have it. Some of the patients who suffer from claustrophobia can have MRI scan in upright or open MRI machines.

Problem 2-3:   Non-radiological neuro-investigations. How to interpret non-radiological neuro-investigations in a smart way?

Most diagnostic investigations of neuro-surgical conditions involve neuro-radiological imaging. However a number of other investigations are used in neuro-surgery for diagnosis and monitoring. Therefore some knowledge of the underlying principles of

Problem based tool box:

Lumbar puncture and CSF

EEG	**NCS**
EMG	**AEP**
SSP	**VEP**

these investigations will help maximise their utility, diagnostic value and interpretation.

2-3-1 *How can I perform and interpret CSF examination?*

CSF analysis is usually required for diagnostic purposes to rule out potential life-threatening conditions such as bacterial meningitis or subarachnoid haemorrhage. CSF fluid analysis can also aid in the diagnosis of various other conditions, such as demyelinating diseases and carcinomatous meningitis. To obtain CSF for analysis a lumbar puncture (L/P), cisternal puncture or ventricular puncture is required. L/P is the most commonly used method to obtain CSF and it should never be performed before thorough neurological examination and it should never delay life-saving treatments. L/P should only be used after ruling out mass lesions on CT scan. L/P is also sometimes performed for therapeutic reasons, such as the treatment of pseudotumour cerebri (Benign Intracranial Hypertension — BIH), communicating hydrocephalus after SAH, normal pressure hydrocephalus (NPH), to relax the brain during surgery, e.g. during clipping of intracranial aneurysm, for infusion test in NPH, for intrathecal injection of antibiotics, baclofen, ziconamide, morphine, and chemotherapeutic agents and to control CSF leakage from post-operative wounds or assist neurosurgical repair of CSF fistulae, e.g. after transsphenoidal, translabrynthine and transnasal surgery. L/P is absolutely contraindicated in:

1- Unequal pressures between supra- and infra-tentorial compartments, usually inferred by characteristic CT findings: midline shift, loss of suprachiasmatic and basilar cisterns, posterior fossa mass, loss of superior cerebellar cistern, and loss of quadrigeminal cistern.

2- Infected skin over the needle entry site.

L/P should also be avoided in the presence of: increased intracranial pressure (ICP) and coagulopathy. CT is always recommended before L/P and L/P should only be performed if the perceived benefits outweighed its risks in patients who are fully consciousness, had no focal neurology and had no papilloedema. CT should always be performed before L/P in all patients over 60 years, immunocompromised, CNS lesions, a seizure within one week of presentation, reduced level of consciousness, and focal neurological findings or papilloedema seen on physical examination.

2-3-2 *How L/P is performed?*

Explain the procedure of L/P to the patient carefully, including its risks and benefits. In experienced hands, L/P is a relatively safe procedure; post-L/P headaches, infection, intrathecal bleed, radicular pain, nausea, photophobia and intraspinal haematomas can occur.

Patient position is extremely important for successful L/P. The patient is asked to lie on his/her side or sitting up, with the back arched toward the examiner and as close to the edge of the coach as possible and then curl into a ball. This involves the patient flexing his/her neck and lower spine, whilst drawing up his/her thighs toward the chest. The shoulders and pelvis should be vertically aligned without any tilt. In 94% of adults the spinal cord terminates at L1. In 6% of adults the spinal cord extends to L2/L3. Therefore L/P is generally performed at or below L3/L4 interspace. As a general anatomical rule, a line drawn between the posterior iliac crests often corresponds closely to L3-L4 (Figure 2-30). The interspace is identified after palpation of the spinous processes at each lumbar level.

To avoid infection, the examiner puts on a mask and sterile gloves and the skin is cleansed with alcohol or iodine-based disinfectant and the area is draped with sterile drapes. A local anaesthetic, commonly 1% lignocaine, is injected into the subcutaneous area — this should be ideally done

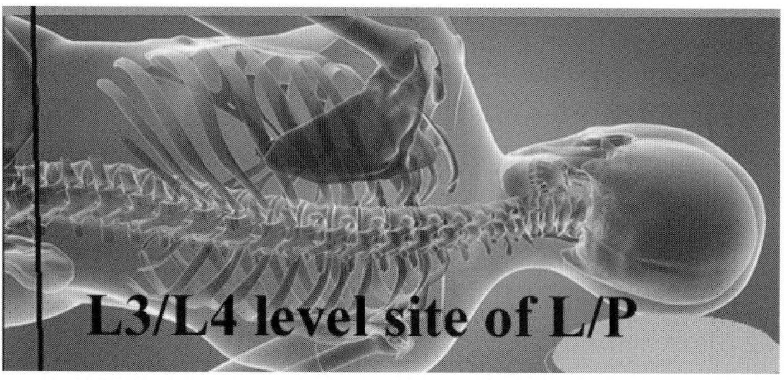

Figure 2-30: Site of L/P needle at L3/4 level.

at least five minutes prior to insertion of the lumbar puncture needle. The lumbar puncture needle is typically a 20–22 gauge needle (use 18-16 gauge for therapeutic L/P) and it is inserted into the target area and slowly advanced. The bevel of the needle is maintained in a horizontal position (with the flat portion of the bevel pointing up) and it should be parallel to the direction of the dural fibres. In most cases the needle is advanced 4–5 cm before the subarachnoid space is reached — this is characteristically recognised by a sudden decrease in resistance (give-way) and sometimes a "popping" sound may be heard. Once the subarachnoid space has been reached, a manometer can be attached to the needle to record the opening pressure. Fluid is then usually obtained for collection in three subsequent universal containers. Five millilitres of CSF in each container is usually sufficient. In most cases CSF will be colourless, but it can often be blood stained. To differentiate between true blood-stained CSF, e.g. secondary to SAH and traumatic tap, observe the intensity of colour in the three samples; if the CSF becomes clear with each subsequent sample, it is most likely to be traumatic and traumatic tap does not have xanthochromia.

2-3-3 *What should CSF analysis include?*

In all CSF samples sent to the laboratory the following tests are performed: cell count, CSF glucose, CSF protein, smear Gram stain examination and culture. In special circumstances on the request of the treating physician the following tests are also performed: acid-fast bacilli smear and culture, antigen tests and serology (e.g. cryptococcal antigen, latex agglutination, limulus lusate tests), PCR (polymerase chain reaction) tests to amplify DNA or RNA of micro-organisms, antibody tests, immunoelectrophoresis, and cytology.

2-3-4 *What is the differential of abnormal CSF analysis?*

Table 2-2 summarises the different CSF findings in the most common conditions compared to normal CSF analysis. When interpreting the glucose level in CSF it is important to compare it to blood glucose level (BGL). Therefore it is important to send blood for BGL at the same time as the L/P.

2-4-1 *How can I interpret an EEG?*

EEG (electroencephalography) is recording of electrical brain activity produced by the firing of neurons. Clinically EEG refers to recording of brain's spontaneous electrical activity over a short period of time (20–40 minutes) as recorded from multiple electrodes placed on the scalp. The main diagnostic application of EEG is in the case of epilepsy, as epileptic

Table 2-2: CSF analysis results

Condition	Cells	Glucose	Protein (g/L)	Others
Normal	0–5	2/3 BGL	0.15–0.45	Normal pressure,* clear
Bacterial meningitis	Polymorph-leukocytosis	Very low	1–10	High pressure, turbid, bacteria
Viral CNS infection	Monocytosis	Normal	0.4–1.0	Normal, clear colourless
Subarachnoid haemorrhage	RBCs	Normal	Raised	High ICP, red, xanthochromia
Tuberculosis infect	Lymphocytosis	Low	0.6–7	High ICP, yellow, acid-fast bacteria
Guillain-Barre syndrome	0–5	Normal	0.5–10	Normal ICP, clear

* Normal pressure = 70–180 mmH$_2$O.

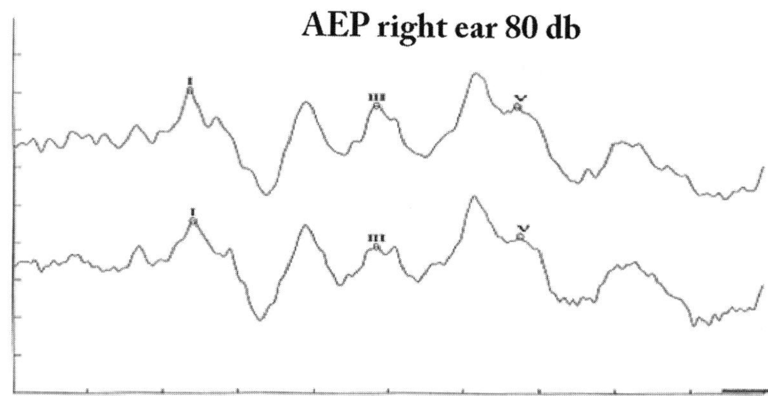

Figure 2-31: AEP during removal of an acoustic neuroma, this generated by summation of EEG activity in response to auditory clicking stimulus.

activity can create clear abnormalities on a standard EEG study.[3] A secondary clinical use of EEG is in diagnosis of coma, encephalopathies, and brain death. EEG was used in the past to diagnose tumours, stroke and other focal brain disorders, but it is no longer used for this purpose with the advent of CT and MRI scanners. EEG is still used intra-operatively to locate an epileptic focus during resective epilepsy surgery.

Evoked potentials (EP), e.g. somatosensory potentials (SSP), visual evoked responses (VER) and auditory evoked potentials (AEP) (Figure 2-31) are derivatives of the EEG technique, which involves averaging the EEG activity time-locked to the presentation of a stimulus. Event-related potentials (ERP) refer to averaged EEG responses that are time-locked to more complex processing of stimuli; this technique is used in cognitive science, cognitive psychology, and psychophysiological research.

2-4-2 *How is EEG generated?*

EEG reflects correlated synaptic activity caused by post-synaptic potentials of cortical neurons. The ionic currents involved in the generation of fast action potentials may not contribute much to the averaged field potentials representing the EEG.[3] Scalp electrical potentials that produce EEG are generally thought to be caused by the extracellular ionic currents caused by dendritic electrical activity, whereas the fields producing magneto encephalographic signals (MEG)[4] are associated with intracellular ionic currents. The electric potentials generated by single neurons are far too small to be picked up by EEG or MEG. EEG activity therefore always reflects the summation of the synchronous activity of thousands or millions of neurons that have similar spatial orientation, radial to the scalp. Currents that are tangential to the scalp are not picked up by the EEG. The EEG therefore benefits from the parallel, radial arrangement of apical dendrites in the cortex. Because voltage fields fall off with the fourth power of the radius, activity from deep sources is more difficult to detect than currents near the skull.

2-4-3 *What are the different types of EEG waves?*

Scalp EEG activity shows oscillations at a variety of frequencies. Several of these oscillations have characteristic frequency ranges, spatial distributions and are associated with different states of brain functioning (awake and various sleep stages). These oscillations represent synchronised activity over a network of neurons. The neuronal networks underlying some of these oscillations are understood (e.g. thalamocortical resonance underlying sleep spindles), while many others are not (e.g. the system that generates the posterior basic rhythm). Figure 2-32 depicts the different types of EEG waves and Table 2-3 summarises their significance.

2-5-1 *How can I interpret results of nerve conduction studies (NCS)?*

NCS are measuring the conduction velocity of electricity along a nerve to diagnose peripheral neuropathy and peripheral nerve entrapment syndromes. NCS are used mainly for evaluation of paraesthesia (numbness, tingling, burning) or weakness of the arms and legs. The type of study required is dependent in part on the symptoms presented. A physical examination and thorough history also help to direct NCS, e.g. if the sensory deficit extends beyond the wrist there is no point looking for carpal tunnel (CTS) or cubital tunnel (UNC = ulnar nerve compression) syndromes. Some of the common disorders which can be diagnosed by nerve

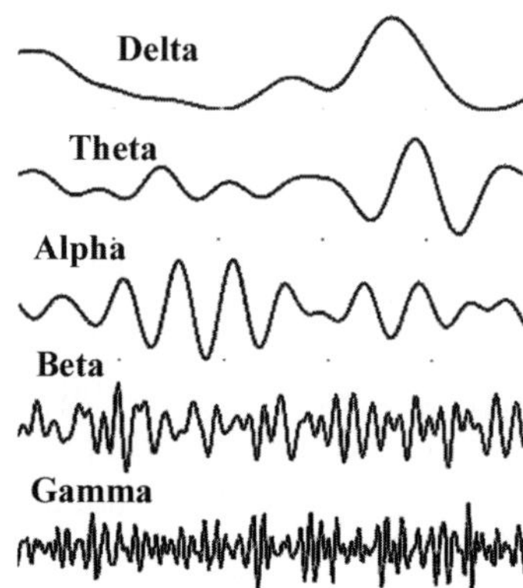

Figure 2-32: Different EEG waves and rhythms.

Table 2-3: Types of EEG waves and rhythms and their significance

EEG wave/ rhythm	Location	Significance
Delta up 4 Hz	Frontal in adults during slow wave sleep and posterior in children and babies.	Can be seen in subcortical lesions, diffuse lesions, deep midline lesions and metabolic encephalopathies.
Theta 4–7 Hz	Seen in young children, drowsiness or arousal in adults.	Seen in focal subcortical lesions, deep midline lesions, metabolic encephalopathies, hydrocephalus.
Alpha 8–12 Hz	Seen posteriorly during relaxation eyes closed.	Can be seen in coma.
Beta 12–30 Hz	Seen bilaterally more frontally in active busy states.	Can be seen with benzodiazepines.
Gamma 30–>100 Hz	Seen in certain cognitive and motor functions.	

conduction studies include CTS, UNC, peripheral neuropathy, Guillain-Barré syndrome, Facioscapulohumeral muscular dystrophy, and radiculopathy. NCS include sensory NCS, motor NCS, F-wave study and H-reflex study.

2-5-2 *Motor NCS*

Motor NCS are performed by electrical stimulation of a peripheral nerve and recording from a muscle supplied by the nerve. The time it takes for the electrical impulse to travel from the stimulation to the recording site is measured. This value is called the latency and is measured in milliseconds (msec). The size of the response (amplitude) is also measured. Motor amplitudes are measured in millivolts (mV). By stimulating in two or more different locations along the same nerve, the nerve conduction velocity (NCV) across different segments can be determined. Calculations are performed using the distance between the different stimulating electrodes and the difference in latencies.

2-5-3 *Sensory NCS*

Sensory NCS are performed in a similar fashion to motor NCS by electrical stimulation of a peripheral nerve and recording from a purely-sensory portion of the nerve, such as on a finger. Like the motor NCS, sensory latencies are on the scale of msec. Sensory amplitudes are much smaller than the motor amplitudes, usually in the microvolt (μV) range. The sensory NCV is calculated based upon the latency and the distance between the stimulating and recording electrode.

2-5-4 *What is F-wave study?*

F-wave is the second of two voltage changes observed after electrical stimulation is applied to the skin surface above the distal region of a nerve. F-waves are particularly useful for evaluating conduction problems in the proximal region of nerves. It is called F wave because it was initially recorded in the foot muscles. In a typical F-wave study, a strong electrical stimulus is applied to the skin surface above the distal portion of a nerve so that the impulse travels both distally (towards muscle fibres) and proximally (back to motor neurons of spinal cord), are also known as orthodromic and antidromic respectively. When the orthodromic stimulus reaches the muscle fibre, it elicits a strong M-wave indicative of muscle contraction. When the antidromic stimulus reaches the motor neurons, a small portion of the motor neurons backfires and orthodromic wave travels back down the nerve towards the muscle. This reflected stimulus evokes small proportion of the muscle fibres causing a small, second wave called the F-wave. Because a different population of anterior horn cells is stimulated by each stimulus, each F-wave has a slightly different shape, amplitude and latency. NCV is derived by measuring the limb length in millimetres from the stimulation site to the corresponding spinal segment (C7 spinous process to wrist crease for median nerve). This is multiplied by two as it goes to the cord and returns to the muscle (2D); 2D is divided by the latency difference between mean F and M waves and one millisecond subtracted (F − M − 1). The formula for NCV during F-wave study is 2D/(F − M − 1) mm/msec.

2-5-5 *H-reflex study*

H-reflex study uses stimulation of a nerve and recording the reflex electrical discharge from a muscle in the limb. This test evaluates conduction between a limb and spinal cord, but afferent impulses are in sensory nerves while efferent impulses are in motor nerves.

2-5-6 *What is the normal F-wave response?*

A normal F-wave response has a latency of 25–32 msec in the upper limbs and 45–56 msec in the lower extremities and with repeated stimulation normal F-wave should persist more than 50% of the time (80–100%).

While interpretation of NCS is complex, slowing of NCV usually indicates damage to the myelin sheath, slowing across the wrist for motor and sensory latencies of the median nerve indicates CTS, and slowing of all nerve conductions in more than one limb indicates peripheral polyneuropathy.

References

1. Hart D, Wall BF. UK population dose from medical X-ray examinations. *Eur J Radiol* 2004; 50: 285–291.

2. De Coene B, Hajnal JV, Gatehouse P *et al.* MR of the brain using fluid-attenuated inversion recovery (FLAIR) pulse sequences. *Am J Neuroradiol* 1992; 13: 1555–1564.

3. Abou-Khalil B, Musilus, KE. *Atlas of EEG and Seizure Semiology*. Elsevier, 2006.

4. Creutzfeldt OD, Watanabe S, Lux HD. Relations between EEG phenomena and potentials of single cortical cells. I. Evoked responses after thalamic and epicortical stimulation. *Electroencephalogr Clin Neurophysiol* 1966; 20: 1–18.

Chapter 3: Trauma (Head and Spinal Injured Patients)

Problem 3-1:   Head injuries and head trauma. How to manage a patient presenting with a head injury?

Any patient presenting with head injury should be assessed carefully to detect any intracranial pathology and provide appropriate therapy to prevent secondary brain damage. It is also important to keep a high index of suspicion to avoid missing associated spinal injuries.

Problem based toolkit:

Acute subdural haematoma

Cerebral contusion

Chronic subdural haematoma

Diffuse axonal injury

Epidural haematoma

PCS3-1-1:

A 20-year-old female driver of a car that was involved in a collision with another vehicle. The impact was sustained at the driver's side of her vehicle. An ambulance arrived and she was found with no eye opening, no verbal response and no motor response (GCS = 3) at the scene of the accident. She had an airway obstruction and was intubated at the scene. There was no spontaneous respiration. Distal pulses were felt and blood pressure was 160/70. Pulse was 95/min. Her cervical spine was then cleared by X-ray with no fractures. aPO_2 on 8L oxygen/minute = 5.5 kPa, $aPCO_2$ = 4.8 kPa and chest was clear. CT of head demonstrated traumatic subarachnoid haemorrhage with blood in lateral ventricles. Extensive skull fractures of vertex and base of skull which crossed midline to left carotid canal. After resuscitation her pupils were reactive to light but sluggish, her neurological status improved to eye opening spontaneously, extending to pain and no verbal response (GCS = 7). Na 142, K 4.3, Ur 4.6, Creat 69. Patient was managed on the neuro-intensive care unit with ventilation and ICP monitoring.

3-1-2 *What is the incidence of head injuries?*

The incidence of head injuries vary from country to country depending on road safety and health safety at work, e.g. head injuries in the UK affect 6–10 per 100,000 of the population and 20% of head injuries attending emergency departments in the UK end up admitted to hospital with 0.2% mortality. To reduce morbidity, secondary brain injury and mortality from head injuries several guidelines and protocols were developed and implemented. The National Institute of Clinical Excellence (NICE)[1] and the Scottish Intercollegiate Guidelines Network (SIGN)[2] are just a few to list in this short synopsis.

3-1-3 *What is the rationale of head injury management?*

The rationale of head injury management is to prevent secondary brain damage and maximise the best chances of recovery from primary brain damage that occurred at the time of the head injury. The main causes of secondary brain damage are: hypoxia, hypotension and raised intracranial pressure. The main causes of raised intracranial pressure after primary head injury are: extradural haematoma (EDH) (Figure 3-1), acute subdural

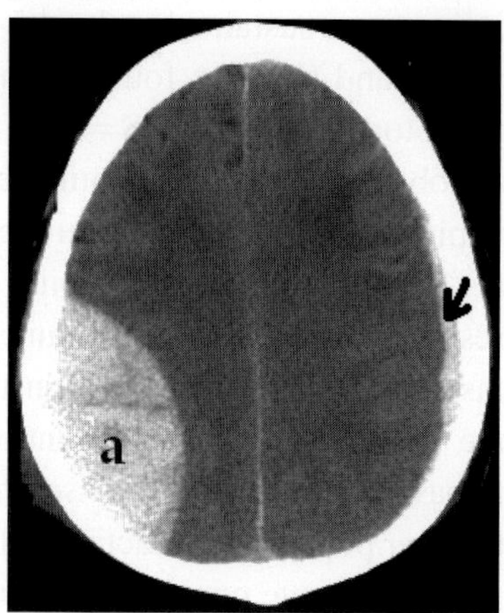

Figure 3-1: Extradural haematoma (EDH) (a) after a head injury. Axial CT-image demonstrating right parietal high density bilenticular clot (a). There is also a very thin small acute subdural on the left side (arrow).

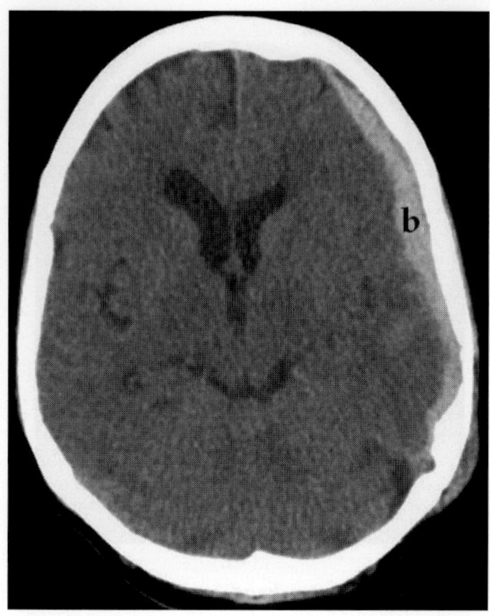

Figure 3-2: Acute subdural haematoma (ASDH) (b) after a head injury. Axial CT-image showing high density blood clot concave towards the brain and convex towards the inner table of the skull (b).

haematoma (ASDH) (Figure 3-2), burst lobe and contusions (Figure 3-3) or brain oedema (Figure 3-4).

3-1-4 *When would you refer a patient to hospital after a head injury?*

When referring a patient to hospital accident and emergency room you need to take full history and perform full neurological examination. In the history you need to know the circumstances and timing of the injury, whether the patient lost consciousness or not, what was the last thing the patient had remembered before the injury, and what was the first thing he/she remembered after the injury. Amnesia prior to the injury is called pre-traumatic or retrograde amnesia. Amnesia after the injury is called post-traumatic or antegrade amnesia. History of persistent headaches, nausea and vomiting, weakness, sensory disturbance, loss of vision, hearing, sense of smell or balance, diplopia, seizures or speech impairment are important to note. Clinical examination should include assessment of

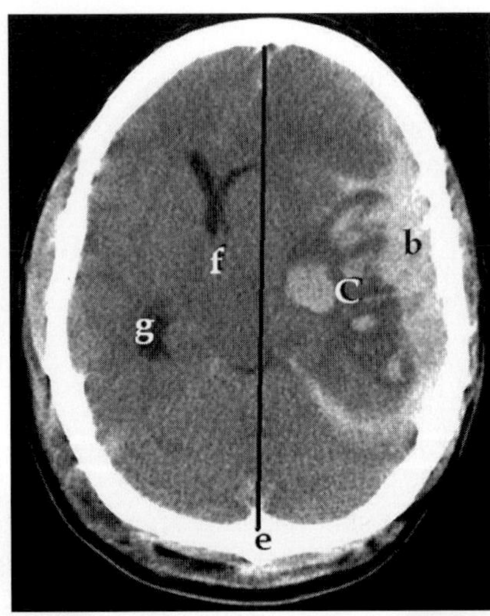

Figure 3-3: Burst temporal lobe after head injury (brain contusion) (C). Axial CT-image demonstrating mixed density area in the brain (C). This was associated with acute subdural clot (b) on the left and over the tentorium with shift of the ventricles (f + g) from the midline (e).

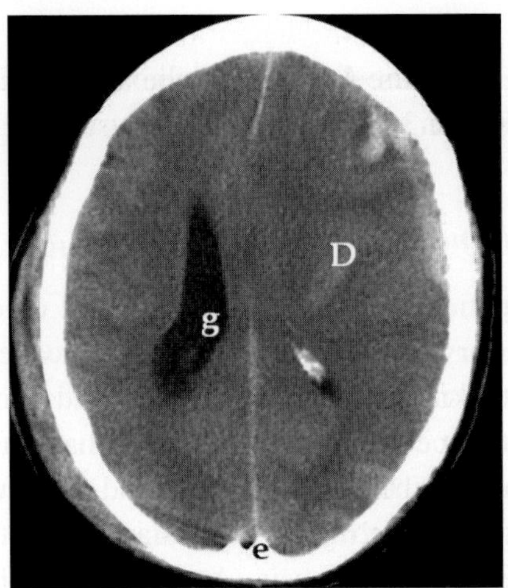

Figure 3-4: Diffuse axonal injury (DAI) of the left hemisphere (D) with small acute subdural haematoma after head injury causing brain swelling as shown on axial CT-image and complete effacement of the left lateral ventricle and dilatation of the contralateral ventricle (g) due to brain shift and obstruction of the III ventricle.

level of consciousness, short-term memory, speech and language, vision, hearing, motor power, sensory function and co-ordination. It is also important to note any external bruises on the face and the scalp. Bruising around the mastoid is called battle sign and indicates a temporal skull base fracture and may be associated with blood in the middle ear (haemotympanum), conductive hearing loss, facial palsy or otorrhoea (CSF leak through the ear) or even paradoxical rhinorrhoea (CSF leak through the nose if the tympanic membrane was intact and CSF flows through the fracture into the middle ear, via the Eustachian tube into the nostril). Bilateral black eyes or panda eyes indicate anterior cranial fossa basal skull fracture and may be associated with CSF rhinorrhoea. Scalp lacerations may overly depress a skull fracture that needs wound cleaning and fracture elevation. The level of consciousness is assessed by the Glasgow Coma Scale (GCS).

Refer a patient who had a head injury to the emergency room using an emergency ambulance service if:

1. The person presents with an altered level of consciousness. Fully conscious individuals should be able to open their eyes spontaneously, should be orientated in time place and person and should be able to obey simple commands. Any person who is not fully conscious at the time of examination after head injury must be referred to an emergency room.
2. There has been a seizure since the head injury.
3. There was evidence of a basal skull fracture, such as CSF leak from the nose or ear, black eyes with no damage around the eyes (panda eyes); bleeding from one or both ears; haemotympanum (blood behind the ear drum); or bruising around both or one mastoid (battle sign).
4. There was evidence of focal neurological deficit, such as double vision, speech impairment, problems with balance, loss of muscle power; or sensory disturbance of the extremities.
5. Any person with deteriorating level of consciousness.
6. Presence of associated other injuries such as chest or abdominal trauma; limb or pelvic trauma; or there was significant vascular injury.
7. If the injured did not have access to adequate transportation to hospital.

A head injured patient should be referred to hospital if any of the following is present:

a- Impaired consciousness (not fully conscious) at any time since injury.
b- Amnesia for the incident or subsequent events.
c- Presence of any neurological symptoms, e.g. severe and persistent headache, nausea and vomiting, irritability or altered behaviour, seizure, speech impairment, limb weakness or double vision.
d- Clinical evidence of a skull fracture, e.g. CSF leak from nose or ear, periorbital haematoma (panda eyes), battle sign, or haemotympanum.
e- Significant extracranial injuries.
f- A mechanism of injury suggesting: high energy injury (e.g. road traffic accident, fall from height), possible penetrating brain injury, possible non-accidental injury (in a child) or continuing uncertainty about the diagnosis after first assessment.
g- Presence of medical co-morbidity, e.g. anticoagulant treatment (warfarin), antiplatelet therapy (aspirin, clopedigrol, persantin), drug abuse or alcohol abuse.
h- Presence of adverse social factors, e.g. absence of caregiver to supervise the patient at home.

3-1-5 *When can a person be sent home after minor head injury?*

1. Clinical history and examination indicated a low risk of brain injury and the referral criteria were not met.
2. They had appropriate support structures and competent supervision at home.
3. They had received verbal and written head injury advice (Table 3-1).

Table 3-1: Head injury advice

Seek medical attention if you develop any of the following:

Change in level of consciousness, e.g. drowsy, sleepy, confused
Increased or persistent headaches, nausea or vomiting
If you develop any weakness, speech problem or sensory disturbance
If you develop blackouts, fits, seizures or any convulsions
Asymmetry of the pupils

3-1-6 *When are skull X-rays indicated after head injury?*

Skull X-rays should be performed if any of the following apply and if CT is not being performed:

a.   If the patient is alert and orientated and obeying commands and

  o   the mechanism of injury has not been trivial; or
  o   consciousness has been lost; or
  o   the patient has amnesia or has vomited; or
  o   scalp has a full thickness laceration or a boggy haematoma; or
  o   the history is inadequate.

b.   If the level of consciousness was impaired.

3-1-7 *When does a CT become indicated?*

CT scan should be undertaken in a patient who has any of the following features:

1.   The patient's eye opens only to pain or does not converse.
2.   A deteriorating level of consciousness or progressive focal neurological signs.
3.   Confusion or drowsiness followed by failure to improve within at most four hours of clinical observation.
4.   Radiological/clinical evidence of a fracture, whatever the level of consciousness.
5.   New focal neurological signs which are not getting worse.
6.   Full consciousness with no fracture but other features, e.g.:

  o   severe and persistent headache.
  o   nausea and vomiting.
  o   irritability or altered behaviour.
  o   development of a seizure.

3-1-8 *When do X-rays of the cervical spine become essential?*

Imaging of the cervical spine, including the cervico-thoracic junction should be carried out:

- In a fully conscious patient if clinical symptoms or signs or the mechanism of injury indicate the possibility of injury to the spine.
- In a patient with persisting impaired consciousness. In an unconscious patient, not localising pain. CT scanning of the cervical spine down to C2 should be undertaken routinely, at the time of head scanning.

3-1-9 *Which HI-patients should I discuss with a neurosurgeon?*

A head injured patient should be discussed with a neurosurgeon if one or more of the following features existed:

1) When a CT scan in a general hospital shows a recent intracranial lesion.
2) When a patient fulfils the criteria for CT scanning but this cannot be done within an appropriate time frame locally.
3) Irrespective of the result of any CT scan, if the patient fulfils any of the following criteria:

   a) Persisting coma after initial resuscitation.
   b) Confusion which persists for more than four hours.
   c) Deterioration in level of consciousness after admission (sustained drop of one point on the motor or verbal subscales, or two points on the eye opening subscale of the GCS).
   d) Progressive focal neurological signs.
   e) Seizure without full recovery.
   f) Compound depressed skull fracture.
   g) Definite or suspected penetrating injury.
   h) CSF leak or other signs of a basal skull fracture.

3-1-10 *Who should be admitted to hospital after head injury?*

A patient should be admitted to hospital for neurological observation if:

1) The level of consciousness is impaired.

2) The patient is fully conscious but any of the following risk factors are present:

   a) Continuing amnesia (for at least five minutes after injury).
   b) Continuing nausea and/or vomiting.
   c) Seizure at any time after injury.
   d) Focal neurological signs.
   e) Irritability or abnormal behaviour.
   f) Clinical or radiological evidence of a recent skull fracture or suspected penetrating injury.
   g) Abnormal CT scan.
   h) Severe headache or other neurological symptoms.

3) The patient has significant medical problems, e.g. anticoagulant use.
4) The patient has social problems or cannot be supervised by a responsible adult.

Patients admitted to hospital should have their neurological observations performed every 15 minutes four times, if remains stable every half an hour four times, if remains stable every hour four times, if remains stable every two hours four times and then every four hours thereafter. Any of the following examples of neurological deterioration should prompt urgent re-appraisal by a doctor:

1) The development of agitation or abnormal behaviour.
2) Sustained decrease in conscious level of at least one point in the motor or verbal response or two points in the eye opening response of the GCS.
3) The development of severe or increasing headache or persisting vomiting.
4) New or evolving neurological symptoms or signs, such as pupil inequality or asymmetry of limb or facial movement.

3-1-11 *What is concussion and contusion?*

Concussion is transient loss of consciousness following non-penetrating closed head injury without gross or microscopic brain damage, while contusion is intra-parenchymal brain haemorrhage with much less mass effect on CT than its actual size and usually reaches the surface of the brain. Concussion is divided into three grades as follow:

- Grade 1: No loss of consciousness and confusion without amnesia.
- Grade 2: No loss of consciousness and confusion with amnesia.
- Grade 3: Loss of consciousness.

3-1-12 *How to manage a patient with traumatic cranial haematomas?*

3-1-12i *Extradural (epidural) haematoma (EDH):*

The classical history of an EDH (Figure 3-1) is that a patient was concussed with brief loss of consciousness followed by a lucid interval that can be from minutes to hours during which the patient appears normal, followed by sudden deterioration in level of consciousness. The classical history occurs in less than 27% of EDH. In 85% of patients the source of bleeding was the middle meningeal artery, in the young (less than 30 years of age) 40% of EDH was associated with skull fracture of the cranial vault, while in those over 30 years skull fracture was found in almost all patients. It is associated with ASDH in 20% and the mortality rate from EDH was 20–55% but with new head injury guidelines and early treatment the mortality from EDH was reduced to 5–10%.

3-1-12ii *Subdural haematomas (SDH):*

SDH used to be classified according to their age into acute (ASDH Figure 3-2) if discovered within 72 hours, subacute (SASDH) if it was three days to three weeks old and chronic (CSDH) if it was more than three weeks old. However, most patients do not remember the onset of head injury and therefore this classification went by the wayside after CT and MRI brain was introduced. The most relevant classification clinically is to classify these lesions into:

- Hyperdense SDH (HSDH) where the clot is higher density than the brain on CT and takes the shape of the brain as demonstrated in

Figure 3-2. If this lesion was symptomatic its removal requires craniotomy. If it was more than 1 cm thick it generally requires to be removed. Its volume can be measured by the formula: (thickness × height × length)/2. If the volume was > 80 ml removal is also recommended. Other factors that influence the decision making process is mass effect in the form of midline shift and the GCS. If a HSDH is removed before four hours of the ictus the survival can be expected in up to 70% compared to only 10% if the surgical evacuation was delayed more than four hours or the pupil was unreactive. In more than 79% of patients who had a HSDH evacuated surgically develop raised ICP and therefore monitoring ICP is desirable in these patients after surgery.

- Mixed density SDH (MSDH) where the density of the clot is a mixture of high and isodense in appearance. This usually treated in the same fashion as HSDH if the majority was hyperdense and as CSDH if the majority was hypodense in appearance.
- Isodense SDH (IDSH) when the density of SDH is the same as that of the brain. This can be a challenging diagnosis and keeping a high index of suspicion is essential to pick up these lesions. Always look for indirect signs such as midline shift, effacement of the lateral ventricle or effacement of the ipsilateral sulci. Intravenous contrast injection will often show enhancement of the SDH membrane and makes visibility easier. These lesions can be evacuated through one or two burr holes.
- Hypodense SDH (CSDH) (Figures 3-5 and 3-6) when the lesions had lower density than the brain. This can be drained via one or two burr holes. If the brain surface did not come to the surface during drainage, it is advisable to leave a subdural drain *in situ* to drain any residual clot on one hand and avoid tension pneumocephalus. The latter can arise if the CSDH was drained while the head is elevated and the cavity was filled with air at room temperature that will heat up during the next few hours. The air will then expand according to Boyle's law leading to tension pneumocephalus. Routine scans are not required after drainage as removal of 20% of the fluid normalises the ICP and 78% would have residual collection by day 10 and 15% by day 40 post-drainage. The important step is to leave the dura within the burr hole open and make a small pocket in the subgaleal space for it to be absorbed. More than three quarters can be drained adequately by a single burr hole.

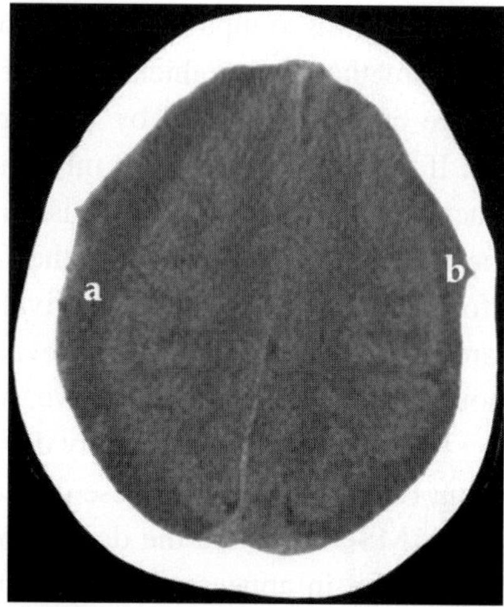

Figure 3-5: Bilateral CSDH (a and b) demonstrated on CT.

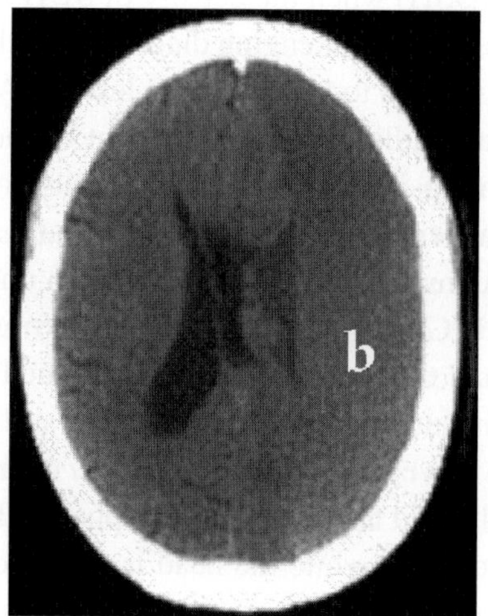

Figure 3-6: CSDH (b) demonstrated on CT.

3-1-13 *How to manage dural fistulae and CSF leaks?*

CSF rhinorrhoea or otorrhoea indicates that there was a breach of the dura mater. This often occurs in association with skull base fractures involving the ACF, sphenoid or temporal bone. It is often difficult to be sure that

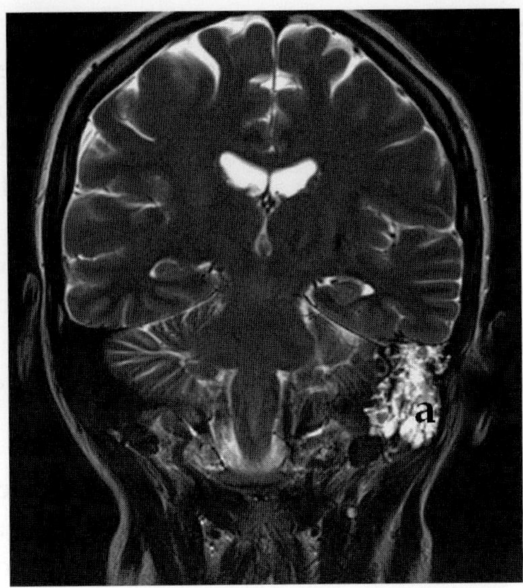

Figure 3-7: MRI T2-weighted showing CSF (a) in the left mastoid air cells.

blood stained nasal or ear discharge contains CSF. Glucose and protein estimations in the discharge are often positive even in the absence of CSF. The best test to confirm the presence of CSF is to measure B2-transferrin (B2T). B2T is present only in the CSF and aqueous humour of the eye.[3] So if you are in doubt collect the fluid and send it for B2T measurement. The reason why CSF leaks are treated seriously is the high risk of recurrent meningitis in these patients, often due to Streptococcus pneumonia that still carries high mortality.[4,5] Prophylactic antibiotics are not indicated here because they merely change the type of organism rather than prevent meningitis.[6] CSF leaks can be diagnosed and localised using fine slice CT to demonstrate the bony defect and MRI scan that demonstrates CSF leakage (Figure 3-7) or brain hernia through the fistula.[7] Persistent CSF leaks and those complicated by meningitis require dural repair.

3-1-14 *Categorisation of head injury severity*

There are many classifications of head injuries used in the past to determine the risk of significant intracranial brain injury such as contusion, EH, SDH and DAI. However, the most important findings are level of consciousness, pupillary responses and limb responses. The initial assessment should include the assessment of airways, breathing and circulation, followed by primary survey looking for life-threatening conditions that require treatment on the spot, these are haemothorax, haemoperitonium, cardiac tamponade, tension pneumothorax and intracranial haematomas. Then you must perform complete history and physical examination paying special attention to LOC, pupils, limbs, and cranial nerves, detecting in the process any lacerations, cephalohaematomas, panda eyes, battle sign, CSF leakage, haemotympanum, LeFort or orbital rim fractures, proptosis, or carotid bruit.

- Low risk HI: Asymptomatic HI, there is no loss of consciousness, patient is fully conscious and oriented and there is no clinical or radiological evidence of skull fracture. The risk of significant intracranial pathology in this group is < 9/10,000. Skull X-ray is normal in 99.6% and they can be discharged home provided there is a responsible adult who can observe the patient, they have means to return to hospital, and have been given written head injury advice (Table 3-2).

Table 3-2: Post-head injury advice to those discharged home

If you are affected by any of the following after leaving the hospital, you should get someone to take you to your nearest hospital A&E as soon as possible:

1. Unconsciousness, or lack of full consciousness (for example, problems keeping your eyes open).
2. Any confusion (not knowing where you are, getting things muddled up).
3. Any drowsiness (feeling sleepy) that goes on for longer than one hour when you would normally be wide awake.
4. Any problems understanding or speaking.
5. Any loss of balance or problems walking.
6. Any weakness in one or both arms or legs.
7. Any problems with your eyesight.
8. Very painful headache that will not go away.
9. Any vomiting — getting sick.
10. Any fits (collapsing or passing out suddenly).
11. Clear fluid coming out of your ear or nose.
12. Bleeding from one or both ears.
13. New deafness in one or both ears.

- Moderate risk HI: If there is history of loss of consciousness, progressive headache or vomiting, post-traumatic seizures, post-traumatic amnesia, there is unreliable history, or there are signs of basal skull fracture or penetrating facial injury. These patients can only be discharged home if they fulfill all the following criteria: Normal CT brain, initial GCS > 13, GCS 15 at discharge, there is a responsible adult who can look after them and bring them back if necessary, there are no complicating factors such as non-accidental injury (NAI) or domestic violence and they are given written head injury advice (Table 3-2).

- High risk HI: Any patient with reduced level of consciousness, has neurological deterioration, develops focal neurological deficit, has penetrating head injury or depressed skull fracture is at high risk for brain injury.

In patients with GCS > 13 admit the patient for the following instructions:

Activity level:	Bed rest with head elevated by 30–45 degrees. Neurological observation every two hours if concerned hourly.
Feeding:	Nil by mouth till fully alert — advance as tolerated.
Analgesia:	Simple analgesics such as tramadol or codeine.
Antiemetic:	As required.

In patients with GCS 9–13 admit the patient for the following instructions:

Activity level:	Bed rest with head elevated by 30–45 degrees. Neurological observation every one hour, consider high dependency.
Feeding:	Nil by mouth till fully alert — advance as tolerated.
Analgesia:	Simple analgesics such as tramadol or codeine.
Antiemetic:	As required.
Fluids IV:	100 ml/h normal saline with 20 mmol/L KCl. If not awake by 12 hours repeat the CT brain.

In patients with GCS < 9 transfer the patient to dedicated neurosurgical facility, prior to transfer consider the following problems:

- If there was a concern about hypoxia or airway protection during inter-hospital transfer, intubate and artificially ventilate the patient.
- If there were any seizures administer anticonvulsants.
- If there was concern about neck injuries immobilise the spine.
- If there was concern about raised ICP administer mannitol 2 g/kg of 20% and keep the $PaCO_2$ between 3.5–4 Kpa during transfer.

When should you intubate and artificially ventilate a head injured patient? This should always be performed for the following reasons:

- To protect the airways if GCS < 8 or there was maxillo-facial injury.
- If there was evidence of raised ICP, e.g. pupillary dilatation, asymmetric pupillary reaction, decerebrate/decorticate posture or progressive neurological deterioration.
- To carry out safe inter-hospital transfer.
- To properly assess a combative or agitated patient by CT.

3-1-15 *What are the indications of monitoring ICP?*

If you plan to treat raised ICP then you must monitor it closely to see the response to therapy. The following are some of the indications of ICP monitoring:

— Severe head injury GCS < 8.
— Following evacuation of mass lesion.
— Ventilated patients with abnormal CT.
— Multiple injuries.

ICP monitoring should be avoided in awake patient and in the presence of coagulopathy. ICP monitoring is not without risks: there is a risk of infection of about 1–2%, bleeding in up to 2.8% and malfunction in 6–40%. ICP monitoring can be performed by inserting a transducer in the subdural space, ventricle or brain parenchyma, e.g. Camino bolt, Codman transducer,

Spielberg transducer, etc. Most units would treat any ICP of 25 mmHg or more to maintain cerebral perfusions pressure (CPP) of > 70 mmHg. CPP is measured by subtracting mean ICP from mean arterial BP. Causes of raised ICP include reduced venous return, e.g. severe neck flexion or due to head down position, venous thrombosis, sustained seizures, intracranial pathology such as EDH, SDH, brain oedema, DAI or ischaemia.

3-1-16 *What is the relationship between ICP and CPP?*

The CPP remains constant when mean arterial BP (maBP) is 60–160 mmHg in normal individuals, however in head injured patients and SAH autoregulation is lost and the CPP would be directly related to maBP (Figure 3-8).

3-1-17 *How to treat raised ICP?*

Start off with simple measures such as adjusting the head and neck posture, checking the ventilator settings and controlling any seizures or pyrexia.

If simple head and neck position does not normalise ICP, the second tier manoeuvres are instituted: increasing maBP, e.g. will lead to increased CPP, reducing body temperature to 32–35 degrees reduces cerebral metabolism and reduces ICP in the process, however watch out for reduced cardiac output (CO), pancreatitis and renal impairment.

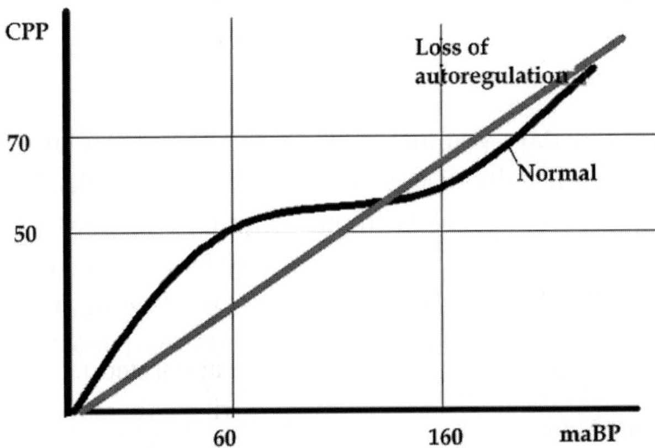

Figure 3-8: The relationship between CPP and maBP in normal and abnormal autoregulation.

Hyperventilation and reducing $PaCO_2$ to 3 Kpa in the short term will lead to vasoconstriction that reduces intracranial blood volume and reduced ICP. However, if hyperventilation is maintained for more than a few days cerebral ischaemia will occur. Surgical decompression of the skull vault reduces ICP, however the key is to include subtemporal decompression for it to work.

Finally induced barbiturate coma reduces cerebral metabolism and the ICP, however, this can lead to hypotension.

Mannitol is used to reduce ICP and impart cerebral protection, the dose is 2 g/kg of 20% IV over 20 minutes, thereafter the smallest effective dose, it is used before the CT if there was clinical evidence of raised ICP or mass lesion, or in sudden deterioration. It is also used to assess salvage-ability. After CT mannitol is used in mass lesion with raised ICP just before and during surgery. Mannitol will not work during hypotension and raised plasma osmolality (> 300 mosmol/L).

The role of exploratory burr holes is questionable in the current century because of the wide availability of CT scan and the speedy interhospital safe transfer of patients. However, rarely this may have to be used when a patient suddenly deteriorates with pupillary dilatation after a lucid interval when it is not practical or possible to get a CT. Burr hole then can be made in the temporal area 2 cm in front and above the tragus, then frontal just behind the hairline at least two finger breaths from the midline and finally a parietal burr hole over the parietal eminence.

Things you should not worry about:

Over the next few days you may experience one or more of the following symptoms, which usually disappear in the next two weeks. These include a mild headache, feeling sick (without vomiting), dizziness, irritability or bad temper, problems concentrating or problems with your short term memory, tiredness, lack of appetite or problems sleeping. If you feel very concerned about any of these symptoms in the first few days after discharge, you should go and see your own doctor.

If these problems do not go away after two weeks, you should go and see your doctor anyway. We would also recommend that you seek a doctor's opinion about your ability to drive a car or a motorbike.

Problem 3-2: Spinal trauma and traumatic spinal cord syndromes. How to manage a patient following spinal trauma?

To manage spinal trauma correctly you need to keep a high index of suspicion as the main objective in spinal trauma management is to prevent secondary damage and maximise the chances of recovery from the primary injury.

Problem based tool box:

Spinal trauma/fractures/shock

Anterior/Central Cord
  syndrome

Brown-seqaurd syndrome

Jefferson's/Hangman's/
  Odontoid fractures.

  Traction/Braces/Collars

PCS3-2-1:

A 61-year-old, right-handed advocacy female worker presented to the Accident and Emergency department following a road traffic accident (RTA) in which she, the pedestrian, was hit at around 30 mph by a car. She was hit on the left side, fell to the ground and sustained head and neck injuries. Immediately after the impact she lost consciousness for less than one minute and awoke to find herself lying on the ground unable to move or feel sensation in any of her limbs. After a few minutes she was able to move her left arm and leg but continued to be unable to move or feel her right limbs. She was experiencing pain in the occipital region of the head which was later found to be a small left-sided laceration. She did not have any other pain. She did not feel nauseous or experienced visual, hearing, swallowing or speech difficulties. She did not have any further loss of consciousness. She had hypothyroidism, depression, gastro-oesophageal reflux and left hip replacement in 2009. She was on Levothyroxine 75 μg OD, Omeprazole 20 mg OD, Fluoxetine 20 mg OD, Paracetamol 1 g PO, Movicol 1 sachet oral OD, Fragmin 500 units SC, Codeine Sulphate 60 mg PO, Cyclizine 50 mg PRN, Chlorepheriamine 4 mg PO, Diazepam 2 mg PO, Oromorph 20 mg PO, and Prochlorperazine 12 mg PO/IM.

On examination she was fully conscious and respiratory rate was 21, heart rate was 60 bpm, blood pressure was 126/46 mmHg, and O_2-saturation of 100% on room air. Cranial nerves I to XII had no abnormality. Examination of the limbs revealed the signs summarised in Table 3-3.

Table 3-3: Examination findings of the limbs

	Right upper limb	Left upper limb	Right lower limb	Left lower limb
Tone	Normal	Normal	Normal	Normal
Power	4	5	4	5
Reflexes	All present	All present	All normal	All normal
Sensation	Normal	Reduced pinprick in C7,8 and T1	Normal	Reduced pinprick L2 to S1

Differential Diagnosis

This is a case of C4 hemiparesis and contralateral hemisensory loss with sensory level at C7 after spinal injury (Brown Sequard syndrome). Anatomically she had a lesion at C6/7 on the right side of the spinal cord. The differential is between cord haematoma, contusion or bone/disc compression. Cervical spine X-rays (Lateral, AP and open-mouth view), pelvis and chest, bloods for FBC, Urea and Electrolytes, clotting factors, blood glucose, and urinanalysis were all within normal limits.

CT scan of the cervical spine demonstrated a fracture of C4 facet. MRI of the cervical spine demonstrated disruption of the C3/4 disc with compression of the spinal cord and disruption of the posterior ligaments. The patient had been given IV fluids, catheterised and given analgesics. She underwent C3/4 decompression and fixation. The fractures were reduced by externally using a halo brace. By the tenth day after the accident the patient was making excellent progress in the right direction. The strength of her left side had returned to normal and she had no sensory symptoms on the left. She continued to have reduced sensation to pain in the right upper limb but the weakness had decreased. There is uncertainty about the extent of the recovery, a patient with brown-Sequard syndrome will make.

3-2-2 What is the incidence and early management of spinal injuries?

It is thought that about one in 10,000 each year sustains a traumatic spinal injury and the majority of these patients do not develop neurological complications. However it is essential that patients who sustain spinal cord injury are identified and managed appropriately in order to avoid further neurological injury. It is thought that 85% of cord injuries occur at the time of the trauma but correct management can ensure that the other 15% occurring thereafter can be prevented. Spinal injuries are caused by falls in 41.7%, road traffic accidents in 36.8%, sports injuries in 11.6%, industrial accidents in 4.2%, and assaults in 2.7%. About half of all cervical spinal injuries result in spinal cord injury. These injuries are more common among males at a mean age of 30 years. A high index of suspicion is needed to detect spinal injury. Spinal injury is suspected in any patient who had significant trauma, unresponsive patients and presence of spinal pain. At the scene patients should have their airways, breathing and circulation maintained and their spine immobilised. Immobilisation can be achieved with sandbags and straps, hard cervical collar, and spinal board. This is maintained in hospital, in addition to maintaining oxygenation, passing a nasogastric tube, urinary catheter, and maintaining temperature. The cervical spine must be stabilised in hospital using sandbags and straps, a hard collar such as a Philadelphia collar, skull traction or halo vest. Soft collars are not recommended because they do not prevent spinal movements. To examine the spine "logrolling" techniques have to be used to avoid secondary spinal cord injuries. When dealing with spinal trauma musculoskeletal and neurological injuries need to be considered.

3-2-3 *What are the types of spinal cord injuries?*

1- **Complete lesion:** Complete cord or nerve injury occurs when the spinal cord, nerve root or peripheral nerve is completely transacted with complete loss of function of the injured neurological structure. There has been no study so far to show that early surgery for complete spinal cord lesion makes any difference to recovery.

2- **Incomplete lesions:** These lesions include partial section, neuropraxia or compression. These lesions present with incomplete loss of function:

    a.   Brown Sequard Syndrome (BSS).
    b.   Central Cord Syndrome (CCS).
    c.   Anterior Cord Syndrome (ACS).

The American Spinal Injury Association categorised traumatic spinal cord injuries into five types:

A) Complete spinal cord injury where no motor or sensory function is preserved.

B) Incomplete spinal cord injury where sensory but no motor function is preserved below the neurological level and includes the sacral segments S4-S5. This is typically a transient phase and if the person recovers any motor function below the neurological level, that person essentially becomes motor incomplete.

C) Incomplete spinal cord injury where motor function is preserved below the neurological level and more than half of key muscles below the neurological level have a muscle grade of less than 3.

D) Incomplete spinal cord injury where motor function is preserved below the neurological level and at least half of the key muscles below the neurological level have a muscle grade of 3 or more.

E) Normal where motor and sensory scores are normal.

3-2-4 *What is spinal shock in trauma?*

Shock in spinal injuries is not uncommon; shock could arise because of excessive blood loss related to trauma (hypovolaemic shock) or transient complete loss of reflexes (spinal shock). Hypovolaemic shock occurs because of hypotonia, and blood loss and it is treated as part of ABC and resuscitation except in spinal trauma a systolic blood pressure >90 mmHg would be acceptable because of the vasodilatation associated with loss of autonomic vasomotor responses. Pneumatic boots are useful to increase venous return in these patients. If these measures are insufficient vasopressers can be used. Spinal shock on the other hand can last from few hours to months and is characterised by flaccidity and loss of reflexes.

3-2-5 *How to evaluate the spine radiologically?*

1) Lateral X-ray of cervical spine:

This needs to be complete and able to visualise C1 to T1 (Figure 3-9). If only top of C6 is visible (Figure 3-10), caudal traction might be sufficient

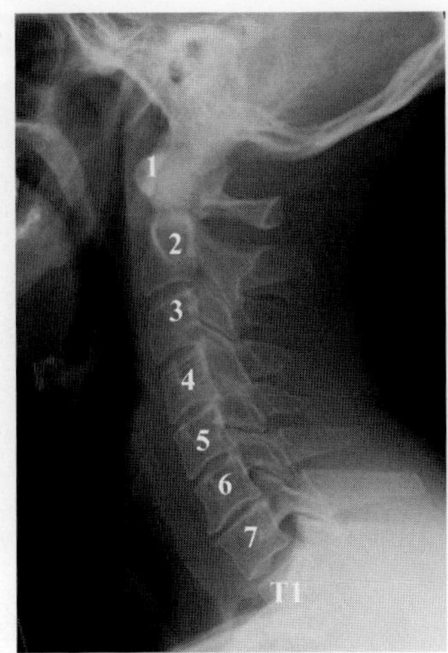

Figure 3-9: Adequate lateral C-spine X-ray demonstrating C1 to T1.

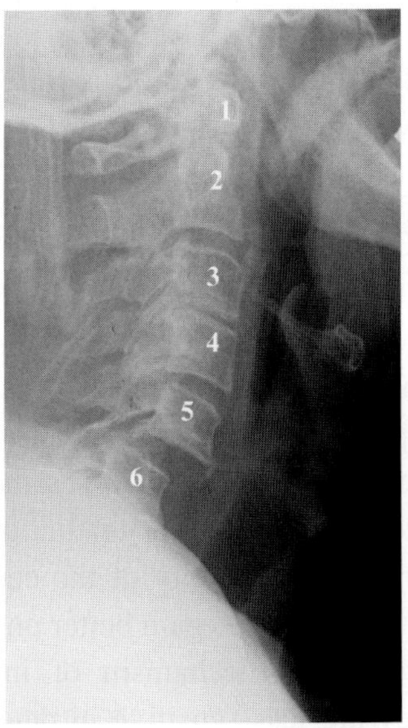

Figure 3-10: Incomplete lateral C-spine X-ray demonstrating C5/6 subluxation but C7 is not seen.

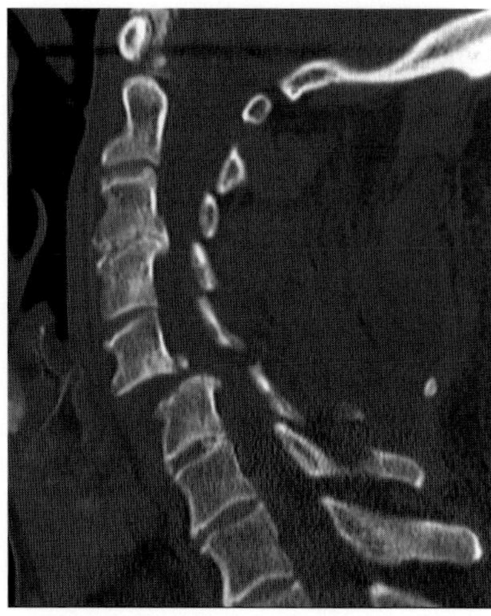

Figure 3-11: CT reconstruction of C-spine demonstrating that C7 and T1 were fine in the same patient shown in Figure 3-10.

to reveal the rest and the right thing to do is to repeat these X-rays with caudal traction. Otherwise perform fine cuts CT scan with 3D reconstruction (Figure 3-11).

2)   Anterio-posterior C-spine X-ray.
3)   Open mouth view to X-ray the odontoid process (Figure 3-12).

The American Association of Neurological Surgeons (AANS) reviewed around 40,000 trauma patients who were asymptomatic for cervical spine injury and suggested that no radiographic assessment was required as the procedure exposes patients to unnecessary radiation and discomfort when in a collar. If a fracture or abnormality of the cervical spine was found after trauma a CT scan is required to gain better understanding of the fracture's orientation, extent and mechanism of injury. Radiographs are inadequate because they are less sensitive in detecting fractures, with a sensitivity of 19–31% and as high as 96% of the lateral C-spine X-rays could be incomplete.[8] However, CT scan of the spine exposes that patient to a higher radiation dose than C-spine X-ray (2.5 mSv for CT compared

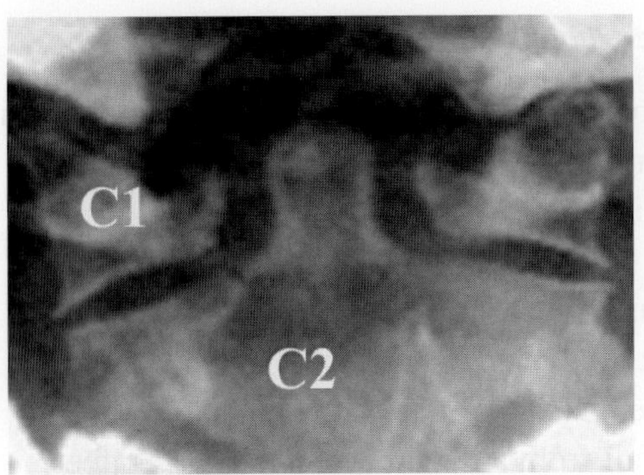

Figure 3-12: Open mouth view of the odontoid process — C1 =Atlas, C2 =Axis.

to 0.04 mSv from a single radiograph of the cervical spine). MRI is an important investigation that can be employed to study acute neurological symptoms and ligamentous injury. MRI demonstrates spinal cord compression, haemorrhage or contusion. MRI has 100% sensitivity for spinal cord injury and ligamentous damage but around 55% sensitivity for detection of spinal fractures. MRI also offers information about the prognosis of the injury. Increased amounts of oedema and haemorrhage are associated with poorer recovery. MRI is contraindicated in patients with pacemakers, aneurysm clips, ocular implants, middle ear implants and neurostimulators.

3-2-6 *How to manage patients with suspected cervical spinal injury after radiological evaluation?*

After the X-rays were taken, and the X-rays were complete, patient had no focal neurology and (s)he had no spinal pain:

a. If the X-rays were radiographically normal, no further action is required and the C-spine can be cleared.
b. If the X-rays demonstrated < 3 mm subluxation, perform flexion/ extension X-rays. If they were normal, no further action is required. If the subluxation reduces or exacerbates, immobilise the spine.

3-2-7 *When are whole spine X-rays required?*

Because a number of patients suffer multiple spinal injuries, a high index of suspicion is required. Here are some of the indicators associated with multiple spinal injuries:

1-   Unconscious patient.
2-   Thrown out of a vehicle.
3-   No adequate history available.
4-   History of fall from a height (greater than six feet).
5-   Complaining of spinal pain in multiple locations.

3-2-8 *When will you perform an emergency MRI scan?*

Emergency MRI will be indicated to demonstrate soft tissue injury including spinal cord injury. If the MRI scan will change the management of the patient then it should be done;

1-   Incomplete spinal cord lesion to rule out compressive lesions.
2-   Deteriorating neurological deficit.
3-   If the radiological abnormality differs from patient's signs and symptoms location.
4-   Suspected acute disc.

3-2-9 *When will emergency surgery be required?*

No scientific study had demonstrated any benefit from emergency surgery in patients who had complete cord lesions. Therefore indications for emergency spinal surgery in trauma include:

1-   Progressive neurological deficit.
2-   Retro-pulsed bone fragment.
3-   Acute anterior disc syndrome.
4-   Penetrating injury.
5-   Irreducible locked facets.
6-   Vital nerve compression.

3-2-10 *What are indications for steroids in spinal trauma?*

Following the NASCIS II trial high dose methylprednisolone was shown to increase limb motor function following spinal cord injury. However since that time, a number of studies suggested that the trial data was not reproducible and steroid treatment led to significant increase in infections. As a result steroids are not used routinely. The recommended protocol was to infuse 30 mg/kg of methylprednisolone IV over 15 minutes within eight hours of the injury. After 45 minutes of the bolus dose, the infusion is continued at a dose of 4.5 mg/kg for 23 hours.

3-2-11 *What is Brown Squard Syndrome (BSS)?*

BSS is caused by penetrating injuries, epidural compression as in the aforementioned PCS3-2-1, and radiation. The classical BSS is characterised by ipsilateral weakness and loss of proprioception and contralateral loss of pain, temperature and touch sensation (Figure 3-13).

An example of an incomplete BSS is the patient case study in PCS3-2-1. Another example is a 25-year-old patient who was stabbed in the neck and found to be ataxic with loss of proprioception (Figure 3-14).

Ninety per cent of these patients become independent.

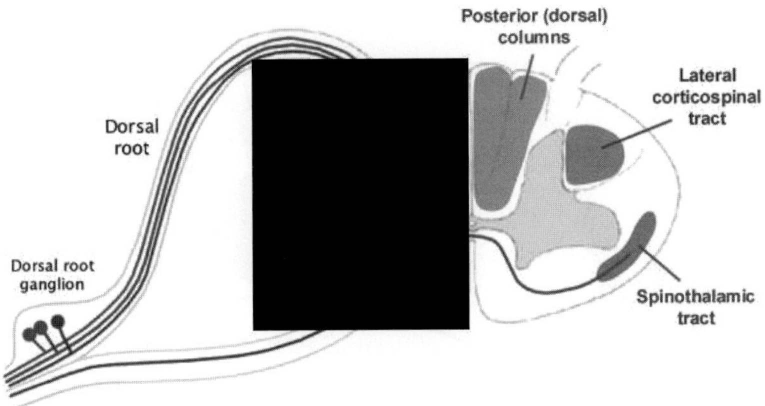

Figure 3-13: Schematic representation of BSS.

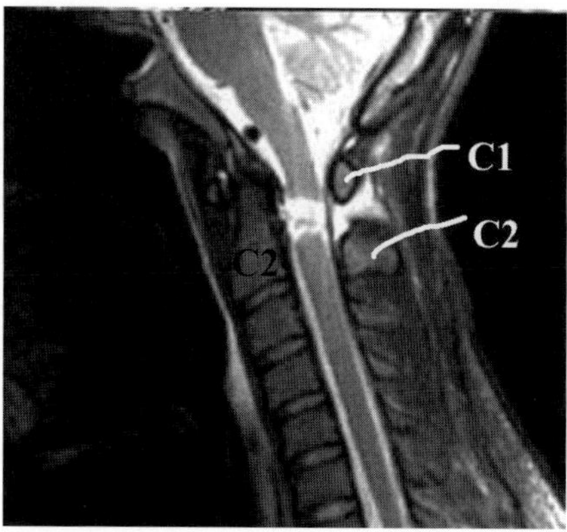

Figure 3-14: MRI scan demonstrating stabbing and severance of the posterior column. C1 = post-arch of atlas, and C2 = spinous process of C2.

3-2-12 *What is central cord syndrome (CCS)?*

CCS is often found after hyperextension injury in a narrow spinal canal. Elderly patients with cervical spondylosis who had narrow spinal canal, go out drinking, walking back home, tripping over and falling face down, coming to hospital with bruised face and tetraparesis worse in the upper limbs and affecting more the extensor muscles. Patients may exhibit variable sensory changes and urinary retention (Figure 3-15). Only 50% of patients may walk independently after CCS.

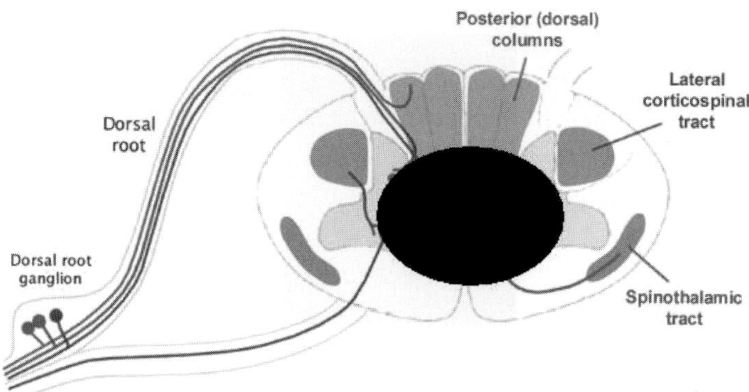

Figure 3-15: Schematic presentation of CCS.

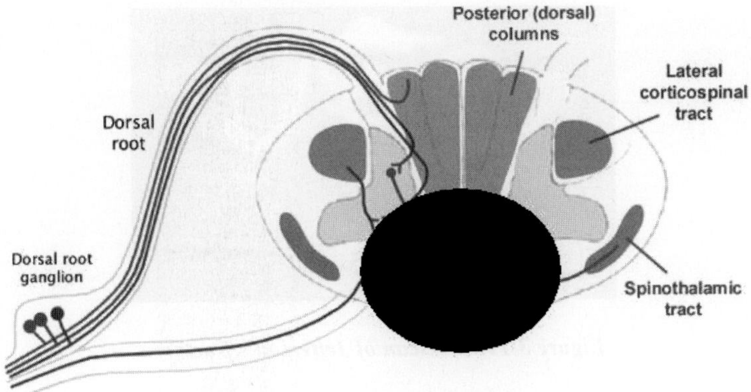

Figure 3-16: Schematic presentation of ACS.

3-2-13 *What is Anterior Cord Syndrome (ACS)?*

The causes of ACS are anterior cord compression, such as that following acute disc prolapse or retropulsed bone fragment, and occlusion of the anterior spinal artery. It results in tetraplegia or paraplegia and dissociate anaesthesia (loss of pain sensation, preserved proprioception) (Figure 3-16). Surgery is often performed but only 10–20% recovers the lower limb functions after ACS.

3-2-14 *What are the different types of C-spine fractures?*

1- *Atlanto-occipital subluxation (AOS):*

AOS represents 1% of all cervical spinal traumas. Patients often do not have any neurological deficit, the fracture however is unstable and patients should be immobilised in a halo brace for three to four months. If it did not heal spontaneously, it should be internally fixed using occipito-cervical fixation.

2- *C1 fractures:*

They represent 3–13% of all cervical spinal injuries, 56% of C1 fractures were isolated and 44% were associated with C2 fractures. Blow out fractures of C1 were called Jefferson's fractures (Figure 3-17). They are caused by

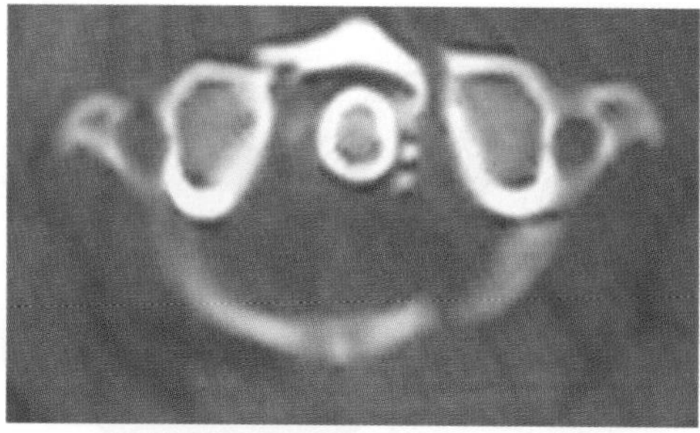

Figure 3-17: CT scan of Jefferson's fracture.

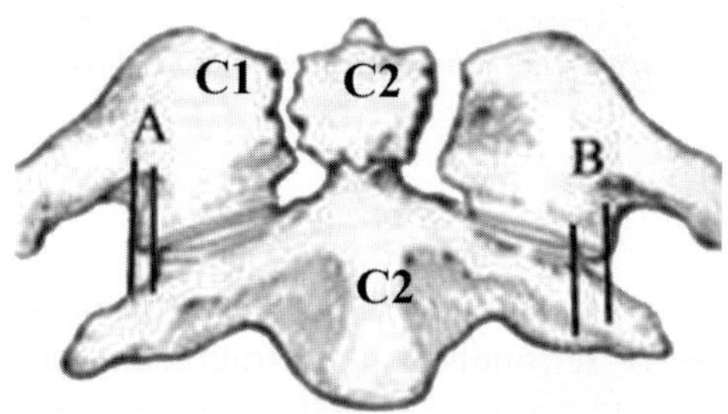

Figure 3-18: Schematic representation of diagnosis of C1 fracture on open mouth view by adding the overhang A + B (rule of Spence).

axial loading and are associated with normal neurology. However, these fractures are unstable and require immobilisation. The diagnosis is made on the open mouth view when the overhang of C1 condyles exceeds 6 mm (Figure 3-18). Fractures of C1 have an excellent prognosis.

3- *Atlanto-Axial Rotary Subluxation (AARS):*

AARS is characterised by torticollis of 20 degrees lateral flexion and 20 degrees rotation. This deformity was described as cock-robin torticollis. The treatment is reduction followed by immobilisation in a halo brace. Reduction is performed by gradual skull traction (Figure 3-19).

4- *Hangman's fractures:*

It is traumatic bilateral fracture of the pedicles of C2 and often associated with disruption of C2/3 disc (Figure 3-20).

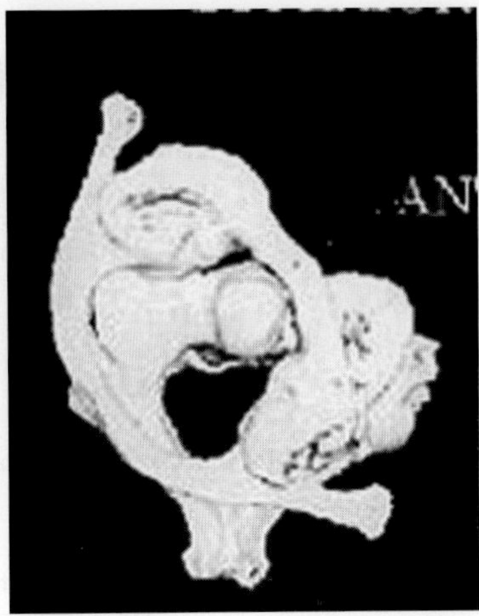

Figure 3-19: Three-dimensional CT reconstruction of AARS.

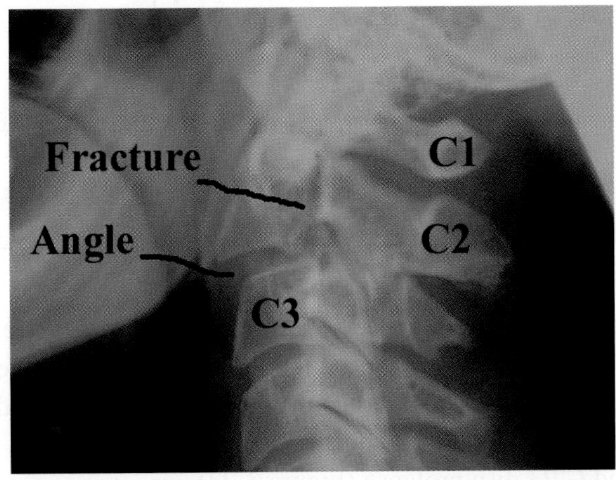

Figure 3-20: Hangman's fracture associated with C2/3 disc disruption and posterior angle.

These fractures occur because of hyperextension injury associated with axial loading and can be classified according to the fracture displacement and the angle between the odontoid process and the vertical axis of the cervical spine (Figure 3-21 and Table 3-4).

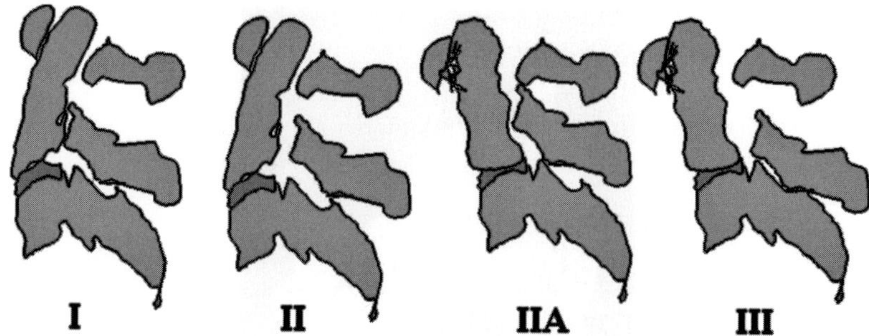

Figure 3-21: Schematic representation of Hangman's fractures.

Table 3-4: Effendi's classification modified by Levine and Edwards

Type (%)	# displacement	Angle	Mechanism	Stability
Type I (29%)	3 mm or less	Zero	Hyperextension with axial loading and intact ligaments	Stable
Type II (56%)	> 3 mm	10 degree or less	Hyperextension + axial loading followed by hyperflexion + axial loading	Unstable
Type IIA (6%)	3 mm or less	> 10 degrees	Hyperflexion with axial loading	Unstable
Type III (9%)	> 3 mm	> 10 degrees	Hyperflexion and axial loading	Unstable

For stable type I fractures cervical collar might be sufficient for pain control. For the other types (unstable) reduce and immobilise in a halo brace for 12 weeks. Surgical reduction and fixation is reserved for failed reduction and non-union or associated incomplete spinal cord injury due to associated C2/3 disc prolapse (Figure 3-22).

5- *Odontoid fractures:*

Odontoid fractures occur in 10–15% of cervical spinal injuries. In young adults they are commonly seen after road traffic accidents, falls and ski accidents, whilst in the elderly are common after minor falls. Hence when you are faced with an elderly patient after a fall, look out for three common things that you do not want to miss: fracture of the odontoid peg,

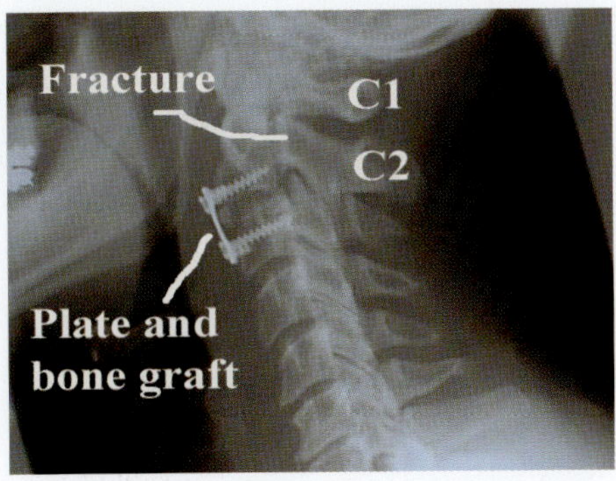

Figure 3-22: Type II Hangman's fracture associated with C2/3 disc prolapse in a 35-year-old who had somersaulted in a racing car and had hyperextension with axial loading followed by hyperflexion with axial loading.

Table 3-5: Classification of odontoid peg fractures

Type (Incidence)	Description	Stability
Type I (5%)	Avulsion fracture of the odontoid tip	Usually unstable
Type II (60%)	Fracture at the base of the odontoid	Unstable
Type III (30%)	Fracture at the base and body	Usually stable
C2 body # (5%)	This is pure fracture of the body of C2	Usually stable

fracture of neck of femur and chronic subdural haematoma. The exact mechanism of odontoid fractures is not completely understood but it almost always involves an element of hyperflexion that may be associated with extensions and lateral rotation. The classical presentation is with neck pain and occipital neuralgia associated with neck spasm. Patients with odontoid peg fractures tend to hold their head in their hands to reduce the pain and may complain of pins and needles in the tips of the fingers.

Odontoid fractures are classified according to their location along the odontoid peg into three types (Table 3-5 and Figure 3-23).

The majority of fractures of C1/2 are associated with no focal neurological deficit due to the fact that the size of C1 ring is wide enough to accommodate the odontoid peg (1/3 of the space), and the spinal cord (1/3 of the space) and sufficient spare space remains to accommodate CSF, and blood vessels. (This rule of thirds is called the rule of Steele.) Unstable

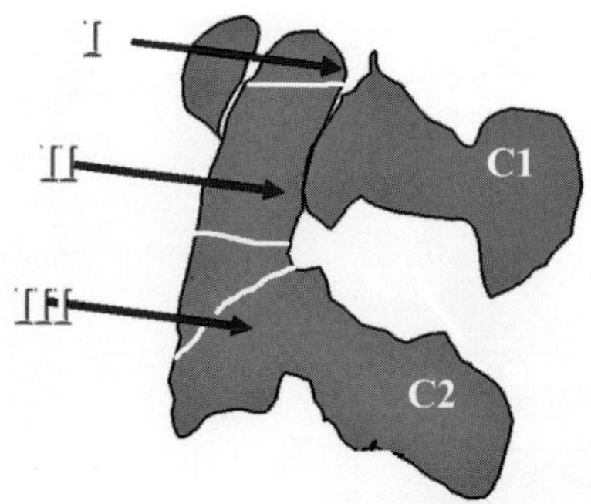

Figure 3-23: Schematic representation of odontoid fractures.

type 1 odontoid fractures are best treated with spinal fixation while other types of fractures are best treated with reduction and halo vest immobilisation for 12 weeks. Failed reduction and non-union are indications for surgical fixation. Factors associated with non-union include widely displaced fracture (6 mm or more), age > 65 years and poor healing environment such as osteoporosis and chronic steroids. Non-union can occur in up to 30% of odontoid fractures. Surgical fusion/fixation was initially performed using Gallie's technique where the posterior arch of C1 is fixed to the posterior elements of C2 using a wire and bone graft. This was later modified by Brooks by passing the wires behind the laminae of C2 to reduce the high failure of Gallie's fusion (10–28%). Further modifications were also reported by Sonttag and others including posterior arch plate and hooks (Figure 3-24). Other techniques include posterior C1/2 transarticular screws, anterior odontoid screws and occipito-cervical fixation in patients who suffered associated C1 fractures.

6- *Subaxial spinal injuries:*

These injuries include the following types:

1- Anterior subluxation associated with hyperflexion (Figure 3-25).
2- Locked facets due to hyperflexion associated with rotation.
3- Burst vertebral body fractures, also called teardrop fracture of the vertebral body. This type of serious fracture needs to be distinguished from teardrop sign often seen in hyperextension injuries seen on lateral C-spine X-rays where the edge of the vertebral body avulsed.

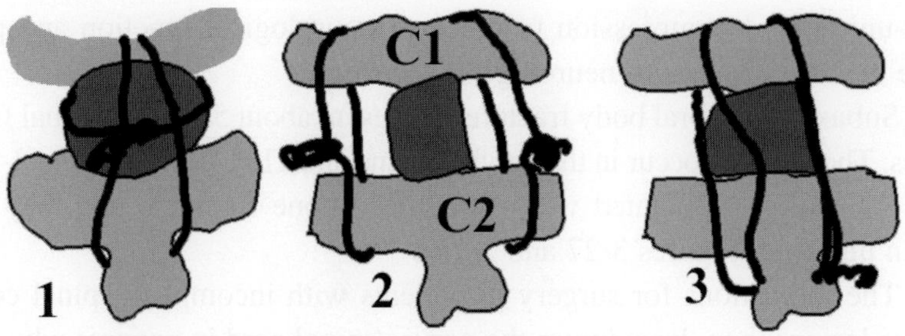

Figure 3-24: Posterior C1/2 fusion (1 = Gallie, 2 = Brooks and 3 = Sonttag).

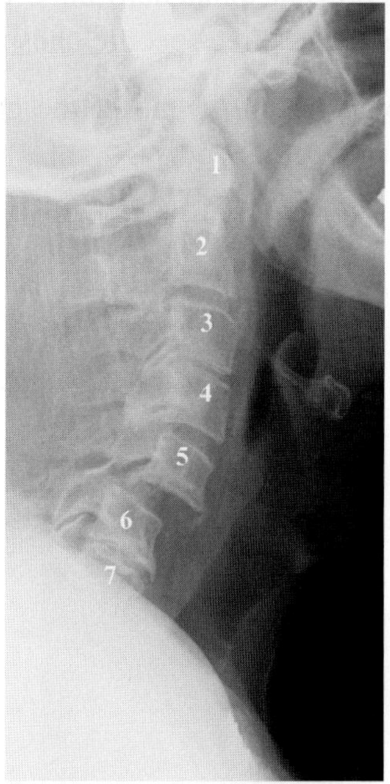

Figure 3-25: Subaxial subluxation of C4/5 in a 50-year-old man involved in a road traffic accident, reduced by 23 pounds of skull traction followed by internal fixation.

4- Clay shoveler's fracture of the spinous process of C7 seen in individuals who shovel the clay above their shoulders.

The treatment of these fractures follows the same general principles of reduction and immobilisation. Surgery is preserved for failed reduction, non-union or decompression to preserve neurological function and provide the best chances of neurological recovery.

Subaxial vertebral body fractures represent about 5% of all spinal fractures. They mostly occur in the cervical spine and Tl1/L2 area (Figure 3-26). They are often associated with retropulsed bone fragment and they are often unstable (Figures 3-27 and 3-28).

The indications for surgery in patients with incomplete spinal cord/ nerve lesions is to decompress the nerves/spinal cord in patients who had deteriorating neurology, acute disc or > 50% spinal canal compromise. In patients with complete cord lesion early surgery may be indicated for early mobilisation or to prevent spinal deformity. The approach of surgery is dependent on the answer to three specific questions:

1- Where was the compression, if one of the goals of surgery was to decompress the nerves/spinal cord?

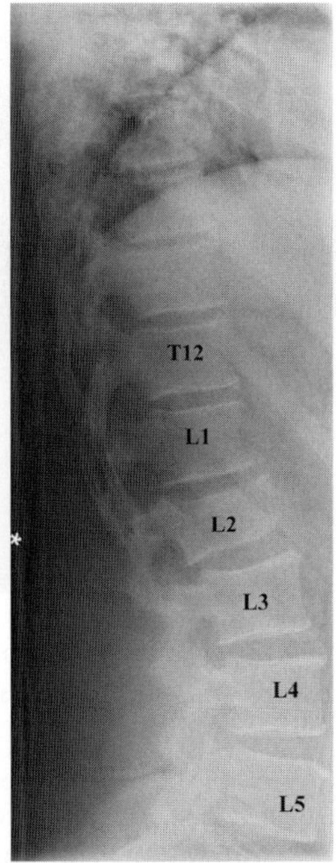

Figure 3-26: Burst fracture of L2 associated with retropulsed fragment after a fall from a horse.

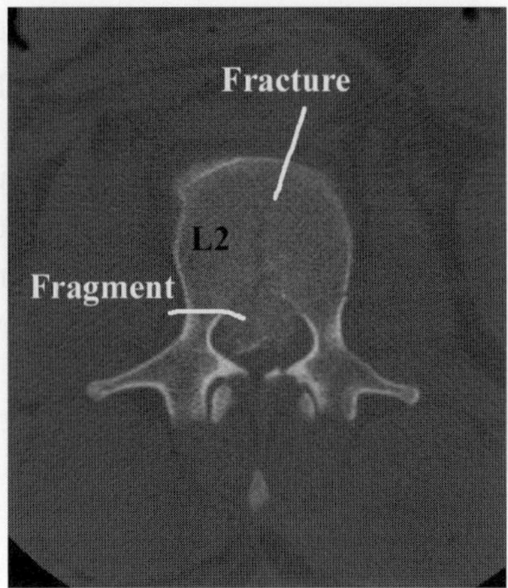

Figure 3-27: Axial CT scan of the same patient demonstrating the retropulsed bone fragment and note the split fracture of L2 body.

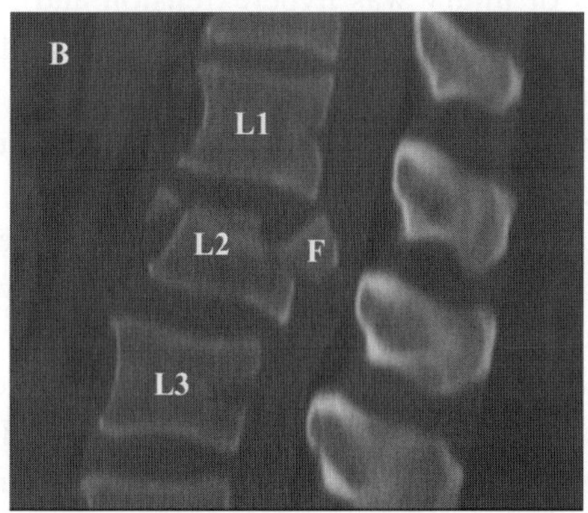

Figure 3-28: Sagittal CT scan of the same patient demonstrating the retropulsed bone fragment (F).

2- What was the mechanism of injury causing spinal instability?

3- What were the risks of each approach compared to the potential benefits?

For example if the mechanism of injury was hyperflexion and there was no decompression necessary, a posterior approach to fix the spine from the back would make sense. If the cause of neurological deficit was anterior compression it would make more sense to decompress the spine from the front to achieve maximum decompression.

Occasionally patients develop cord injury with normal radiology. In these circumstances patients need to be admitted to hospital for observation and immobilisation of the spine. This kind of injury is common in children under 16 years, their diagnosis is often delayed in over 50% and they are prone to repeated injuries.

3-2-15 *How to use skull traction?*

Skull traction is used to reduce cervical fractures or subluxations and to provide immobilisation (Figure 3-29). The location of the pins is 4 cm above the ear pinnas at the level of the external auditory meatus. However move 3 cm posterior to achieve skull traction in slight flexion if the mechanism of injury was hyperextension and 3 cm anterior for slight extension if the mechanism of injury was hyperflexion. It would be better to make small nick incisions in the scalp at the pin sites. To prevent infection of the pin sites, they must be cleaned carefully and regularly. The average starting weight of skull traction is 10 lb + the level, e.g. for C5 fracture start with 15 lb and for C6 fracture start with 16 lb and so on. Perform lateral cervical spine X-rays after two to three hours of traction. Increase the traction by 5 lb increments till the fracture/subluxation is reduced. Remove the cervical collar after the skull traction is placed. Skull traction pins are spring loaded and the pins need to be tightened after three days. The classical set for skull traction is the Gardner-Wells tongs. However, it would make more sense to apply the head ring of the halo vest for skull traction so that the halo vest could be applied for immobilisation once the fracture or subluxation was reduced.

3-2-16 *What are the mechanisms of spinal injuries?*

Several mechanisms of injury can potentially lead to spinal injury. Hyperflexion hinge-like injury occurs more commonly in the lumbar spine but can occur in the lower cervical spine as well. The movement forward is

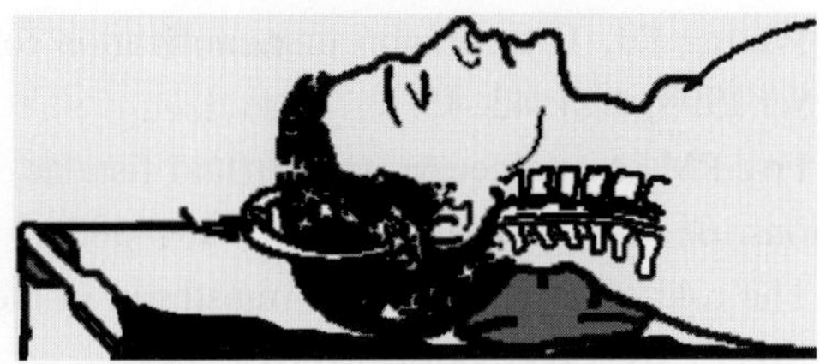

Figure 3-29: Skull traction in cervical spine injuries.

usually limited by the chin coming into contact with the chest in the cervical spine. Hyperextension hinge injuries on the other hand, such as that from a blow to the front of the head, e.g. falling face down, can cause injury to the upper cervical vertebrae. This can result in stable fracture of atlas or axis, or an unstable fracture of C2 pedicle "hangman fracture". A fracture to the odontoid peg of C2 can occur from severe falls or road traffic accidents. Many spinal injuries are not straight forward flexion or extension injury and a degree of rotation may occur during the traumatic event. This commonly happens during falls when the patient impacts onto the head and can result in facet joint dislocation in the cervical spine. Rotation and extension are more likely to result in fracture of the pedicles.[9] A burst fracture of the cervical vertebrae can occur if there is vertical compression, such as a heavy object falling from above onto the head or in a diving accident in a shallow or empty swimming pool. Retropulsion of bone fragments into the spinal canal causing spinal cord damage may occur and the energy from the impact is transferred to the cord.[10] Avulsion injuries may occur as in the clay shovler's fracture of C7 when the tip of the spinous process fractures and remains attached to the soft tissues.

References

1. Head injury — Triage, assessment, investigation and early management of head injury in infants, children and adults. NICE, 2007. http://www.nice.org.uk/guidance/index.jsp?action=download&o=36260. http://www.nice.org.uk/Guidance/CG56.
2. SIGN Publication No. 46 (2000) — Early management of patients with a head injury. http://www.sign.ac.uk/guidelines/fulltext/46/.

3. Eljamel MS, Waring DJ. The paragon immunofixation for CSF identification. *Biomed Sci* 1993; 4(2): 43–45.
4. Eljamel MS, Foy PM. Acute cerebrospinal fluid fistulae, the risk of intracranial infections. *Br J Neurosurg* 1990; 4(5): 381–385.
5. Eljamel MS. The role of surgery and B2-transferrin in the management of CSF fistulae. MD thesis, Liverpool University, 1991.
6. Eljamel MS. Antibiotic prophylaxis in CSF fistulae. *Br J Neurosurg* 1993; 7(5): 501–506.
7. Eljamel MS, Pidgeon CN, Toland J *et al*. MRI-cisternography in CSF fistulae localisation. *Br J Neurosurg* 1994; 8(4): 433–437.
8. Duane TM *et al*. Is the lateral cervical spine plain film obsolete? *J Surg Res* 2008; 147: 267–269.
9. Vaccaro AR, Madigan L *et al*. Magnetic resonance imaging analysis of soft tissue disruption after flexion-distraction injuries of the subaxial cervical spine. *Spine* 2001; 26: 1866–1872.
10. Hall RM, Oakland RJ *et al*. Spinal cord–fragment interactions following burst fracture: an *in vitro* model. *J Neurosurg Spine* 2006; 5: 243–250.

Your personal notes:

....

....

....

....

....

....

....

....

....

....

Chapter 4: Sudden Headache or Collapse (SAH, ICH, Seizures)

Problem 4-1: Sudden headache and subarachnoid haemorrhage. How to manage a patient presenting with sudden headache?

Any patient presenting with sudden headache should be managed as sub-arachnoid haemorrhage (SAH) unless and until proven otherwise.

Although many patients presenting with sudden headache do not have SAH, missing a SAH can have serious consequences to the patient because of the high rebleeding rate and death.

> **Problem based toolbox:**
> **Aneurysm   AVM Collapse**
> **Orgasmic cephalgia**
> **Subarachnoid haemorrhage**
> **Sudden headache**
> **Thunder clap headache**

PCS4-1-1:

A 67-year-old woman presented acutely with sudden severe headache of an eight-hour duration. She described the headache as a "sudden blow to the head and the worst experience so far". The headache was occipital to start with but now is all over the head. She vomited once and complained of neck stiffness. Apart from hiatus hernia and Omeprazole she had no other past medical history. She was a smoker. Examination revealed that she was fully conscious, with no focal neurological deficit. Fundoscopy was normal, BP and pulse were normal.

4-1-2 What is the differential diagnosis of sudden (acute) headache?

1- SAH — patient should be managed as SAH till proven otherwise.
2- Thunderclap headache.
3- Orgasmic cephalgia.

The classical presentation of SAH is sudden severe headache associated with nausea, vomiting, photophobia, and neck stiffness (meningitic presentation). Some patients however may present in coma, with focal neurological deficit or after seizures.

The headache of SAH is usually severe, often described as "the worst headache of my life" or "like an axe struck at the back of my head" or as an "explosion in my head". The initial headache may be mild and clears off and the patient may not seek medical attention (referred to as sentinel headache or warning headache). The warning headache occurs in 10–40% of patients presenting with SAH.[1] About 10–25% of patients with sudden severe headache have a SAH.[2,3] When sudden severe headache is the only symptom, one in ten patients turned out to have SAH, therefore the absence of other symptoms cannot be used to rule out SAH. Conversely, other symptoms of SAH may accompany other causes of sudden severe headache, so they cannot reliably distinguish SAH from migraine.[3]

4-1-3 *What are the signs associated with SAH?*

Some patients with SAH present in coma after the headache, while other causes of sudden headache hardly ever cause coma. Coma in SAH happens as a result of raised intracranial pressure. cerebral ischaemic damage to brain tissue from intraparenchymal haemorrhage, development of hydrocephalus, or seizures. Assessment of conscious level (GCS) is therefore crucial in the management of these patients. Some patients lose consciousness after SAH and recover fully shortly after. In these patients the mechanism of brief coma is caused by the sudden rise of ICP during the SAH leading to transient cerebral hypoperfusion. Some patients may present after minor head injury as a result of a fall secondary to SAH or road traffic accident secondary to SAH. In these patients it is very difficult to disentangle trauma and spontaneous SAH. These patients should therefore be treated and investigated thoroughly to rule out a cause of SAH and you can only avoid missing SAH in patients who appear on the surface to have a head injury is by keeping a high index of suspicion and thinking outside the box.

Focal cranial nerve deficits may also occur in SAH, e.g. third nerve palsy with diplopia, ptosis or pupillary dilatation from aneurysmal SAH following expanding PComA aneurysm, but could also be due to superior cerebellar artery (SCA) aneurysm. Sixth nerve palsy may occur due to raised ICP and often is a false localising sign. Partial or complete ophthalmoplegia may occur in aneurysms located in the cavernous sinus. Focal neurological deficits due to intracerebral haemorrhage or ischaemia may also follow SAH, e.g. dysphasia in dominant MCA aneurysms.

Fundoscopy is essential in SAH as it may reveal haemorrhage and arterial disease. Three types of intraocular haemorrhages may occur in association with SAH. These may occur alone or in various combinations in 20–40% of patients with SAH.[4]

1. Subhyaloid haemorrhage: This bleed is in the preretinal layer and takes the shape of half circle. It is detected in 11–33% of cases as bright red blood near the optic disc that obscures the underlying retinal vessels. It may be associated with a higher mortality rate.
2. Intraretinal haemorrhages: Occur in small number of patients.
3. Vitreous haemorrhage: Occurs in 4–27% of patients with SAH. It is often missed on initial examination. Most vitreous haemorrhages clear spontaneously within six to 12 months, but patients should be followed up for complications of elevated intraocular pressure. If the haemorrhage was bilateral and obscured the red reflex it may lead to blindness (Terson's syndrome).

4-1-4 *What is the epidemiology of SAH?*

The incidence of SAH is approximately eight per 100,000 of the population.[5] It is therefore estimated that there will be 4800 new cases of SAH diagnosed in the UK alone per year. The mean age at presentation is 61 years with a female preponderance (64% females); 85% of the patients are over 45 years of age.[6] SAH accounts for 3% of patients presenting to emergency departments with headaches and represent around 20 admissions per year to a general hospital covering 300,000 population.[7] As family doctors will encounter only a few cases of SAH during a lifetime career, a high index of suspicion is paramount to early and referral of patients with suspected SAH.

4-1-5 *What are the risk factors for SAH?*

Patients who are at risk of developing cerebrovascular disease are also predisposed to develop SAH. Cerebrovascular disease risk factors include smoking, hypertension, diabetes mellitus, and advancing age. There are however, specific conditions that predispose to SAH, these include: auto-somal dominant polycystic kidney disease that is associated with multiple intracranial aneurysms, fibromuscular dysplasia, Ehlers-Danlos syndrome, Marfan's syndrome, Psudoxanthoma Elasticum, Moya-Moya disease and bacterial endocarditis. Although the vast majority of SAH patients are non-familial and sporadic in nature, if a patient had two first degree relatives who had had SAH, (s)he is at slightly higher risk of developing SAH. True familial SAH had been reported in few families.

4-1-6 *What causes SAH?*

Although SAH as such is not a final diagnosis in most patients as the vast majority of cases of SAH had an underlying cause, in 10–15% of patients no underlying cause could be detected by our current investigations. These are called idiopathic SAH, or angio-negative SAH. Common causes of SAH include:

1- Ruptured intracranial aneurysm (RIA): In 75–80% of patients, the SAH is caused by RIA. The exact pathophysiology of the development of intracranial aneurysms is still not completely understood. It is likely that aneurysms arise from a complex multifactorial set of circumstances involving a congenital anatomical predisposition enhanced by local or systemic factors that weaken the arterial wall and lead to aneurysmal dilatation (Figures 4-1 and 4-2).

    The majority of aneurysms occur at arterial junctions in the circle of Willis (Figure 4-3). More than 90% of RIAs occur in the anterior circulation, and the rest in the vertebrobasilar system (VBS — site 4 in Figure 4-3). Anterior communicating artery aneurysms (AComAA) are the most common (30% — site 1 in Figure 4-3), followed by posterior communicating artery aneurysms (PComAA) 25% (site 3 in Figure 4-3), and middle cerebral artery aneurysms (MCAA) 20% (site 2 in Figure 4-3).

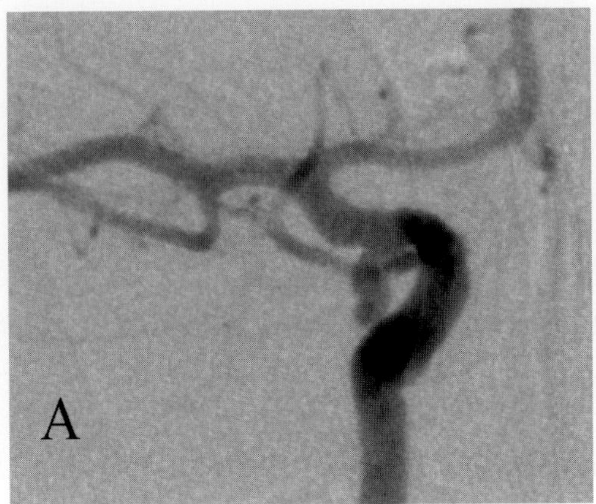

Figure 4-1

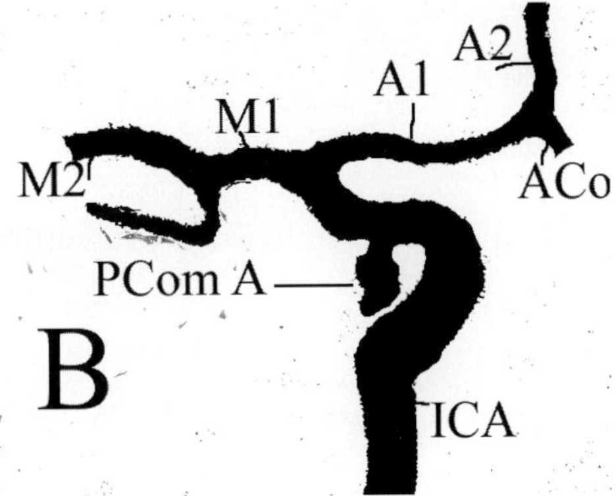

Figure 4-2

Figure 4-1 (A) and Figure 4-2 (B): Intracranial aneurysm — real angiographic picture (A) and schematic presentation (B). ICA = Internal carotid artery, PComA = posterior communicating artery, ACo = anterior communicating artery, M1 = middle cerebral artery (MCA) segment between ICA bifurcation and MCA bifurcation, M2 = MCA segments after its bifurcation, A1 = anterior cerebral artery (ACA) segment between ICA bifurcation to Aco, and A2 = ACA segments distal to ACo.

2- Ruptured arteriovenous malformation (AVM): In about 5% of patients, SAH is caused by an AVM, a condition where a leach of blood vessels cluster together and form abnormal connections that are weak and prone to bleeding (Figures 4-4 and 4-5).

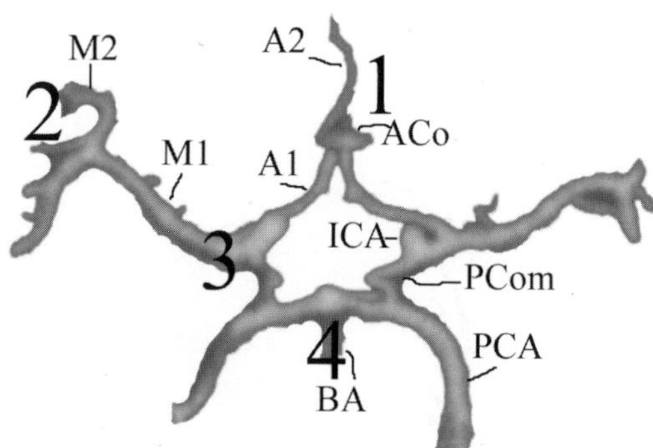

Figure 4-3: *CT angiographic picture of the circle of Willis (BA = basilar artery, PCA = posterior cerebral artery).*

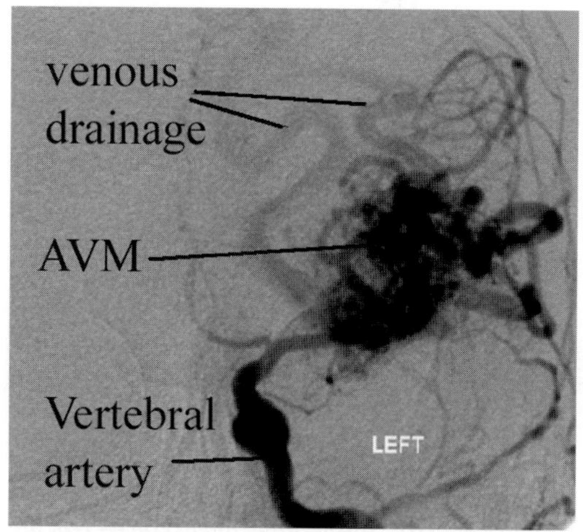

Figure 4-4: *AVM appearance on DSA.*

4-1-7 *What is the natural history of SAH?*

The natural history of SAH is dependent on the underlying cause. In the most common case scenario the underlying cause is RIA. In these patients 10–15% die before reaching a hospital, a further 5% die within the first 24 hours of SAH.[6] Of the survivors 25–30% of patients rebleed within the first four weeks from the SAH, of these; approximately 70% die after the rebleed.[8] By the 30th day of SAH, the overall case fatality rate increases

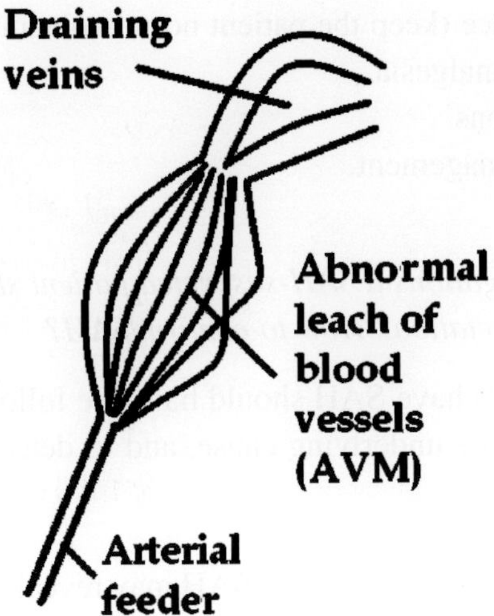

Figure 4-5: Sketch of an AVM.

to nearly 50%.[6,9] After the first six weeks of SAH, the rebleeding rate is about 4% per year. In contrast patients who had an AVM underlying the SAH, the rebleeding rate is about 12% in the first year and 4% per year thereafter. In patients with idiopathic SAH, where a good quality cerebral angiogram was negative, the rebleeding rate is negligible. SAH patients irrespective of the underlying cause may develop delayed cerebral ischaemia or hydrocephalus, e.g. 10% of patients with aneurysmal SAH develop delayed cerebral ischaemia and one in four develop hydrocephalus.

4-1-8 *What is the management of a patient suspected of having SAH?*

Any patient suspected to have had SAH, should have the following:

1- Ensure that the respiratory airways are patent and clear.
2- Ensure that the patient has adequate spontaneous or assisted breathing.
3- Ensure that the patient has adequate circulation.
4- Admit the patient to hospital for:

    a.   Bed rest.
    b.   Neurological observation.

   c.   Fluid balance (keep the patient normovolaemic).
   d.   Adequate analgesia.
   e.   Investigations
   f.   Further management.

4-1-9 *What investigations a SAH-suspected patient should have? What is the interpretation? How to confirm SAH?*

Patients suspected to have SAH should have the following investigations designed to detect the underlying cause, and to detect and manage SAH complications:

1- Full blood count (FBC): FBC in SAH may reveal slightly raised white cell count (WBC). Red cell count (RBC), and platelet count should be normal unless there was concomitant illness such as anaemia, and thrombocytopenia.

2- Blood chemistry: Blood glucose (BGL) may be slightly elevated due to endogenous glucocorticoids release due to the stress of SAH, serum sodium (Na), potassium (K), and blood urea should be normal unless there was a concomitant illness such as renal failure.

3- Urine analysis: There may be slight glucose due to the stress-related hyperglycaemia, or slight protein related to reactive hypertension. Otherwise the urine analysis should be normal unless there is a concomitant illness such as urinary tract infection.

4- Electrocardiogram (ECG): The ECG should be normal unless there is a concomitant heart disease. However, due to the associated reactive hypertension at the onset of SAH, the ECG may demonstrate ST elevation or inversion of T-waves due to subendocardial ischaemia. In a small number of patients the ECG may reveal cardiac arrhythmia or infarction.

5- Clotting factors: Should be normal unless the patient is on anticoagulants (that should be stopped in SAH) or has a concomitant blood diathesis.

6- Chest X-ray: Should be normal unless there is a concomitant lung or heart disease.

7- Computerised Tomography (CT) scan of the head: CT scan of the head is mandatory in patients suspected to have SAH. It should be

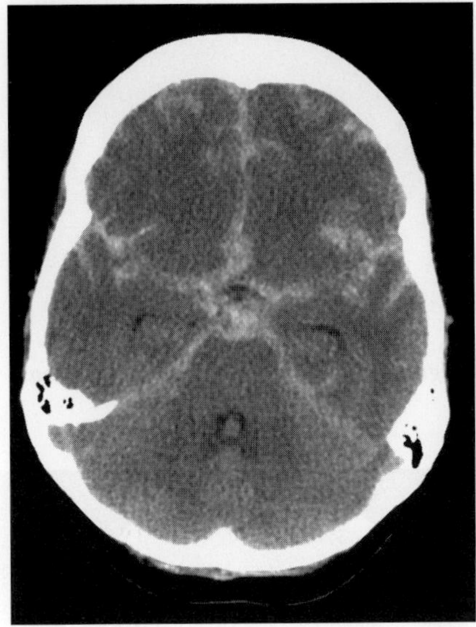

Figure 4-6: Diffuse SAH.

done urgently to confirm the SAH. The longer the scan is delayed the more likely it will be negative. The sensitivity of CT brain exceeds 95% if performed within 48 hours of the SAH.[10] SAH on CT appears as high density in the subarachanoid space (Figure 4-6). Delays in scanning allow the blood in the subarachnoid space to degrade and increase the possibility of a CT appearing as normal. The sensitivity of CT to demonstrate SAH falls sharply after 48 hours to 85% in five days, 50% after one week, 30% after two weeks and almost to nil after three weeks from the haemorrhage.[11] The CT appearances can be very subtle and can be easily missed in particular if the blood is confined to one fissure.[12] A good place to detect bleed is the occipital horns where blood usually produces fluid level (Figure 4-7).

The distribution of the blood on the CT scan may help in localising the location of the aneurysm that bled in patients who harbour multiple aneurysms; 20% of patients with SAH have multiple intracranial aneurysms. For example if the SAH is concentrated in the left Sylvain fissure, a MCAA is most likely. If it is concentrated in the

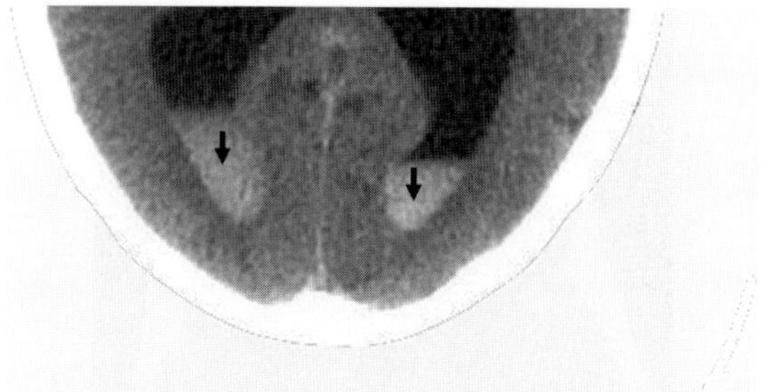

Figure 4-7: Blood in the occipital horn.

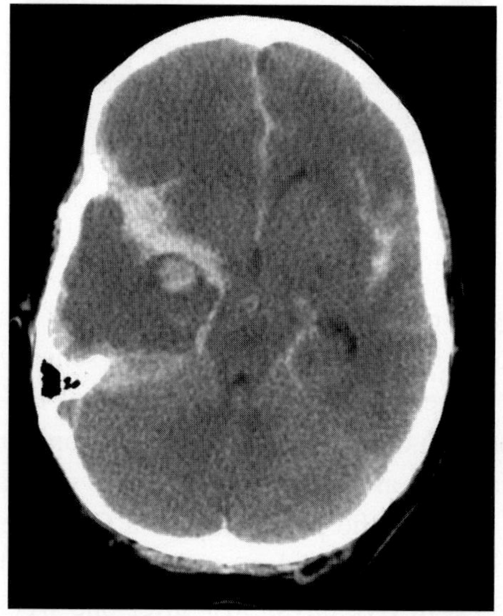

Figure 4-8: SAH with MCAA.

interhemispheric fissure anteriorly, an aneurysm in the ACoA is most likely; If the blood is mainly in the interpenduncular cistern, a basilar tip aneurysm will be more likely. If the blood is in the third ventricle the aneurysm may be in the ACoA, and if it is in the fourth ventricle the aneurysm will be in the vertebrobasilar system. However, when the SAH is diffuse (Figure 4-6) the aneurysm can be anywhere. The CT scan may also show the actual aneurysm (Figure 4-8) or an

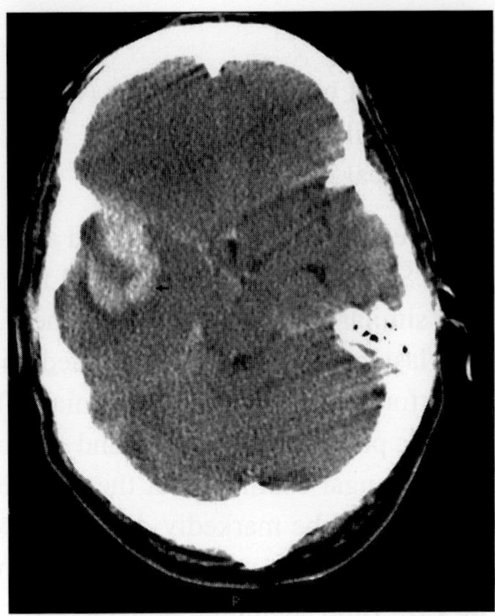

Figure 4-9: Intracerebral haematoma.

associated intracerebral haematoma (Figure 4-9) or acute subdural haematoma (ASDH). ASDH may occur in up to 10% of SAH and often indicate an ICA aneurysm.

8- Lumbar puncture (L/P): If CT brain is negative for SAH, lumbar puncture (L/P) will be required to confirm SAH.[10] L/P will reveal uniformally blood stained CSF with equal intensity in three consecutive CSF bottles, xanthochromia (yellow discolouration of the spinned CSF) appears after six hours from the ictus of SAH due to the degradation of haemoglobin into oxyhaemoglobin and bilirubin.[13] Bilirubin confirms SAH as it can only occur *in vivo*, unlike oxyhaemoglobin that may result from a traumatic tap or prolonged storage or agitation of bloodstained CSF *in vitro*.[14]

To perform L/P the patient must fulfil the following criteria:

i- The management of the patient will be altered significantly by the results of L/P, e.g. to distinguish migraine from SAH or to culture the bug in meningitis.

ii- The CT scan brain is normal.

iii- In the absence of CT brain:

    a.   The patient must be fully conscious (GCS = 15).
    b.   There is no papilloedema.
    c.   There is no focal neurological deficit.

The opening pressure of CSF must be recorded at the time of L/P and three samples of CSF are taken and observed for colour. If all the three samples are similar in colour (blood stained), SAH should be suspected and the last sample should be spinned and protected from light and analysed for bilirubin (xanthochromia). The other samples are also analysed for protein, cell-counts, and glucose (remember to send blood for blood sugar estimation at the same time as in meningitis the CSF glucose will be markedly diminished — haemorrhagic meningitis is rare but it can occur in Haemophylis influenza bacterial meningitis). The CSF fluid should be protected from light to prevent degradation of the bilirubin. The estimation of red cell counts in three consecutive samples of CSF does not reliably distinguish SAH from traumatic tap.[13] However, if you are in doubt, err on the side of SAH and investigate the patient with angiography if the history is suggestive of SAH.

9- Cerebral angiography: This can be achieved using CTA, DSA or MRA.

a- CTA:

CTA can be used to reveal the underlying cause of SAH nowadays due to its speed, tolerability, convenience, and its ability to provide three-dimensional reconstructions of the cerebral circulation. Essentially if SAH is suspected CT is performed to confirm the diagnosis. If the CT demonstrated SAH, proceed to CTA immediately if the patient is stable enough. The sensitivity of CTA is about 95% in detecting intracranial aneurysms compared to conventional DSA and decisions about treatment can be based on CTA alone in most cases (Figure 4-10).

b- DSA:

Digital subtraction angiography (Figure 4-11) becomes necessary in patients who have confirmed SAH with negative CTA or during

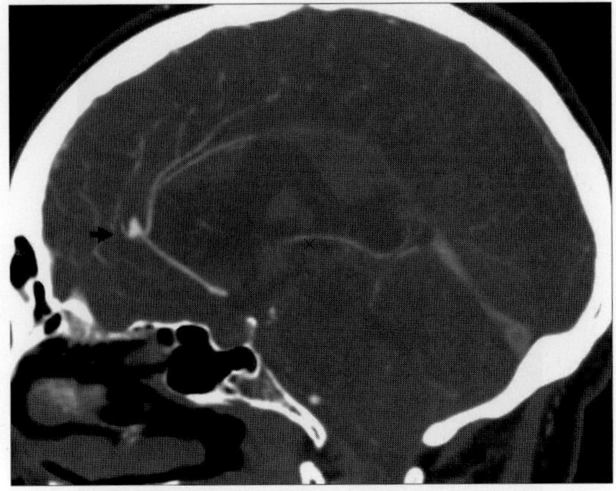

Figure 4-10: CTA of pericallosal artery aneurysm (arrow).

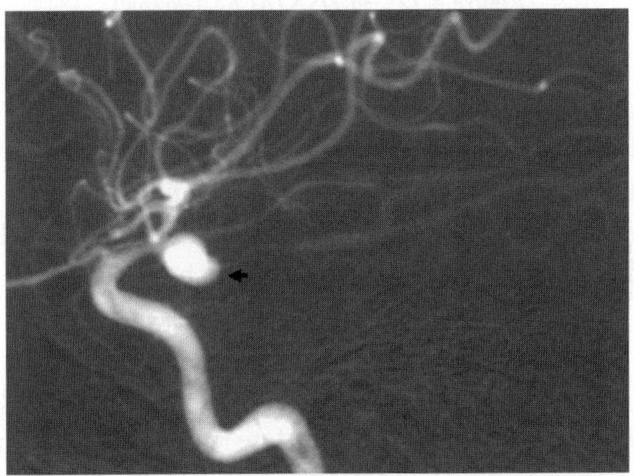

Figure 4-11: DSA left ICA PComAA (arrow).

coiling. 3D-DSA (Figure 4-12) may also become necessary to determine the configuration of the aneurysm before deciding on the best therapy. Repeated cerebral DSA, spinal catheter DSA, or magnetic resonance imaging (MRI) may be necessary to identify alternative causes of SAH in some patients. For patients with purely perimesencephalic bleed (blood around the brain stem), a normal, good quality

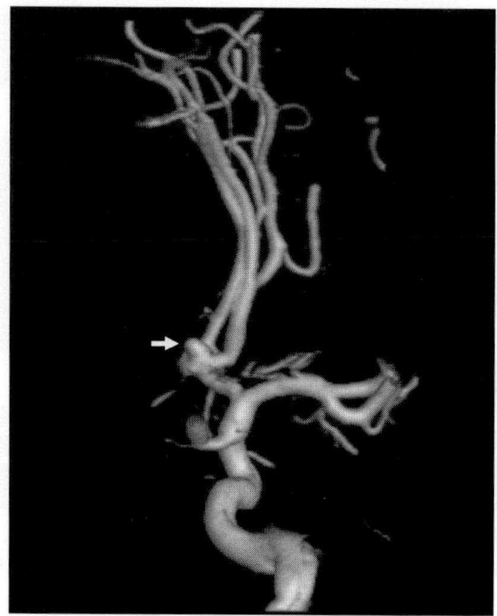

Figure 4-12: 3d-DSA (ACoAA-arrow).

cerebral DSA allows a diagnosis of idiopathic perimesencephalic SAH without the need for further investigation.[13]

10- MRI and MRA: MRI with proton density and fluid attenuated inversion recovery (FLAIR) have been shown to be as sensitive as CT for the detection of SAH.[15] However, MRI is impractical in most acute cases of SAH due to its lack of availability on one hand and the extra safety concerns in the MRI setting. MRI would be very useful in those who present late when CT scan and L/P were negative or undiagnostic. MRI-FLAIR and T2-weighted sequences were shown to be very sensitive in detecting the byproduct of SAH, haemosiderin. An MRI sensitivity of 90% was reported in delayed presentation of SAH compared to 46% with CT at that stage.[16] MRA can also be used to detect an underlying cause of SAH such as aneurysms (Figure 4-13). However its use is limited due to its low sensitivity, e.g. as low as 35% detection rate was reported in aneurysms of < 5 mm.[17]

The following flow chart depicts the investigations of suspected SAH patients.

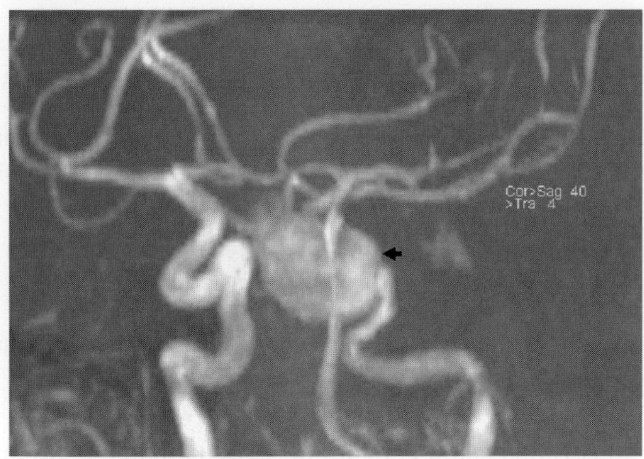

Figure 4-13: MRA demonstrating a large ICA aneurysm (arrow).

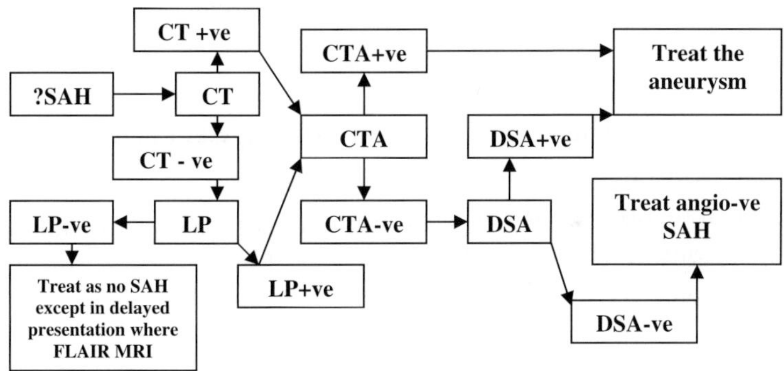

There are advantages and disadvantages of CTA and DSA in SAH which is given in Table 4-1.

4-1-10 *How to manage a patient with confirmed SAH?*

1- *Medical management:*

Patients with SAH should be managed initially as follows:

a- Admit to hospital for neurological observation.
b- Bed rest.

Table 4-1: Comparison of CTA and DSA in SAH

	CTA	DSA
Access	Readily available	In specialist centres only
Risk	Almost zero	1.8% risk of stroke (CVA)
Invasiveness	Non-invasive	Invasive
Sensitivity	95%	>95%
Timing	Can be obtained straightaway after SAH diagnosis	Requires special arrangement
3D views	Possible	Needs special equipment

c- Intravenous fluids using crystalloids. The patient should be kept normovolaemic with 3 L/24 hours.

d- Analgesia using moderate strength medications, e.g. Tramadol, Codeine, Tylex, Dihydrocodeine or similar analgesics. Avoid strong opiates as they may interfere with neurological observations or lead to depression of respiration. Avoid non-steroidal anti-inflammatory drugs as they interfere with platelet functions.

e- Laxative to counteract and treat constipation, e.g. Lactulose.

f- Antiemetics to treat nausea and vomiting.

g- Oxygen therapy by face mask.

h- Nimodipine orally or intravenously to reduce the risk of ischaemia. Nimodipine is a selective calcium channel antagonist. There is enough scientific evidence that supports the use of Nimodipine to reduce the incidence of a poor outcome from delayed cerebral ischaemia.[18]

i- Referral to specialist centre for urgent investigations and further management of the underlying cause of SAH.

2- *Prevention of rebleeding:*

The risk of rebleeding is more or less evenly distributed during the first four weeks after the aneurysmal rupture, with a cumulative risk of 30% without intervention. Following rebleeding, the prognosis is poor: 70% of patients die or remain severely disabled.[19]

The treatment options for securing the aneurysm is either to coil the aneurysm by packing it with platinum coils that lead to thrombosis of the aneurysm or by clipping the neck of the aneurysm. To coil an aneurysm it has to be accessible to endovascular approaches such as aneurysms located at the bifurcation of the major vessels at the circle of Willis, the neck of the aneurysm preferably narrower than its fundus, no important branches coming off the aneurysm and the aneurysm of adequate size to hold the coils, otherwise the coils may prolapse back into the parent artery and cause complications (Figures 4-14 and 4-15).

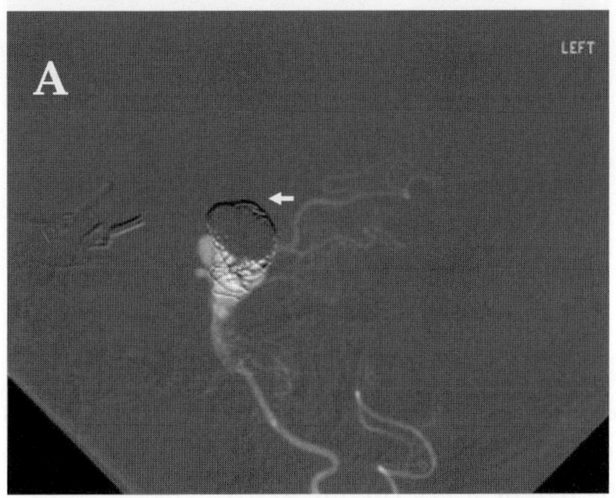

Figure 4-14: Coiled aneurysm-BTAA.

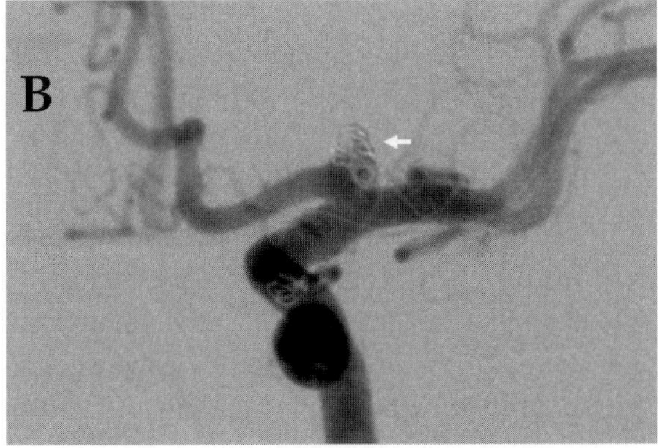

Figure 4-15: Incomplete coiling and prolapse of coil.

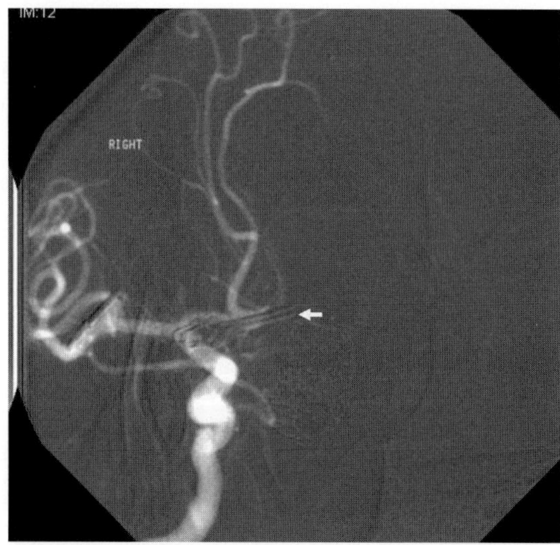

Figure 4-16: Clipped intracranial aneurysm. The two clips are to secure ACoAA (arrow).

Similar rules apply to clipping otherwise clipping will not be possible and wrapping is instituted to avoid damage to some perforators or branches of the parent artery (Figure 4-16).

Over the past decade, endovascular techniques have gained the upper hand in the management of ruptured intracranial aneurysms and have become the first treatment option when available for ruptured posterior circulation aneurysms. In recent years the International Subarachnoid Aneurysm Trial (ISAT) had supported the development of aneurysm coiling for anterior circulation aneurysms as well. Most patients in ISAT were in good clinical condition and had small (< 1 cm) anterior circulation aneurysms. After a year of follow-up, coiling conferred an absolute risk reduction over clipping of about 7% for dependency or death, with the benefit sustained up to seven years.[20] While ISAT had led to sweeping changes in aneurysmal SAH management, there were several shortcomings of the study, e.g. the coiling was performed by expert neuro-radiologists who were at the top of their game, while clipping was performed by sub-specialists and generalist surgeons, and only a fraction of the eligible patients who were suitable for the trial were recruited and enrolled.

However, complete aneurysm occlusion was more likely to be achieved with clipping. The durability of coiling beyond seven years is still awaited. If coiling is not appropriate, clipping of the aneurysm is undertaken. Clipping is usually performed within 72 hours of SAH to minimise the rebleed risk and enable aggressive treatment of any subsequent delayed cerebral ischaemia.

3- *Post coiling/clipping management:*

The main complications of aneurysmal SAH are:

a- Rebleeding can be prevented by clipping or coiling. However, if the patient has incomplete occlusion of the ruptured aneurysm or multiple aneurysms, the patient is still at risk of rebleeding (Figure 4-17).

b- Delayed cerebral ischaemia: one in ten of patients with aneurysmal SAH may develop vasospasm and delayed cerebral ischaemia (Figure 4-18).

c- Hydrocephalus due to blockage of CSF absorption at the arachnoid villi (Figure 4-19) or by intraventricular blood clot blocking the III or

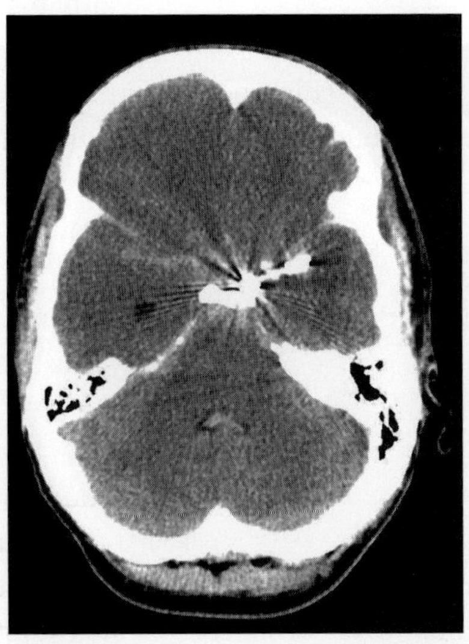

Figure 4-17: Rebleeding following coiled ICA bifurcation aneurysm (notice the artefact from the coils in the left Sylvain fissure, blood in the subarachnoid cisterns and IV ventricle).

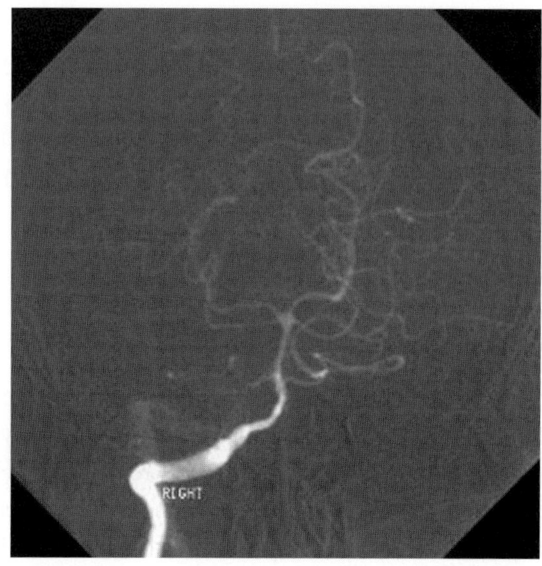

Figure 4-18: Vasospasm after aneurysmal SAH. The basilar and its branches vasospastic.

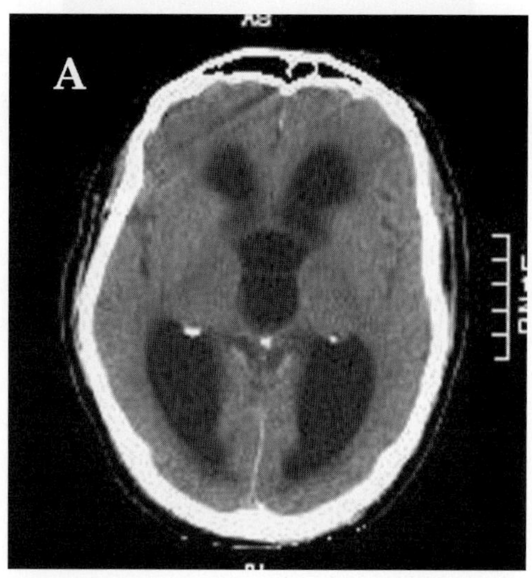

Figure 4-19: Post-SAH hydrocephalus.

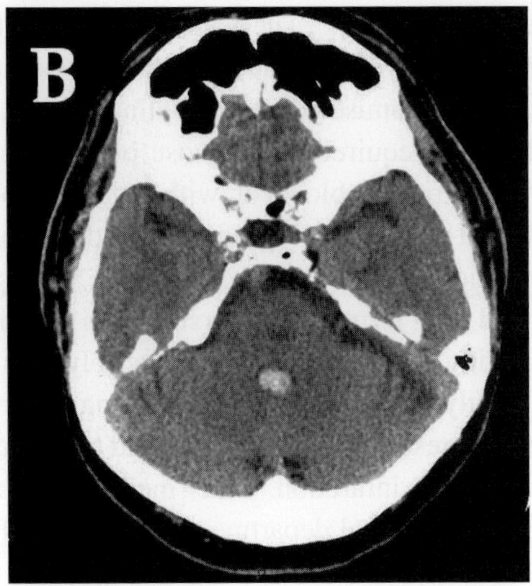

Figure 4-20: Blood clot in the fourth ventricle.

IV ventricles. One in four patients with SAH had acute hydrocephalus at presentation (Figure 4-20).

The principal causes of post-treatment deterioration are distal vessel compromise as a result of treatment, delayed cerebral ischaemia, hydrocephalus, cerebral salt wasting syndrome, infective or thromboembolic complications. The former is minimised by careful attention during the procedure. Aspirin or heparin may be beneficial to minimise the risk of an early intraluminal thrombosis in patients who have undergone coiling. Delayed cerebral ischaemia (peak incidence day 4–10 post-SAH) due to vasospasm should be managed prophylactically (normal or hypervolaemia and Nimodipine) and therapeutically by HHH- therapy (HHH-therapy stands for hypertension, hypervolaemia, haemodilution). A target systolic blood pressure of around 160 mmHg and CVP of 8–10 cm are desirable in HHH-therapy, using fluids and ionotropes as required. Should clinical features of vasospasm become evident, the blood pressure is further augmented to evaluate whether improvement occurs or not. Transcranial doppler sonography is used in some centres to detect impending cerebral ischaemia by means of increased blood flow velocity, but the positive and negative predictive value of these tests are disappointing.[21] The value of angioplasty or papaverine injection in patients with symptomatic vasospasm is yet to be proven and would require further randomised controlled clinical trials.

Repeat CT brain is required to diagnose or exclude hydrocephalus. Patients with intraventricular blood or with extensive blood clot in the basal cistern will be at risk of developing acute hydrocephalus, and should be treated with ventricular or lumbar drainage of CSF. A small percentage of patients will need long term CSF diversion with a shunt.

Careful monitoring of fluid balance and electrolytes is also mandatory. Hyponatraemia, mostly due to cerebral salt wasting syndrome, should not be managed with fluid restriction since it can lead to worsening of cerebral ischaemia and subsequent infarction. Other medical complications should be dealt with according to local departmental and hospital protocols.

4-1-11 *What is the prognosis after aneurysmal SAH?*

Almost all SAH-deaths that occur after hospital admission happen within the first three weeks after SAH, mostly due to rebleeding. Around one-third of survivors become dependent, often with cognitive impairment, and two-thirds have a reduced quality of life.[22] The three strongest predictors of poor outcome of aneursmal SAH are impaired conscious level on admission,[23] increasing age and large volume of blood on the initial CT brain (Fisher grades):

1- The level of consciousness is the main factor in determining the grade of SAH in the World Federation of Neurological Surgeons (WFNS) grading system of SAH and is a strong predictor of outcome after SAH (Table 4-2).
2- The Fisher grade of SAH on the CT scan also predicts delayed cerebral ischaemia and the outcome of SAH (Table 4-3).[24]

The first clinical grading system used in SAH to predict prognosis is the Hunt and Hess scale in 1968[25] (Table 4-4).

In good grade SAH patients, a favourable outcome can be achieved in 90% of patients. However, the prognosis in poor grade SAH patients is generally poor (67% mortality and 25% with favourable outcome).[25,26]

Table 4-2: The WFNS grades of SAH and the outcome of SAH[23]

Grade	GCS	Hemi/mono-paresis or dysphasia	Prognosis odd ratio for poor outcome (95% CI)
I	15	Absent	
II	13–14	Absent	2.3 (1.3 to 4.1)
III	13–14	Present	6.1 (2.9 to 12.8)
IV	7–12	With or without	7.7 (4.3 to 13.7)
V	3–6	With or without	69.2 (30.6 to 156.3)

Table 4-3: Fisher grades of SAH on CT

Grade	Description	Signs of vasospasm
I	No blood detected on CT	0
II	Diffuse or vertical layers < 1 mm thick	0
III	Localised clot or vertical layer of 1 mm or thicker	96%
IV	Intraventricular or intracerebral clot and diffuse SAH	0

Table 4-4: Hunt and Hess grades of SAH

Grade	Description	Survival rate
I	Asymptomatic; or minimal headache and slight nuchal rigidity.	70%
II	Moderate to severe headache; nuchal rigidity; no neurologic deficit except cranial nerve palsy.	60%
III	Drowsy; minimal neurologic deficit.	50%
IV	Stuporous; moderate to severe hemiparesis; possibly early decerebrate rigidity and vegetative disturbances.	20%
V	Deep coma; decerebrate rigidity; moribund.	10%

A recent national SAH audit in the UK showed that the six months outcome of 2168 patients was 62% had favourable outcome (good recovery or moderate disability). The percentage of patients with good recovery did not differ between patients who were clipped or coiled. Only 19% of patients who underwent no repair had favourable outcome.[27]

Late rebleeding can occur in patients with successfully occluded aneurysms from *de novo* aneurysms, or from regrowth of the aneurysm that caused the first bleed. The risk of late rebleeding is a concern after coiling. The ISAT trial showed 0.7% risk of rebleeding between one month and one year after coiling. This risk of late rebleeding is also noted to be higher when compared to clipping[20] which is around 2–3% in ten years after clipping.[28]

Epilepsy develops after discharge in 14–20% of patients following SAH. The risk factors for epilepsy after SAH include the presence of acute subdural haematoma, cerebral infarction, or disability at discharge. The ISAT trial had shown that the risk of epilepsy is slightly higher for patients treated by clipping when compared to those treated by coiling.[20]

Cognitive deficits and psychosocial dysfunction in the first year after SAH are common in patients who make good recovery. Although improvement occurs up to 18 months after SAH, many patients and their partners experience reduced quality of life. In a survey of 610 patients who were interviewed after a mean period of 8.9 years after SAH and treated by surgical clipping, 26% of the employed patients had stopped working, and another 24% worked shorter hours or had a position with less responsibility, 60% of the patients reported changes in personality, and only 25% reported complete recovery without psychosocial or neurological problems.[29]

Your personal notes:

....

....

....

....

....

....

....

....

....

....

Problem 4-2:   Collapse and sudden focal neurological deficits. How to manage a patient presenting with sudden focal neurological deficit or collapse?

Focal neurological deficit (FND) is a manifestation of a wide range of neurological disorders and any patient presenting with FND needs urgent investigation to confirm the underlying aetiology.

<table>
<tr><td colspan="2"><u>Problem based tool box:</u></td></tr>
<tr><td>Stroke</td><td>TIA</td></tr>
<tr><td colspan="2">Focal neurological deficit</td></tr>
<tr><td colspan="2">Blood supply of the brain</td></tr>
</table>

PCS4-2-1:

A 65-year-old man presented with acute speech impairment that lasted for few hours. Few days later he developed sudden flaccid right hemiplegia and drowsiness. His hemiplegia was flaccid and associated with weakness of the lower half of the face. He was hypertensive on antihypertensive therapy. He had a CT scan of the brain (Figure 4-21).

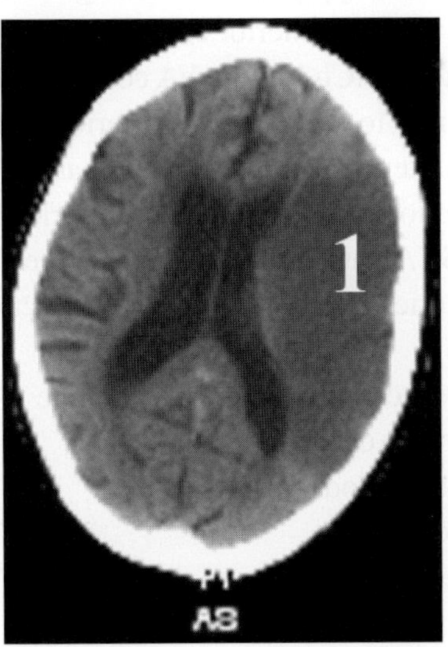

Figure 4-21: CT scan of the brain demonstrating a large low density area (1) of the left hemisphere. This was infarct in the middle cerebral artery (MCA) territory.

4-2-2 *What is the differential diagnosis?*

A patient presenting with sudden onset FND may had suffered from:

1-   Transient ischaemic attack (TIA).
2-   Cerebrovascular infarct.
3-   Spontaneous intracranial haemorrhage.
4-   Spontaneous arterial dissection.
5-   Cerebral venous sinus thrombosis.
6-   Todd's paresis after focal seizure.
7-   Hemiplegic migraine.
8-   Haemorrhage secondary to other underlying pathology.

4-2-3 *What is CVA (cerebrovascular accidents: strokes, infarcts, TIAs)?*

CVAs occur as a result of an occlusion of blood supply to part of the brain. The brain is supplied by two internal carotid arteries (ICA) and two vertebral arteries (VA). The ICA on each side divides into anterior (ACA) and middle cerebral arteries (MCA). Branches of the ICA include meningohypophysial artery (MHA) supplying the meninges and the pituitary gland, the ophthalmic artery (OA), posterior communicating artery (PComA) and anterior choroidal artery (AChA). The VA contributes to the anterior spinal artery (ASA), gives rise to the posterior inferior cerebellar artery (PICA) before joining its counterpart VA to form the basilar artery (BA). The BA gives rise to the anterior inferior cerebellar arteries (AICA), the superior cerebellar arteries (SCA) and the posterior cerebral arteries (PCA). Any blockage of these arteries leads to infarction. Infarctions can be due to:

1-   Thrombosis or embolism of large arteries due to atherosclerosis.
2-   Embolism of cardiac or carotid origin.
3-   Occlusion of small blood vessels.
4-   Other determined cause.
5-   Undetermined cause.

Investigations include brain imaging and blood biochemistry and haematology looking for diabetes mellitus, high cholesterol, etc. CT scan is of

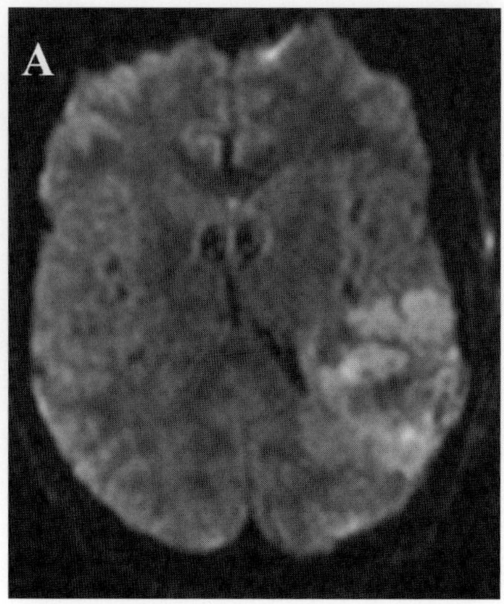

Figure 4-22: Diffusion MRI demonstrating an infarct.

no value in TIAs after the first week of presentation. CT scan is often normal in the first 24 hours. MRI using diffusion protocols may demonstrate infarction in the first 24 hours (Figure 4-22).

On imaging infarcts are labelled according to their vascular territory, e.g. left MCA infarct (Figure 4-21), ACA infarct, lacunar infarct or cerebellar infarct (Figure 4-23).

4-2-4 *What are the risk factors for cerebral infarct?*

CVA is the second commonest cause of death worldwide. Risk factors include hypertension, previous stroke or TIA, diabetes mellitus, hypercholesterolaemia, cigarette smoking, atrial fibrillation and advanced age. Control of hypertension protects against stroke (odds ratio 0.63, CI 0.55–0.72)[30] Smoking cessation is also advisable in patients who suffered TIAs to prevent stroke, high cholesterol can be reduced by statins, atrial fibrillation with anticoagnulants, and antiplatelets to prevent further strokes (aspirin or clopidegrol).[31] Patients who present within three hours with thrombotic or embolic stroke benefit from thrombolysis. Endarterectomy is used to treat ICA stenosis in patients with TIAs and decompressive

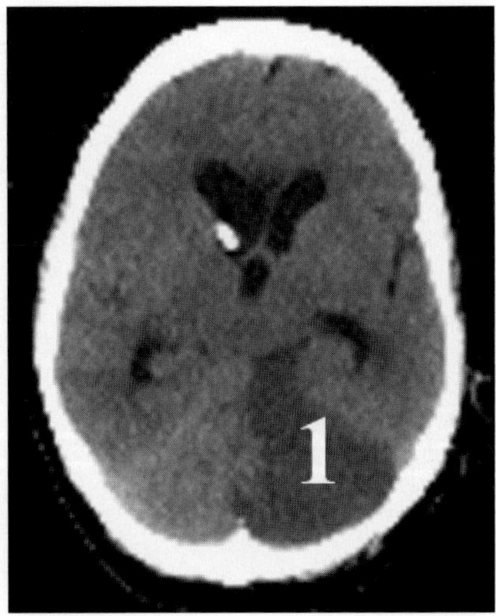

Figure 4-23: CT scan demonstrating left cerebellar infarct (1). Note the hyperdense object in the right frontal horn is the tip of an external drain to divert CSF and relief hydrocephalus.

craniotomy (Figure 4-24) is used to salvage patients who develop intracranial hypertension secondary to ICA stroke or those who develop hydrocephalus secondary to cerebellar infarct (Figure 4-23). Sometimes drainage of the ventricles is required to drain hydrocephalus using external ventricular drain.

4-2-5 *How to manage spontaneous intracerebral haematoma (SICH)?*

Haemorrhagic stroke leads to spontaneous intracerebral haematoma. SICH forms 20% of all strokes and has the highest morbidity and mortality. CT scan is the most common modality of investigation (Figures 4-25 and 4-26).

Causes of SICH include AVMs, aneurysms and tumours (Figures 4-27 and 4-28).

Treatment should be directed towards the underlying pathology. However, significant haematomas that cause neurological deterioration respond to surgical decompression particularly in the cerebellum and

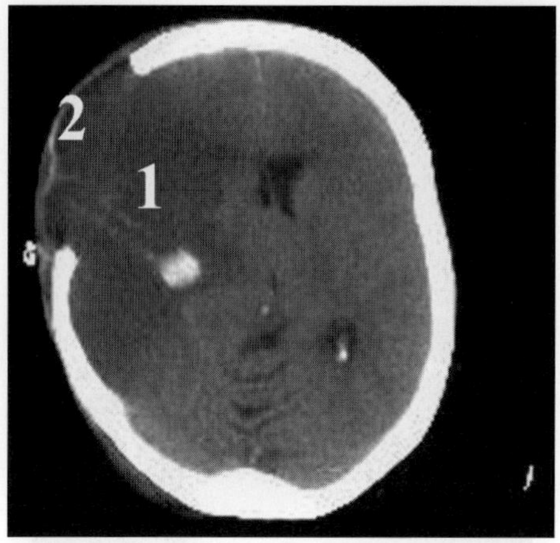

Figure 4-24: Decompressive craniotomy (2) after MCA infarct (1).

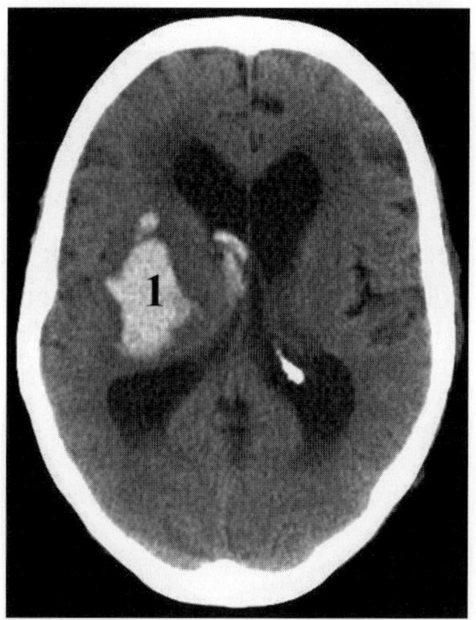

Figure 4-25: CT scan of brain demonstrating SICH in the right striatum (1).

cerebral lobes. Adverse prognostic factors include advanced age, reduced conscious level, co-morbidity, intraventricular bleed and hydrocephalus. If the patient was stable a multicentre randomised controlled trial found a policy of early surgical intervention was not indicated in patients with SICH.[32]

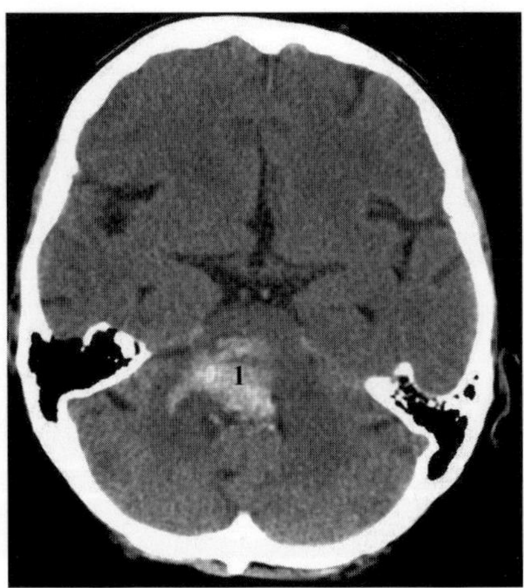

Figure 4-26: CT scan of brain demonstrating SICH in the cerebellum and brain stem (1).

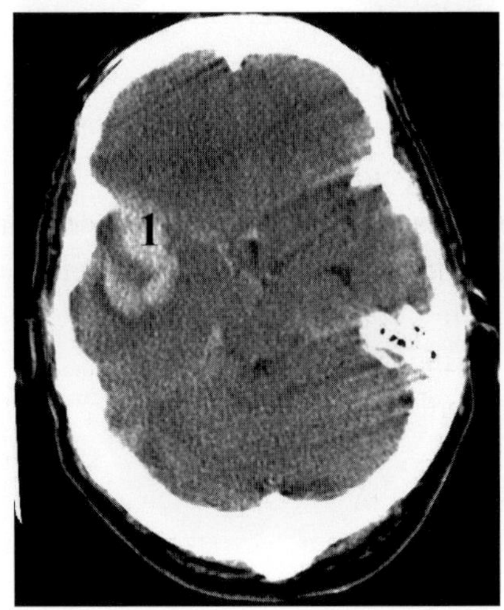

Figure 4-27: CT scan demonstrating SICH (1) associated with SAH due to MCA aneurysm.

4-2-6 *How to manage spontaneous arterial dissection?*

Spontaneous carotid (SCD) and vertebral (SVD) dissections are more common than reported in the literature. They present with ipsilateral

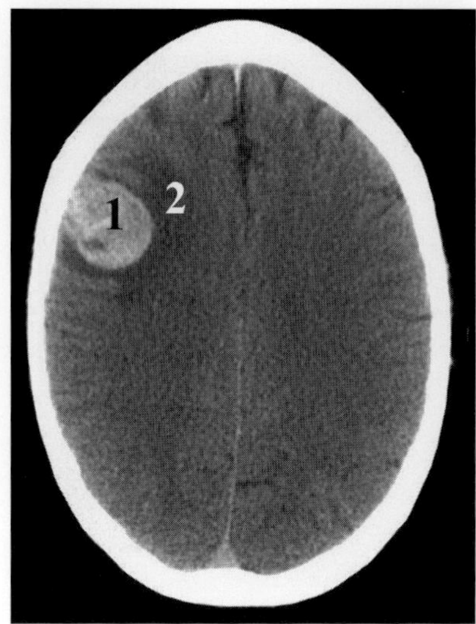

Figure 4-28: Small SICH in the right frontal region (1) surrounded with low density (2) on axial CT of patient. The underlying pathology was metastatic malignant melanoma.

headache associated with sudden onset focal neurological deficit. SCD also associated with ipsilateral Horner's syndrome (partial ptosis, miosis and lack of sweating) and carotid bruits. The diagnosis could be made by DSA (string sign, Figure 4-29), carotid duplex doppler or MRI/MRA.

Once considered uncommon, SCD is an increasingly recognised cause of stroke that preferentially affects individuals between 20–40 years.[33,34] The incidence of SCD has been reported to be 2.6 to 2.9 per 100,000. Patients with SCD may have hereditary connective tissue disorders or family history of stroke. These include Marfan's syndrome, vascular Ehlers-Danlos syndrome, autosomal dominant polycystic kidney disease, pseudoxanthoma elasticum, fibromuscular dysplasia, and osteogenesis imperfecta type I. Carotid dissection is more common after severe violent trauma to the head or neck. An estimated 0.67% of patients admitted to hospital after major accidents were found to have blunt carotid injury; 76% had intimal dissections, pseudoaneurysms, or both. The mechanism of injury for most internal carotid injuries is rapid deceleration, with resultant hyperextension and rotation of the neck, which

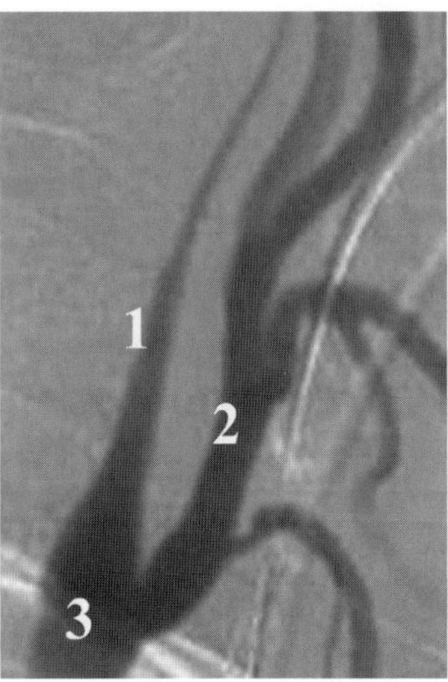

Figure 4-29: DSA of the right carotid artery (1 = internal carotid artery with string sign, 2 = external carotid artery (normal), and 3 = common carotid artery).

stretches the ICA over the upper cervical vertebrae, producing an intimal tear. After such an injury, the patient may remain asymptomatic, have a hemispheric TIA, or suffer a stroke. The goal of treatment is to prevent the development or continuation of neurological deficits. Treatments include observation, anticoagulation, stent implantation and carotid artery ligation. There is no controlled study for the best treatment or management of SCAD. Empiric treatment in acute SCAD to prevent secondary embolism is partial thromboplastin time (PTT)-guided anticoagulation by intravenous heparin followed by anticoagulation with Warfarin. Carotid surgery for treatment of SCAD is not recommended with the possible exception of persisting severe stenosis of the proximal ICA. Carotid angioplasty by balloon dilatation and stenting is used in selected patients of severe cerebral haemodynamic impairment by bilateral SCAD. The duration of secondary prophylaxis by anticoagulation is best guided by Doppler sonography follow-up, and should be continued until normalisation of blood flow or until at least one year after the vessel is occluded. There is no evidence that pseudoaneurysms increase the risk for embolic complications, and there is no evidence for surgery or continuation of anticoagulation in patients with pseudoaneurysms makes much difference. Patients should be advised to avoid exercises that involve excessive head movements (bungee jumping, trampoline jumping, and chiropractic manoeuvres). The patient should be informed that recurrent rate is low in non-familial cases. Doppler sonography is a low-cost and highly sensitive method for patients at risk.

4-2-7 *How to manage cerebral venous sinus thrombosis (CVST)?*

Another example of haemorrhagic stroke is infarction secondary to CVST. It is a rare form of stroke that results from thrombosis of dural venous sinuses. The incidence is about four to five per million and 75% of the affected patients are females. However, CVST is difficult to diagnose and its incidence is likely to be higher than that reported in the literature. Symptoms include headache, visual disturbance, motor weakness or seizures. The diagnosis is based on the demonstration of obstructed venous sinuses by thrombus. Sometimes a thrombus is seen in the confluence of dural sinuses (Torcula) as a triangular filling defect (delta sign). CT and CT venogram (CTV) (Figure 4-30) is more sensitive than MRI and MR venogram (MRV) (Figure 4-31). CTV's sensitivity is about 75–100%. D-dimer may be positive in some cases. Cerebral venous

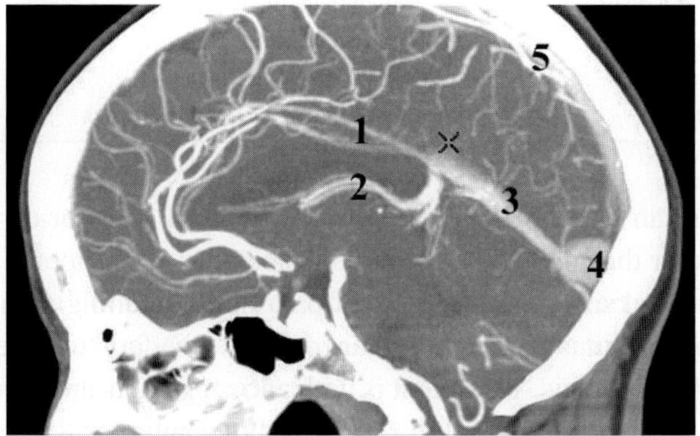

Figure 4-30: Image of normal CTA and CTV demonstrating: 1 = internal cerebral veins, 2 = veins of Rosenthal, 3 = straight sinus, 4 = Torcula, and 5 = superior sagittal sinus.

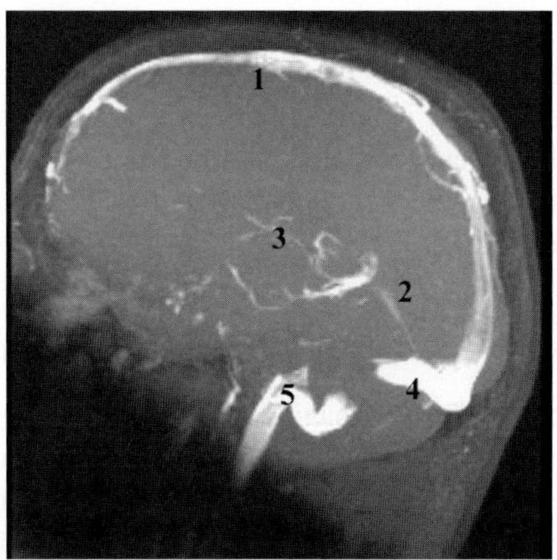

Figure 4-31: MRV demonstrating: 1 = superior sagittal sinus, 2 = straight sinus, 3 = internal cerebral veins, 4 = lateral sinus, and 5 = sigmoid sinus.

Table 4-5: Risk factors for CVST

Risk factor	Comment/Tests
Thrombophilia	Proteins C, S or antithrombin deficiency
Nephrotic syndrome	Chronic renal failure
Chronic inflammation	Inflammatory bowel disease or SLE
Blood disorder	Polycythaemia
Hormones	Pregnancy, OCP
Trauma	Direct injury to sinus
Surgery	Operations near venous sinuses

thrombosis can occur post-operatively when dural sinus or cerebral vein is occluded or thrombosed, e.g. vein of Labe after subtemporal surgery or superior sagittal sinus after surgery of parasagittal meningioma.

Cavernous sinus thrombosis can occur secondary to infection and manifests by proptosis. Treatment is with anticoagulants and rarely thrombolysis. It is important to look for an underlying cause as 85% of patients had one or more risk factors (Table 4-5). CVST is often complicated by raised intracranial pressure, which may warrant surgical intervention such as CSF diversion.

Your personal notes:

Problem 4-3:   Collapse, seizures, fits and funny turns. How to manage a patient presenting with seizure or funny turn?

Epilepsy is not a diagnosis unless an underlying aetiology was excluded. Any patient presenting with seizures needs careful history and examination to establish the semiology and under-lying pathology.

Problem based tool box:	
Epilepsy	**Dysplasia**
Anticonvulsants	**VNS**
Mesial temporal sclerosis	

PCS4-3-1:

A four-year-old child presented with seizures, otherwise the child was normal on examination. His blood tests were normal except his blood glucose was low. This was corrected and had an MRI (Figure 4-32) that demonstrated mushroom gryri. These gyri occurred after perinatal asphyxia and was associated with epilepsy.

PCS4-3-2:

A 50-year-old woman presented with three successive tonic-clonic seizures associated with drowsiness. No other relevant findings. She had

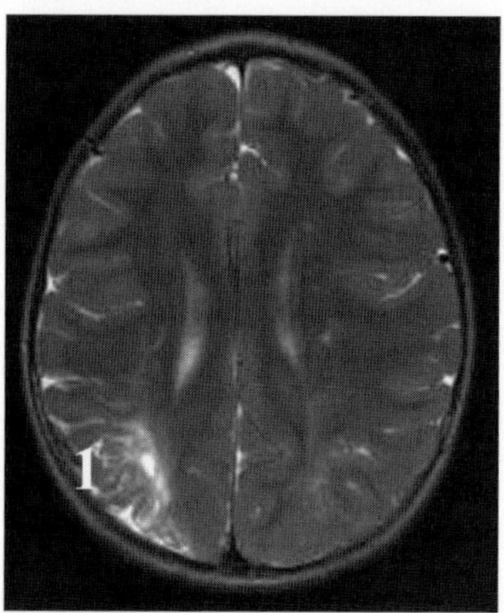

Figure 4-32: T2-weighted axial image demonstrating mushroom gyri (1).

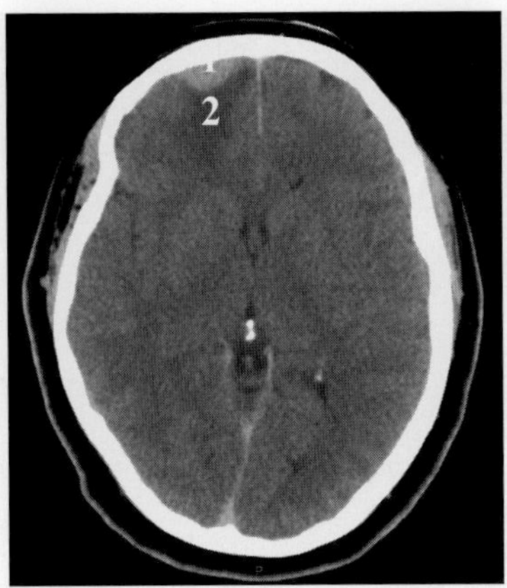

Figure 4-33: CT scan with contrast demonstrating dural based lesion (1) with peritu-moral oedema (2). This was secretory meningioma.

CT on admission and was loaded with Phenytoin IV at 15 mg/kg body weight followed by 100 mg PO every eight hours. CT scan demonstrated a dural based right frontal lesion with surrounding cerebral oedema (Figure 4-33).

PCS4-3-3:

A 64-year-old woman presented with right focal seizures of the face and hand. Otherwise she was completely normal on examination. She had an MRI that demonstrated intrinsic lesion in the left temporal lobe (Glioblatsoma multiforme) (Figure 4-34).

4-3-4 *How are seizures classified?*

Epilepsy is classified according to its semiology as follows:

1- **Focal seizures**:

- Simple partial with no loss of consciousness.
- Partial complex seizures associated with loss of consciousness.

2- **Secondary generalised**: Focal spreads into generalised.

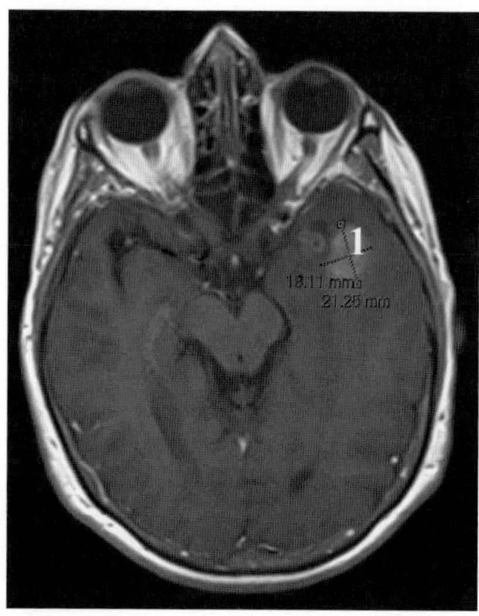

Figure 4-34: Axial T1-weighted image with gadolinium demonstrating intrinsic lesion (1) in the left temporal lobe.

3- **Generalised seizures** (associated with loss of consciousness):

- Absence attacks (petit mal).
- Tonic-clonic (grand mal).

The incidence of epilepsy is about 50 per 100,000 population; 80% of epilepsies are controlled by anticonvulsants (AEDs) but are not cured by AEDs. About 20% however fail medical therapy.

4-3-5 *How do AEDs work and what are the principles of AED therapy?*

Seizures occur secondary to sudden and excessive depolarisation of neurons. AEDs control but not cure seizures by inhibiting the release or function of excitatory neurotransmitters, by stimulating the release or function of inhibitory neurotransmitters or by direct stabilisation of the cell membranes. Aim for monotherapy with a drug with proven efficacy and long-term safety data. Start with low dose and gradually escalate over about a month (enzyme induction). Increase dose up to maximum tolerated dose (if fits persist). Assess dose selection by therapeutic drug monitoring using blood levels. Around 80% otherwise healthy patients are fit free at one year, i.e. provided they have no structural lesion or concomitant metabolic illness that caused the epilepsy. It is desirable to withdraw therapy in such patients because of undesirable side effects of any long term AED therapy, particularly unwanted effects on cognition/behaviour (especially in children). Therefore consider withdrawal of AEDs after three to four years if fit freedom was achieved but should reduce the dose gradually over several months and expect 20% relapse in the first year after withdrawal of AEDs, and a further 20% relapse over the next five years. However, subsequent relapse is rare after six years.

4-3-6 *What are the rules regarding epilepsy and driving?*

The government agency that issued the driving license should be informed by the patient about any development of seizures. The UK rules that no high goods vehicle (HGV) license will be issued to someone with history of seizures. However driving a car is possible on or off treatment as long as there have been no seizures for 12 months or no daytime seizures for the previous three years. These rules may change from one jurisdiction to another and you need to check your local jurisdiction rules before advising the patient.

4-3-7 *What are the common AEDs used?*

Valproate, carbamazepine and phenytoin are the most commonly used AEDs in primary generalised tonic-clonic seizures, partial seizures, and secondary generalised seizures. Valproate and ethosuximide are used in absence attacks and valproate in atyoical absences, myoclonic and atonic seizures (Table 4-6).

4-3-8 *How to investigate a patient presenting with seizures?*

Patients presenting with seizures should have the following investigations:

1- Brain imaging is essential to exclude structural lesion. MRI would be the best investigation. Almost all intracranial pathologies cause epilepsy (Table 4-7).

Table 4-6: AEDs commonly used in epilepsy

AED	Class of AED	Half life	Important side effect
Carbamazepine	Tricyclic	10–15 h	Hyponatraemia, rash, ataxia
Phenytoin	Hydantoin	6–24 h (22 h)	Gum hyperplasia, rash, sedation neuropathy, ataxia, hirsutism
Valproate	Carboxylic acid	5–20 h	Hepatic dysfunction, hair loss, coagulopathy, weight gain
Phenobarbitone	Barbiturates	5 days	Sedation, anaemia
Clonazepam	Benzodiazepines	35 h	Sedation, hypotonia
Ethosuximide	Succinimide	53 h	Ataxia, sedation, SLE, headache
Vigabartin	GABA inhibitor	20–30 h	Ataxia, weight gain
Lamotrigine	Membrane stabiliser	24–34 h	Skin rash
Gabapentin	GABA analogue	5–7 h	Dizziness, drowsiness
Topiramate	Membrane stabiliser	19–23 h	Fatigue, confusions, nausea

Table 4-7: Structural causes of epilepsy

Pathology	Risk of epilepsy
All types of head injuries	2–2.5%
Mild head trauma	1.5%
Moderate head injury	2.9%
Severe head injury	17%
Missile head injury	53%
Traumatic haematomas	25%
Traumatic cerebral contusions	26–31%
Chronic subdural haematoma	7%
Depressed skull fracture	10–15%
Cerebral abscess	37%
Glioblastoma multiforme	30–60%
Oligodendrogliomas	70–90%
Astrocytomas	86%
Cerebral metastases	21%
Arteriovenois malformation	47%
Subarachnoid haemorrhage	7%
Spontaneous haematoma/stroke	10–15%
Meningitis	2.4–13%
Encephalitis	10–22%

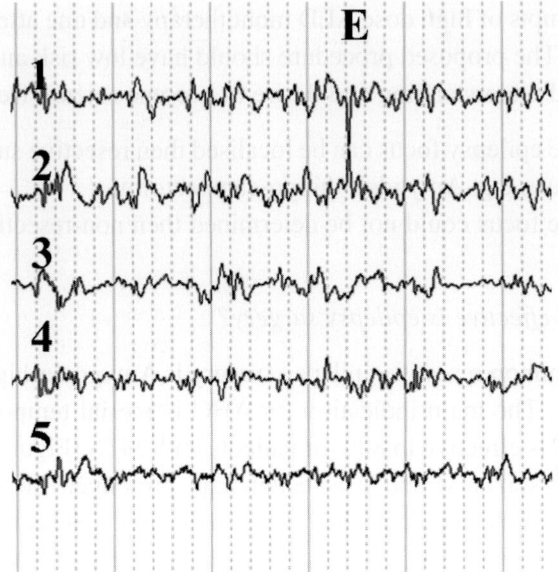

Figure 4-35: EEG localisation of epileptic focus between lead 1 and 2, the inverted depolarisation at time (E) pointing to the focus of the seizure.

2- EEG — electroencephalogram:

EEG is essential to distinguish seizures from pseudoseizures and to localise the focus of the epilepsy (Figure 4-35).

4-3-9 *What are the indications for surgery in epilepsy?*

The first line of treatment of epilepsy is AEDs. Surgery is indicated in the following conditions:

1- Focal lesions such as tumour or vascular malformation: Treatment should be directed at treating the underlying lesion, e.g. meningiomas can be resected. AVM can be either resected or treated with stereotactic radiosurgery.
2- Medically refractory epilepsy is another indication for surgery: Epilepsy is considered medically refractory if it was not controlled by

two attempts of high dose AED monotherapy and one attempt at poly-therapy. The proposed procedure should have low risk and the patient had good understanding and desire to become seizure free.

a. If the epilepsy focus can be localised then resective surgery would be best, e.g. Amygdalo-hippo-campectomy.
b. If the focus could not be determined then non-resective surgery.

4-3-10 *How effective is epilepsy surgery?*

The most common resective epilepsy surgery is Amygdalo-hippo-campec-tomy (AHC). The main indication for AHC is mesial temporal sclerosis (MTS). AHC is effective in 80% of patients with MTS (Figure 4-36) (Egel grade I = no seizures) and it is better than prolonged medical therapy using AEDs,[35] 58% of patients had no seizures after AHC compared to 8% in the AED arm (p < 0.001) and the surgical group had better quality of life compared to the AED group (p < 0.001). There were no deaths in the surgical arm compared to one in the AED arm. AHC is more cost effec-tive than prolonged AEDs after 8.5 years and quality adjusted life years improved from 0.65 to 0.89 after AHC. Lesionectomy controls epilepsy in 50–70% of patients. These may include cavernoma, AVM, cortical dys-plasia, Tuberous sclerosis, cerebral tumours and gliotic scars. The first

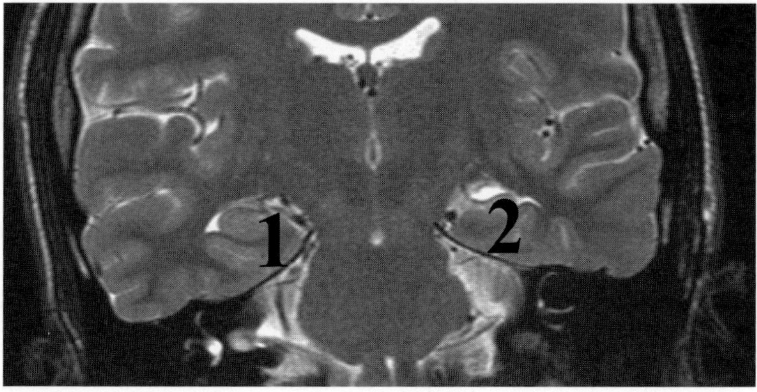

Figure 4-36: Images of left mesial temporal sclerosis (2) and normal right mesial temporal lobe.

epilepsy surgery was performed by Sir Victor Horsley in 1886. AHC was first performed by Baldwin 1952, Hemispherectomy by McKenzie in 1938 and corpus callostomy by Erickson in 1940.

4-3-11 *What other therapeutic options are available apart from resective surgery for epilepsy?*

Medically refractory epilepsy can also be treated by neurostimulation: vagus nerve stimulation (VNS), deep brain stimulation (DBS) and stereotactic radiosurgery (SRS).

1- *VNS in epilepsy:*

The left vagus nerve is mainly sensory and its stimulation had been used to treat epilepsy and treatment refractory depression. Two double-blinded studies [E03 (1994) and E05 (1998)] were conducted in patients with epilepsy, with a total of 313 treatment-resistant completers. In this difficult to treat group, the mean decline of overall seizure frequency was about 25–30% compared to baseline.[36] VNS is indicated adjunctive therapy in reducing the frequency of seizures in adults and adolescents over 12 years of age with partial onset seizures, which are refractory to AEDs. Data from uncontrolled observations suggest that, contrary to a tolerance effect, improvement in seizure control is maintained or may improve over time. Infection leading to device removal was noted in 2%, left vocal cord paralysis in 1%, lower facial muscle paresis in 1%, and pain and accumulation of fluid over the pulse generator requiring aspiration in 0.5%.

2- *DBS for epilepsy:*

High-frequency electrical stimulation of the anterior nucleus of the thalamus (ANT) and of brain structures that project to the ANT was shown to reduce or inhibit seizure activity in animal models of epilepsy. The SANTE® (Stimulation of the Anterior Nucleus of the Thalamus in Epilepsy) study is a prospective, randomised, double-blind pivotal study to evaluate the use of DBS therapy for patients with medically refractory epilepsy with partial-onset seizures, a form of epilepsy that does not respond well to AEDs. The results of the study showed improvement over time with median (mid-point) reduction in seizure frequency of 41% at one year, 56% at two years, and 68% at three years of DBS therapy, in conjunction with AEDs, compared to baseline. Of the original 110 patients who received DBS implants in the trial, 91 remain active in the study, including some who have received DBS therapy for more than five years.[37]

3- *SRS for epilepsy:*

SRS is an established treatment for many lesions that cause epilepsy, e.g. AVMs. Its use in other forms of epilepsy such as MTS had been reported. The beneficial effects of radiosurgery are not displayed immediately. Most patients achieve seizure reduction at nine to 12 months and complete cessation of seizures between 18 and 24 months after SRS. Typically, a transient increase in partial seizures (auras) is noted at approximately the same time as complex seizure-decrease. SRS should be reserved to non-surgical candidates who are not fit for resective surgery and are medically refractory, e.g. hypothalamic hamartomas. These are rare lesions with a prevalence of one to two in 100,000 individuals; they are commonly associated with precocious puberty, developmental cognitive delay, and gelastic (laughing) seizures. Recent reports suggest that SRS may be an excellent treatment option for patients with hypothalamic hamartomas. However, you should be mindful of the long-term complications of SRS. The true incidence of long-term complications following SRS is not yet known. There are however reported cases of "radiation-induced" malignancies associated with SRS.

References

1. de Falco FA. Sentinel headache. *Neurol Sci* 2004; 25(suppl 3): s215–217.
2. Landtblom AM, Fridriksson S, Boivie J *et al*. Sudden onset headache: a prospective study of features, incidence and causes. *Cephalgia* 2002; 22: 354–360.
3. Linn FH, Wijdicks EF, van der Graaf Y *et al*. Prospective study of sentinel headache in aneurysmal subarachnoid haemorrhage. *Lancet* 1994; 344: 590–593.
4. Manschot WA. Subarachnoid haemorrhage. Intraocular symptoms and their pathogenesis. *Am J Ophthalmol* 1954; 38: 501–503.

5. Linn FH, Rinkel GJ, Algra A *et al.* Incidence of subarachnoid haemorrhage: role of region, year and rate of computer tomography: a meta-analysis. *Stroke* 1996; 27: 625–629.

6. Pobereskin LH. Incidence and outcome of subarachnoid haemorrhage: a retrospective population based study. *J Neurol Neurosurg Psychiatry* 2001; 70: 340–343.

7. Al-Shahi R, White PM, Davenport RJ *et al.* Subarachnoid haemorrhage. *Br Med J* 2006; 333: 235–240.

8. Rosenorn J, Eskesen V, Schmidt K *et al.* The risk of rebleeding from ruptured intracranial aneurysms. *J Neurosurg* 1987; 67: 329–332.

9. Hop JW, Rinkel GJ, Algra A *et al.* Case-fatality rates and functional outcome after subarachnoid haemorrhage: a systematic review. *Stroke* 1997; 28: 660–664.

10. Van der Wee N, Rinkel GJE *et al.* Detection of subarachnoid haemorrhage on early CT: is lumbar puncture still needed after a negative scan? *J Neurol Neurosurg Psychiatry* 1995; 58: 357–359.

11. Boesiger BM, Shiber JR. Subarachnoid haemorrhage diagnosis by computed tomography and lumbar puncture are fifth generation CT scanners better at identifying subarachnoid haemorrhage? *J Emerg Med* 2005; 29: 23–27.

12. van Gijn J, van Dongen KJ. The time course of aneurysmal haemorrhage on computed tomograms. *Neuroradiology* 1982; 23: 153–156.

13. van Gijn J, Rinkel GJ. Subarachnoid haemorrhage: diagnosis, causes and management. *Brain* 2001; 124: 249–278.

14. Williams A. Xanthochromia in the cerebrospinal fluid. *Pract Neurol* 2004; 4: 174–175.

15. Noguchi K, Ogawa T, Inugami A *et al.* MR of acute subarachnoid haemorrhage: a preliminary report of fluid-attenuated inversion-recovery pulse sequences. *Am J Neuroradiol* 1994; 15: 1940–1943.

16. Ogawa T, Inugami A, Fujita H *et al.* MR diagnosis of subacute and chronic subarachnoid haemorrhage comparison with CT. *Am J Roentgenol* 1995; 165: 1257–1262.

17. White PM *et al.* Intracranial aneurysms: CT angiography and MR angiography for detection prospective blinded comparison in a large patient cohort. *Radiology* 2001; 219: 739–749.

18. Pickard JD, Murray GD, Illingworth R *et al.* Effect of oral nimodipine on cerebral infarction and outcome after subarachnoid haemorrhage: British aneurysm nimodipine trial. *Br Med J* 1989; 298: 636–642.

19. van Gijin J, Kerr RS, Rinkel GJ. Subarachnoid haemorrhage. *Lancet* 2007; 369: 306–318.

20. Molyneux AJ, Kerr RS, Yu LM *et al.* International subarachnoid aneurysm trial (ISAT) of neurosurgical clipping versus endovascular coiling in 2143 patients with ruptured intracranial aneurysms: a randomised comparison of effects on survival, dependency, seizures, rebleeding, subgroups, and aneurysm occlusion. *Lancet* 2005; 366: 809–817.

21. Rabinstein AA, Friedman JA, Weigand SD *et al.* Predictors of cerebral infarction in aneurysmal subarachnoid haemorrhage. *Stroke* 2004; 35: 1862–1866.

22. Hackett ML, Anderson CS, for the Australasian Cooperative Research on Subarachnoid Haemorrhage Study (ACROSS) Group. Health outcomes 1 year after subarachnoid haemorrhage: an international population-based study. The Australian Cooperative Research on Subarachnoid Haemorrhage Study Group. *Neurology* 2000; 55: 658–662.

23. Annemarie W, van Heuven, MD, Sanne M *et al.* Validation of a prognostic subarachnoid haemorrhage grading scale derived directly from the Glasgow coma scale. *Stroke* 2008; 39: 1347–1348.

24. Fisher CM *et al.* Relation of cerebral vasospasm to subarachnoid haemorrhage visualized by computerized tomographic scanning. *Neurosurgery* 1980; 6: 1–9.

25. Whitfield PC, Moss H, O'Hare D *et al.* An audit of aneurysmal subarachnoid haemorrhage: earlier resuscitation and surgery reduces inpatient stay and deaths from rebleeding. *J Neurol Neurosurg Psychiatry* 1996; 60: 301–306.

26. Hutchinson PJ, Power DM, Tripathi P *et al.* Outcome from poor grade aneurysmal subarachnoid haemorrhage — which poor grade subarachnoid haemorrhage patients benefit from aneurysm clipping? *Br J Neurosurg* 2000; 14: 105–109.

27. National Study of Subarachnoid Haemorrhage — final report. The Royal College of Surgeons of England, February 2006.

28. Wermer MJH, Greebe P, Algra A *et al.* Incidence of recurrent subarachnoid haemorrhage after clipping for ruptured intracranial aneurysms. *Stroke* 2005; 36: 2394–2399.

29. Wermer MJH, Kool H, Albrecht KW *et al.* Aneurysm screening after treatment for ruptured aneurysms study group. Subarachnoid haemorrhage treated with clipping: long-term effects on employment, relationships, personality and mood. *Neurosurgery* 2007; 60: 91–98.

30. He J *et al*. Active treatment better than placebo. Active treatment worse than placebo. *Am Heart J.* 1999; 138: 211–219.

31. Diener HC *et al*. Aspirin and clopidogrel compared with clopidogrel alone after recent ischaemic stroke or transient ischaemic attack in high-risk patients (MATCH): randomised, double-blind, placebo-controlled trial. *Lancet* 2004; 364: 331–337.

32. Mendelow AD, Gregson BA, Fernandes HM *et al*. STICH investigators. Early surgery versus initial conservative treatment in patients with spontaneous supratentorial intracerebral haematomas in the International Surgical Trial in Intracerebral Haemorrhage (STICH): a randomised trial. *Lancet* 2005; 365(9457): 387–397.

33. Lee VH *et al*. Incidence and outcome of cervical dissection; a population-based study. *Neurology* 2006; 67: 1809–1812.

34. Eljamel MS, Humphrey PRD, Shaw MD. Spontaneous dissection of the cervical internal carotid artery, the role of Doppler/Duplex scanning. *J Neurol Neurosurg Psychiatry* 1989; 52: 1461–1462.

35. Wiebe S, Blume WT, Girvin JP *et al*. A randomized, controlled trial of surgery for temporal-lobe epilepsy. *N Engl J Med* 2001; 345: 311–318.

36. Ben-Menachem E, Hellstrom K, Waldton C *et al*. Evaluation of refractory epilepsy treated with vagus nerve stimulation for up to 5 years. *Neurology* 1999; 52: 1265–1267.

37. Nguyen DK, Spencer SS. Recent advances in the treatment of epilepsy. *Arch Neurol* 2003; 60: 929–935.

Your personal notes:

....

....

....

....

....

....

....

....

....

....

Chapter 5: Raised ICP (Tumours, Abscess and Hydrocephalus)

Problem 5-1:   Raised ICP and primary malignant brain tumours. How to manage a patient presenting with raised ICP due to primary malignant brain tumours (PMBT)?

The main goal in any patient presenting with subacute headache is to exclude causes of raised intracranial pressure that may require urgent treatment. Although many patients presenting with subacute headache do not have raised ICP, missing a patient with raised ICP could have serious consequences to the patient.

Problem based toolkit:

Chronic headache	ICP
Gliomas	GBM
Oligodendroglioma	
Primary cerebral lymphoma	
Choroid plexus papilloedema	

PCS5-1-1:

A 52-year-old woman presented with four weeks history of headache associated with nausea and vomiting. Over the last week she developed photophobia and slurred speech. She felt fatigued and lost her appetite but no weight loss. She had previous history of trauma. She was hypothyroid. She smoked when she was in her teens and drank alcohol socially. Examination revealed she was overweight. She had no finger clubbing, cyanosis or anaemia. She was fully conscious and orientated with MMSE of 30/30. She had no focal neurological deficit and no papilloedema. Rest of clinical examination was normal.

Differential diagnosis:

1- High grade glioma.
2- Metastatic brain tumour.

3- Hydrocephalus.
4- Brain abscess.
5- Infection — meningitis.
6- Chronic subdural haematoma.

Investigations:

- Full blood count, urea and electrolytes were normal.
- Chest X-ray was clear.
- Brain imaging demonstrated intrinsic mass lesion in the right tempo-rofrontal region. The lesion enhanced with contrast in irregular manner (Figure 5-1).

A diagnosis of malignant brain tumour was made and she was treated with steroids (Dexamethasone 4 mg QID, orally with gastric protection) for three days. The patient was told that the MRI scan confirmed an abnormal lesion in the right side of the brain that caused these symptoms. The options of treatment were discussed with the patient and the patient's family.

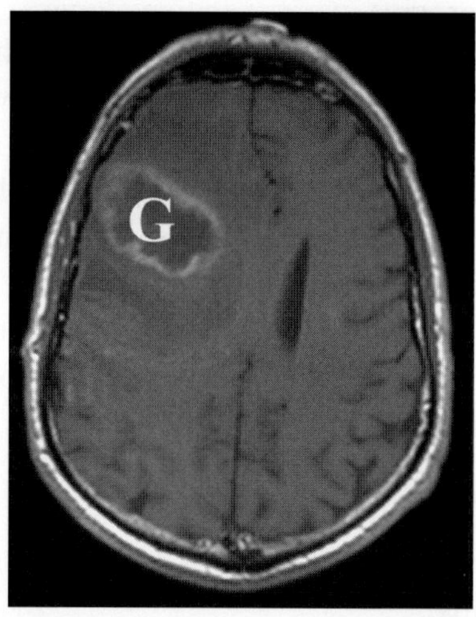

Figure 5-1: MRI scan image (T1) with contrast demonstrating the lesion (G).

Options of management in this case scenario were as follows:

- Stereotactic biopsy to ascertain the histology of the tumour with a risk of bleeding or brain swelling leading to permanent neurological deficit of about 1% and 2% risk of infection.
- Cytoreductive therapy to obtain histological diagnosis and debulk the tumour. Craniotomy to debulk the tumour carries risks including up to 5% risk of permanent neurological deficit and 2% risk of infection.
- Both these options require pretreatment with dexamethazone 4 mg QID.

She underwent debulking of the tumour using fluorescence guided resection technology and the enhancing tumour was removed completely. The pathology confirmed glioblastoma multiforme (GBM) and the patient was treated with 60 Grays external beam radiotherapy.

PCS5-1-2:

A 56-year-old right-handed woman noticed that she bumped into things on the left hand side for four weeks; first event was when she hit her head against a water pipe when bending down. On questioning she reported a one week history of intermittent headaches, with a feeling of pressure in forehead; gradual onset, getting more frequent but not much worse in severity. She had been diagnosed ten years ago with Myasthenia Gravis and she was taking Piridostigmine, Azothioprine, and Diazide. She lived alone and never smoked. On examination she was disorientated with MMSE of 17 out of 30 and had an obvious left homonymous visual field defect. There was no papilloedema and no other focal neurological signs.

Differential diagnosis:

The combination of age, headaches and homonymous visual field defect makes her likely to have a lesion in the right parietal-occipital lobe. The insidious onset makes likely to be a mass lesion rather than a vascular cause. The lack of papilloedema and short history makes likely to be fast growing mass. Therefore high grade glioma would top the list, followed by metastatic lesion, abscess and other rare lesions.

This patient had initially CT scan followed by an MRI scan. Both scans demonstrated a single lesion similar in appearance as that shown in Figure 5-1 but located in the right parietal lobe.

Management:

She was treated with steroids and her neurological status improved markedly. Options of therapy were discussed as in PCS5-1-1 and underwent gross total resection using fluorescence guided techniques followed by temazolamide — radiotherapy as the intra-operative diagnosis was GBM.

5-1-3 *What are the features of raised ICP headaches?*

Raised ICP headache is a generalised ache over the cranium, worst on awakening, may awaken the patient from sleep, aggravated by bending, stooping, or straining and its severity gradually progresses. Initially the headache might be mild and controllable by simple paracetamol, as it progresses even stronger painkillers might have little effect. The reason that raised ICP headache is worse upon a wakening up or may awaken the patient in the middle of the night is due to hypoventilation occurring during sleep, in particular during rapid eye movement (REM) sleep, that leads to accumulation of CO_2 in the blood. Increased CO_2 in the blood leads to cerebral vasodilatation and increased intracranial pressure. The headache is associated with: nausea and vomiting, obscuration (transient loss) of vision with sudden change in posture. (This feature is an indication of markedly elevated ICP and the patient might be at risk of developing impaired conscious level.)

5-1-4 *What are the characteristic features of raised ICP?*

- Headache — typical of raised intracranial pressure.
- Nausea and vomiting.

- Visual disturbances:

    o   Blurring of vision.
    o   Visual obscuration — transient blindness.
    o   Papilloedema in some patients.
    o   Retinal haemorrhages if the rise in ICP has been rapid.

- Brain shifts — often, with depression of conscious level.
- Sixth cranial nerve palsy leading to lateral rectus weakness, as the sixth nerve had a very long intracranial course it is susceptible to injury in raised ICP — false localising sign.
- Third nerve palsy due to ipsilateral uncal herniation — true localising sign, the lesion usually on the same side as the third nerve palsy.
- Hemiparesis due to contralateral shift of the cerebral peduncle leading to pressure against the edge of tentorium — false localising sign, the lesion most often on the same side as the hemiparesis.
- Peptic ulceration.
- Cushing's response: when transtentorial herniation occurs, hypertension and bradycardia develop.
- In infants, slowly increasing intracranial pressure may present as a slowly increasing head size.

5-1-5 *What are the causes of raised ICP?*

- Congenital:

    o   Hydrocephalus.
    o   Dandy Walker Syndrome.

- Acquired:

    o   Tumours:
Gliomas, primary cerebral lymphoma, choroid plexus papilloma, brain metastases, meningiomas, haemangioblastoma, vestibular schwannoma, colloid cysts, pineal tumours, craniopharyngioma, and epidermoid cyst.

    o   Trauma:
EDH, ASDH, CSDH, DAI, cerebral contusion, and brain oedema.

o   Infection/inflammation:

Meningitis, encephalitis, brain abscess, tuberculoma, TB-meningitis, sarcoidosis, and other chronic infections.

o   Vascular:

Spontaneous SAH, SICH, intracranial aneurysm, AVM, infarct, malignant hypertension, and sinus venous thrombosis.

o   Metabolic:

Respiratory failure, hepatic failure, renal failure, intoxication, and some drugs.

5-1-6 *Epidemiology of primary malignant brain tumours:*

Primary malignant tumours of the central nervous system occur in 5–7 per 100,000 of the general population.[1] It is important to note that metastatic brain tumours are more common in the adult population. Metastasis occurs either by haematogenous or direct spread — the commonest primary site being lung, bowel, kidney, breast and malignant melanoma. Studies have shown that one in four cancer patients will have brain metastasis on autopsy[2] and it is not uncommon that many patients present with brain metastasis without ever finding a primary site.[3] Glioblastoma multiforme (GBM) peaks around the age of 65 to 74 years while oligodendroglioma peaks earlier at the age of 35 to 44 years. The average age-at-onset of all primary tumours is around 54 years.

In children the main diagnosis is astrocytoma and medulloblastoma, and 70% of childhood cancers occur in the posterior cranial fossa. In adults 70% of tumours occur above the tentorium with a wider variety of cell types. The WHO in 1993, issued a global classification system for primary brain tumours,[4] which was later modified in 2000 (Table 5-1); 65% of primary CNS tumours are intrinsic in nature.

The aetiology of primary brain tumours had been studied over the years and a number of potential causative factors had been investigated over the years as follows;

- There is some evidence suggesting some inherited genes might increase the risk of developing primary brain tumours. Hereditary

Table 5-1: Modified WHO classification of brain tumours

1	Neuroepithelial (Neuroectodermal)			
	1.1	Astrocytoma		
	1.2	Oligodendroglioma		
	1.3	Ependymoma		
	1.4	Mixed gliomas		
	1.5	Choroid plexus tumours		
	1.6	Uncertain origin		
	1.7	Neuronal and mixed neuronal/glial		
	1.8	Pineal parenchymal		
	1.9	Embryonal		
2	Tumours of Nerve Sheath			
	2.1	Schwannoma		
	2.2	Neurofibroma		
	2.3	Malignant (peripheral) nerve sheath tumour		
3	Tumours of the Meninges			
	3.1	Meningioma		
	3.2	Mesenchymal (not meningothelial)		
		3.2.1-4	Benign	
		3.2.5-10	Malignant	
		3.2.5	Haemangiopericytoma	
	3.3	Primary melanocytic lesions		
4	Lymphoma			
5	Germ Cell Tumours			
	5.1	Germinoma		
6	Cysts and Tumour-like Lesions			
	6.1	Rathke cleft cyst		
	6.2	Epidermoid cyst		
	6.3	Dermoid cyst		
	6.4	Colloid cyst		
7	Tumours of the Sellar Region			
	7.1	Pituitary adenoma		
	7.3	Craniopharyngioma		
8	Local Extension of Regional Tumours			
9	Metastatic			
10	Unclassified			

syndromes including tuberous sclerosis, types 1 and 2 neurofibro-matosis, syndromes involving adenomatous polyps and nevoid basal cell carcinoma are known to have a predisposition to brain tumours. Although these genes are likely to increase the chance of developing brain tumours, they are only responsible for the development of a limited proportion of primary brain tumours. It is estimated that they only contribute to about 2% of tumours diagnosed in children and less than 1% in adults. The majority of primary brain tumours are therefore sporadic.

- Head injury and trauma have been investigated as a potential risk factor for several types of brain tumours. A number of studies were conducted in this area and their findings were not consistent. A large cohort study (n = 228,055) carried out in Denmark, showed no increased risk of glioma or meningioma.

- Some authors reported higher numbers of patients with gliomas suffering from epilepsy or seizures compared to controls. However, seizure is a common symptom of brain tumours and it would be difficult to determine the causality.

- Smoking and alcohol consumption are major risk factors in lung, breast and liver cancers. However there is no evidence to prove that smoking and excess alcohol consumption are responsible for increased risk of developing brain tumours. Most carcinogenic compounds in tobacco do not cross the BBB except N-nitroso compounds. Studies found neither clear association nor significant contribution from smoking tobacco. Review of alcohol brain tumour association found four of a total of eight studies reported a relative risk of less than one for any alcohol use compared to no alcohol use.

- Ionizing radiation is a strong risk factor for brain tumours. In children, therapeutic ionizing radiation is thought to play a role in increasing the risk even though the radiation is relatively low. In adults, who have undergone irradiation for acute lymphoblastic leukaemia during childhood have been reported to have an increased risk of glioma.

- Association between mobile phone use and brain tumour have been under investigation because of its political interest. Most studies showed no association between the use of mobile phones, the duration of mobile phones-use and brain tumours.

Table 5-2: Relative incidence of primary brain tumours compared to other intracranial tumours

Category	Frequency (%)
Glioma (primary malignant brain tumours)	38
Meningiomas	16
Pituitary adenomas	8
Schwannomas	6
Craniopharyngiomas	3
Haemangioblastomas	2
Metastasis	12
Others	15

The relative incidence of brain tumours is summarised in Table 5-2.

5-1-7 What are the different types of primary malignant brain tumours?

1- **Astrocytomas** — These can be divided into several categories as follows:

a. **Pilocystic Astrocytomas (PAs) WHO Grade I**: PAs usually located in the cerebellum, diencephalon (especially the optic nerves and hypothalamus). Children five to 15 years of age are the most affected, with a peak incidence around ten years. Histologically: alternating dense and loose areas, with fusiform "piloid" bipolar astrocytes, and microcysts in loose areas that may coalesce to form large cysts. The presence of nuclear atypia (without mitotic activity) does not convey a worse prognosis. Vascular changes are usually limited to capillary proliferation that may include glomeruloid capillaries and endothelial proliferation. Eosinophilic "Rosenthal fibres" are a characteristic feature. Calcification is possible and always positive on GFAP (Glial Fibrillary Acidic Protein) stain. Prognosis is good and the tumour remains stable but rarely disseminate via CSF pathways and malignant transformation had been reported. On MRI scan these tumours classically look cystic with a tumour nodule. The wall of the cyst is often composed of non-neoplastic tissue, with the tumour limited to a "mural nodule". Enhancement is almost universal, and outlines the

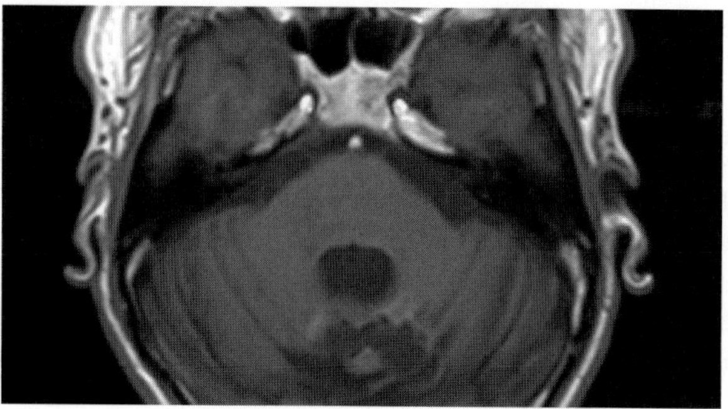

Figure 5-2: MRI of pilocystic astrocytoma.

neoplastic tissue — i.e. part of the cyst wall may not enhance — this is the "classic" cyst-with-nodule appearance (Figure 5-2).

The main treatment is complete surgical excision. Although they are benign tumours, some clinicopathological factors, such as partial resection, optic chiasmatic location, invasion of surrounding structures, and the pilomyxoid variant, have a worse prognosis.[5]

b. **Subependymal Giant Cell Astrocytoma (SGCA) WHO Grade I**: SGCA commonly located in the lateral ventricle, attached to caudate nucleus head. Occurring in 5% to 15% of patients with tuberous sclerosis, nearly all subependymal giant cell astrocytomas are associated with this disorder. Mostly occur in childhood or adolescence; and few tumours are congenital. Due to their anterior location in the lateral ventricle and proximity to the foramen of Monro, symptoms of raised ICP due to obstruction of CSF flow are not uncommon. CT and MRI scans show the demarcated lesion to be contrast-enhancing and without oedema (Figure 5-3).

Calcium is often evident on CT. SGCA show considerable histological variation. Although considered an astrocytic tumour, it often shows a glio-neuronal phenotype. This includes ganglion-like cells and immunoreactivities for glial (S-100 protein, GFAP) and neuronal markers (neurofilament protein, class III beta-tubulin, and neuropeptide staining). Mixed differentiation may also be present on ultrastructure, in addition to glial filament accumulation, microtubules, secretory granules, and even synapses may be present. If

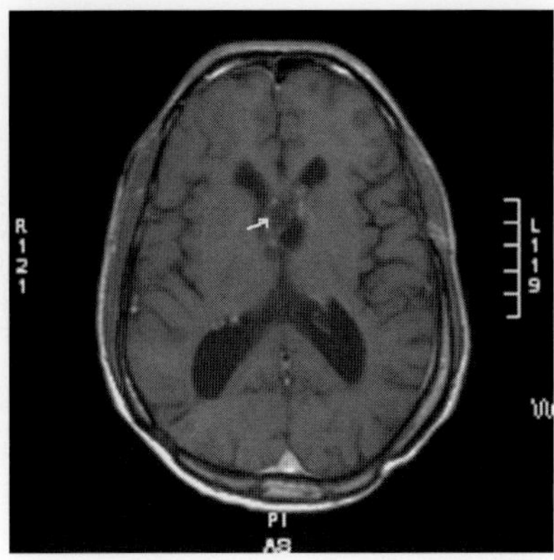

Figure 5-3: Subependymal giant cell astrocytomas.

SGCA is partly resected it may progress later. Rare examples with pleomorphism, mitotic activity, neovascular proliferation or necrosis do not behave in a malignant fashion in this type of tumour. The behaviour of SGCA corresponds to that of WHO grade I tumours. Treatment mainly gross total resection, recurrence is very rare.[6]

c. **Pleomorphic Xanthoastrocytoma (PXA) WHO Grade II–III**: PXA arises from subpial astrocytes and commonly located in the cerebral hemispheres, usually superficial, and often temporal. Children and young adults are the most commonly affected age group. Histologically, PXA is a mixture of unusually pleomorphic cells, ranging from fibrillary to bizarre giant multinucleated cells with intracellular lipid vacuoles ("xanthoma" cells). These xanthoma cells are GFAP positive. PXA may progress in some cases to Grade III (anaplastic astrocytoma) or even Grade IV (GBM). Radiologically, PXA appears as a large hemispheric mass, closely related to the cerebral surface and may have a heterogeneous appearance with cyst formation, variable calcification, and prominent enhancement. The superficial location (Figure 5-4) and presentation in childhood are the most helpful diagnostic features. Dural involvement and a "dural tail" may be seen.[7]

d. **Infiltrating Diffuse Astrocytomas (IDA) WHO Grade II**: IDA often progresses to higher grades and originates from astrocytes. IDA occurs most commonly in cerebral hemispheres in adults and in the

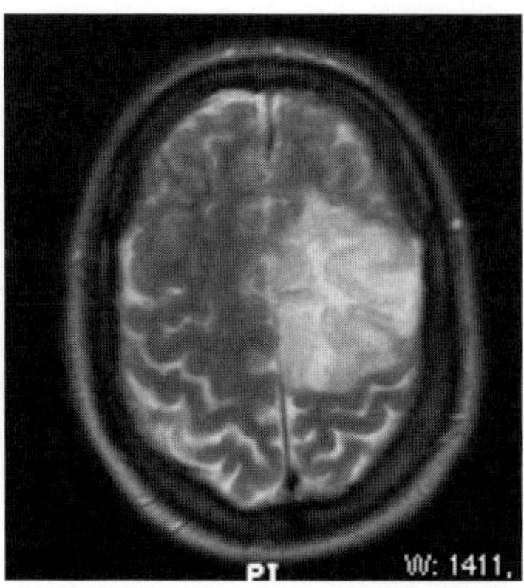

Figure 5-4: PXA of the left posterior frontal cortical region.

pons ("brainstem glioma") in children. They affect adults in their fourth and fifth decades of life (30's and 40's). They appear under the microscope as ill-defined and diffusely infiltrating, with overrun (trap) neurons, and cause enlargement but not destruction of the invaded structures, mitoses, neovascular proliferation, and necrosis are not present in IDA and they stain positive for GFAP. They naturally progress to anaplastic astrocytomas (AA), and then to GBM. On MRI, IDA is usually recognised by causing expansion of the infiltrated portion of the cerebrum or brainstem. Mass effect may be minimal for the overall size of the signal/attenuation abnormality, and the lesion may be surprisingly large at the time of presentation with minimal symptoms (Figure 5-5). Regions of signal and attenuation change usually represent the neoplasm itself — since the intact BBB does not allow enhancement or vasogenic oedema. Haemorrhage is rare, however, calcification can occur. The tumour tends to follow white-matter tracts and may cross the corpus callosum, or follow the peduncles to or from the brainstem.[8]

e.   **Anaplastic Astrocytoma (AA) WHO Grade III**: AA originates from astrocytes. AA occurs in the cerebral hemisphere or the brain stem. The histological features of AA are increased cellularity, pleomorphism, mitotic activity, and nuclear atypia but no necrosis. AA stains positive to GFAP and most likely to progress to GBM. Radiologically

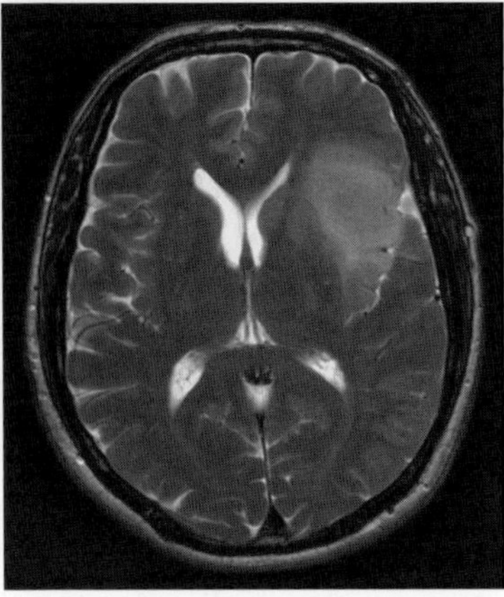

Figure 5-5: Infiltrating diffuse astrocytomas of the insula. The high signal area causing enlargement of the insular cortex and the mass effect is relatively small compared to the size of the tumour with no vasogenic oedema.

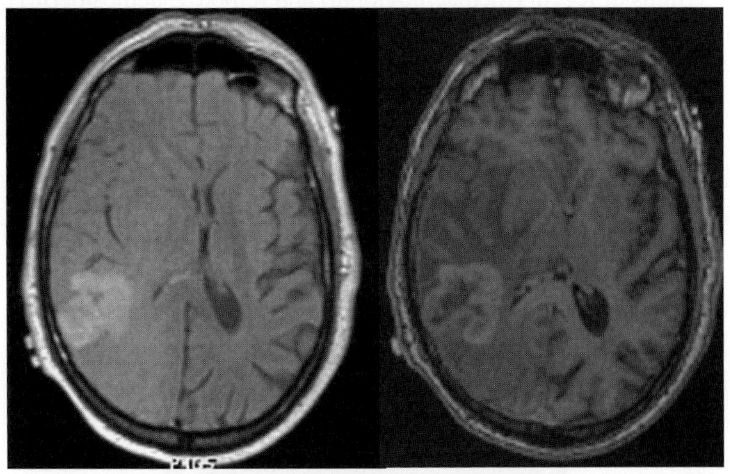

Figure 5-6: AA of right cerebral hemisphere.

AA is variable in appearance of enhancement and surrounding oedema (Figure 5-6). Necrosis (ring enhancement) does not occur, and cyst formation is extremely rare.

AA is considered the least common stage and may represent a short-term intermediate lesion during the transition from WHO grade

II to GBM. The 12-month survival of AA varies from 60% to 73% and the two-year survival from 36% to 50%. Adverse prognostic factors include age > 65 years, Karnofsky performance score of < 70, location in eloquent brain area and partial resection.[9]

f. **Glioblastoma Multiforme (GBM) WHO Grade IV:** GBM originates from astrocytes. It occurs in the cerebral hemispheres, occasionally elsewhere (brainstem, cerebellum, or spinal cord). The mean age at presentation is 45 to 60 years. Histologically, GBM is grossly heterogeneous, with degeneration, necrosis and haemorrhage. GBM has variable GFAP stain, and often present in areas of better differentiation. Radiologically GBM is usually seen as a grossly heterogeneous mass. Ring enhancement surrounding a necrotic centre is the most common appearance (Figure 5-7), but there may be multiple rings with surrounding vasogenic oedema that adds significantly to the mass effect.

   Signs of recent (methaemoglobin) and remote (haemosiderin) haemorrhage are common. Despite its apparent demarcation on enhanced

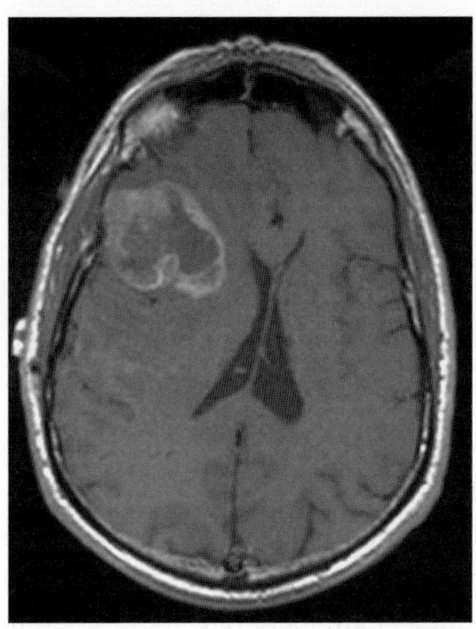

Figure 5-7: MRI scan of GBM of the right frontotemporal region with irregularly enhancing ring.

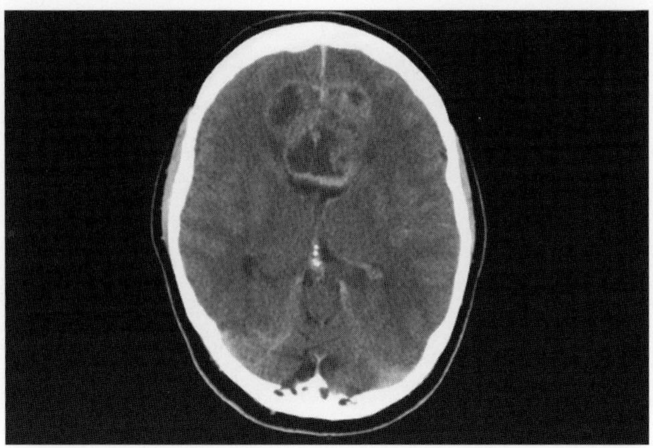

Figure 5-8: Butterfly glioma.

scans, the lesion may diffusely infiltrate into the brain, crossing the corpus callosum in 50–75% of cases (butterfly glioma Figure 5-8).

GBM is locally malignant brain cancer that leads to inevitable death within two years of diagnosis in almost all but very few patients.[10,11] Its ability to invade the brain renders it beyond the reach of the surgical microscope and by the time it manifests clinically, tumour cells have already migrated a long way from what the surgeon can see at operation or what the MRI scan can demonstrate pre- or intra-operatively. Maximal or complete tumour resection of AA or GBM is paramount as the wealth of recent evidence suggests that more extensive resection means longer survival compared to partial resection or biopsy.[12–14] Recent technology had made very little impact on the survival of GBM except for fluorescence guided resection (FGR) that was subjected to randomised controlled trials and had led to 65% complete resection of the enhancing lesion on MRI compared to 35% using standard techniques.[15,16] with significant prolongation of time to tumour recurrence.

Systemic chemotherapy had limited effect because of toxicity and failure to cross the BBB in adequate concentration.[17] Local carmustine implants had been demonstrated to prolong survival in newly diagnosed GBM[18] with median survival of 13.5 months compared to 11.4 months with placebo. However, serious adverse events had been reported with carmustine wafers.

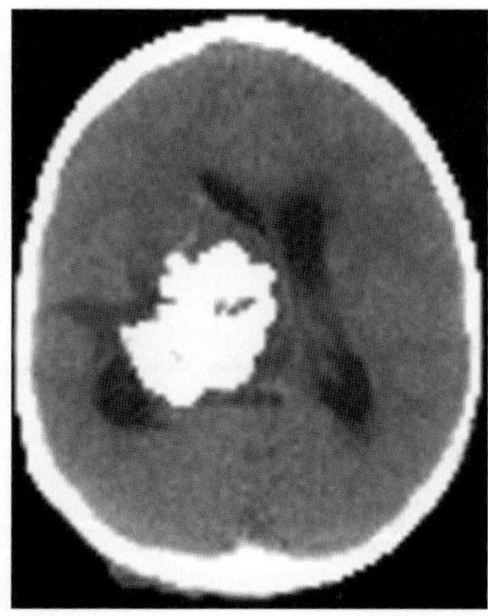

Figure 5-9: Oligodendroglioma on MRI.

2- **Oligodendrogliomas (ODG):**
They arise from oligodendrocytes. ODG are rarer than astrocytomas and are slower growing tumours characteristically seen with a "fried egg" round centred haloed appearance often with calcification (Figure 5-9).

3- **Choroid plexus papilloma** (CPP) (WHO Grade I) and Choroid Plexus Carcinoma (WHO Grade III–IV): They arise from the choroid plexus epithelium. The most common location in adults is the fourth ventricle and in children the left lateral ventricle.[19] It affects children more than adults and 40–50% of papillomas are seen in the first year of life, and 85% in the under five years of age. Carcinomas usually seen only in paediatric age group. They often present with hydrocephalus. CPP have characteristic lobulated gross appearance. Most are well-differentiated and may resemble normal choroid plexus. However, anaplastic transformation can occur. Parenchymal invasion suggests carcinoma, but can be seen with benign tumours. Cytokeratin distinguishes CPP from ependymoma; Prealbumin (transthyretin) may be helpful (although metastases may also stain positive). It is one of CNS tumours that metastasise via CSF seeding (others include ependymomas, and medulloblastoma). On neuroimaging CPP appears well-demarcated intraventricular (or cerebellopontine angle) mass

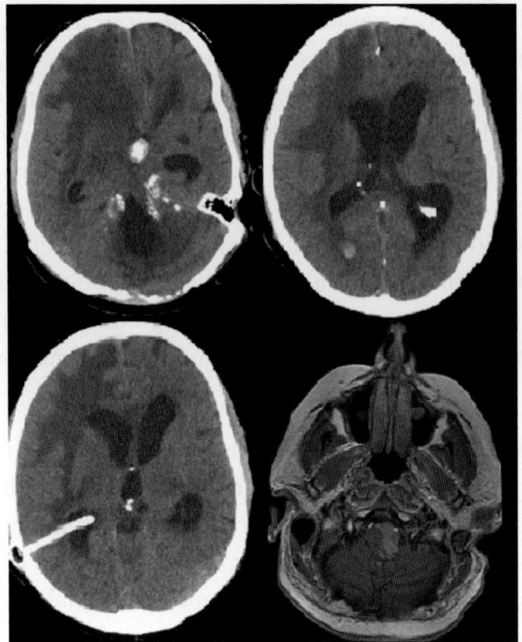

Figure 5-10: CPP of fourth ventricle with calcification and CS dissemination.

with hydrocephalus. Calcification is frequent in fourth ventricular tumours and often attached to the choroid plexus. Hydrocephalus may reflect multiple factors, including CSF over-production, ventricular obstruction, and impaired CSF reabsorption (Figure 5-10).

4- **Neuronal and mixed glial tumours:**

Ganglion Cell Tumours:

i. **Gangliocytoma** (WHO Grade I).

ii. **Ganglioglioma** (WHO Grade I–II).
These tumours arise from large, mature neurons +/− glial component. They may occur anywhere in the neural axis, but especially common in the temporal lobe. They affect any age but most common in the first two decades of life. They present with seizures. Gangliocytomas are composed only of neuronal elements while gangliogliomas also have glial

component. They have varied histological appearance and histology poorly correlated with prognosis. The neuronal component can be verified by synaptophysin, neuron-specific enolase stain and the glial component by GFAP positivity. These tumours are slow-growing lesions. However they have low malignant potential which is restricted to the glial component of ganglioglioma. They appear as well-defined solid or mixed cystic/solid mass with minimal or no mass effect. Calcification is common. Enhancement pattern is variable, but often is in the periphery. They are rarely seen in association with congenital malformations such as Down's syndrome, callosal dysgenesis, and neuronal migration disorders.

iii. **Desmoplastic infantile ganglioglioma** (WHO Grade I).

These tumours originate from large, mature neurons with glial components and together with superficial cerebral astrocytoma may be referred to as desmoplastic supratentorial neuroepithelial tumours of infancy. They present with macrocephaly. They are composed of glial and neuronal differentiation with moderate pleomorphism, infrequent mitoses and abundant desmoplasia characteristic. The neuronal component confirmed by synaptophysin or electron microscopy and GFAP positivity. Treatment is surgical excision with good prognosis. On neuroimaging these tumours appear as very large mass with cystic and solid components. The solid portion tends to be superficial and enhances intensely with contrast. These are related to superficial cerebral astrocytoma, which is distinguished only by its lack of neuronal elements.

iv. **Lhermitte-Duclos** (Dysplastic Gangliocytoma WHO Grade I).

These tumours arise from cerebellar neurons and are considered hamartomas in origin. They arise in the cerebellum in early childhood. They often present with hydrocephalus but may be found as incidental finding on neuro-imaging. Under the microscope they are characterised by derangement of normal laminar cellular organisation of the cerebellum: thickening of outer molecular cell layer, loss of middle Purkinje cell layer, and infiltration of inner granular cell layer with dysplastic ganglion cells. They are synaptophysin-positive. They carry good prognosis with surgical excision. Recurrence is very rare. On neuro-imaging they appear as non-enhancing cerebellar hemispheric mass with characteristic striated

MR appearance and occasionally contained calcification. They have an association with Cowden's disease (mucosal neuromas and breast cancer).

v. **Dysembryoplastic neuroepithelial tumour** (WHO Grade I).
They are thought to arise from external granular layer of the cortex but the histogenesis is uncertain. They are called DNET or DNT and are located in the cortex of the temporal lobe. They can occur at any age but most commonly in children and young adults. They present with partial complex seizures. The diagnosis is based on the presence of: a specific glioneuronal element, consisting of oligodendrocytes in a mucinous matrix in which neurons appear to "float", or glial nodules associated with cortical dysplasia. Neuronal markers (synaptophysin, neuronal specific enolase) and glial markers (GFAP, S-100) are all positive. Despite their benign behaviour, they may have a high MIB-1 labelling index. They remain stable over long periods of time. On neuroimaging they appear as nodular cortical lesions without oedema or mass effect. They may have megagyric or multicystic appearance. Occasionally they may enhance or contain calcification and CT may show calvarial remodelling. They are one of the surgically curable causes of seizures.

vi. **Central neurocytoma** (WHO Grade I).
They arise from neurons and arise within the ventricles (lateral more than the third) often attached to septum pellucidum. They affect young adults (mean age: 25–30 years). They present with hydrocephalus and raised ICP. They have uniform appearance of small, round cells mimicking oligodendroglioma. Electron microscopy may demonstrate neuronal features. Purely neuronal origin is demonstrated by neuronal markers (synaptophysin, neuronal specific enolase) and negativity to glial markers (GAFP). They are slow growing, benign tumours with no extraventricular extension. Surgical resection is usually curative. On CT and MRI they appear as well-circumscribed, lobulated intraventricular mass. About 50% have gross calcification, which is best demonstrated on CT. They are isodense or slightly hyderdense on CT and may be isointense to gray matter on both T1- and T2-weighted MR images. MR often demonstrates small "cysts". In the past they were misdiagnosed as intraventricular oligodendroglioma.

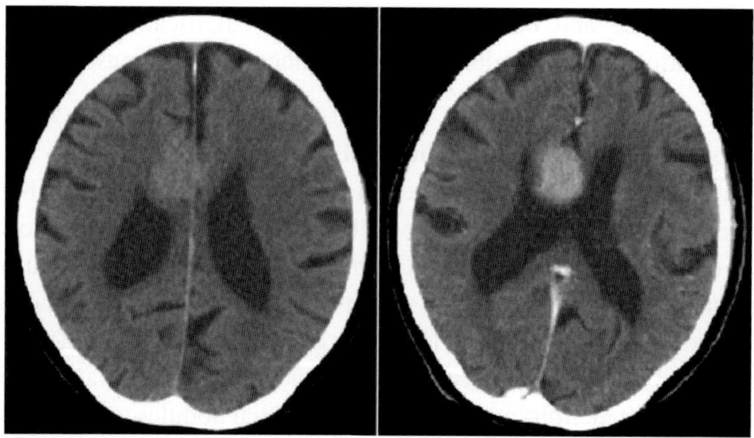

Figure 5-11: CT scan of PCL (left without contrast, right with contrast) close to corpus callosum and slightly hyperdense.

5- **Primary cerebral lymphoma** (PCL) WHO Grade IV:

PCL arises from microglial cells, usually to B-cell lineage. They are commonly found in the basal ganglia, periventricular, and gray-white junction and may involve the corpus callosum and rarely may arise in leptomeninges (Figure 5-11). The fifth and sixth decades in non-AIDS cases are the most affected but can occur at any age group in relation to AIDS. Some series show male predominance of up to 2:1. PCL may express Epstein-Barr virus surface markers. Their presentations are variable including focal neurological deficit, increased intracranial pressure, cognitive dysfunction, and seizures in common with other intracranial tumours. Under the microscope they appear infiltrative in nature with patchy cellularity characterised by angiocentricity and angioinvasion and round lymphocytes with large round nuclei with prominent nucleoli. They are positive for Epstein-Barr virus PCR in immunocompromised patients. PCL had rapid growth, especially in association with AIDS, they may however disappear temporarily with steroids but recurrence is certain and CSF dissemination is common. On CT/MRI scan they appear as iso- to slightly hyperdense on CT (Figure 5-11); may be iso- or hypointense on T2-weighted MR images. Single or multiple, homogeneously or ring-enhancing lesions may be seen and subependymal, callosal, or CSF spread can be best demonstrated by MR.

5-1-8 *What are the other neuroimaging techniques used in brain tumours?*

1- **Functional MRI (fMRI)**: The disadvantages of anatomical diagnostic CT and MRI are: their limited prognostic value, poor indication of the true extent of tumour particularly in malignant types, and post-treatment changes (gliosis post-surgery and radiation necrosis) limits detection of true recurrence, and cannot distinguish tumours from non-tumours due to similar appearance. fMRI would be helpful in localising eloquent brain areas adjacent to tumours and is useful during surgical planning and surgical excision (Figure 5-12).

2- **MRI — spectroscopy: (MRS)**: MRS measures relative chemical composition of metabolically relevant compounds in a region of brain. It is very useful in distinguishing destructive lesions from neoplastic processes. For example it can distinguish glioma from tumour-like lesions: big infarct or tumefactive demyelination (destructive lesions). In destructive lesions (infarct, demyelination) MRS demonstrates classical spectra with large lactate peak (Figure 5-13) while neoplastic lesions demonstrate atypical spectra with large choline peak (Figure 5-14). The main disadvantage of MRS is voxel size may be large and does not conform with the lesion.

3- **Positron emission tomography (PET)**: PET measures blood flow, glucose metabolism, receptor binding, DNA and protein synthetic processes. Most commonly used tracers in PET are FDG and methionine. PET can distinguish recurrent high grade tumours from radiation

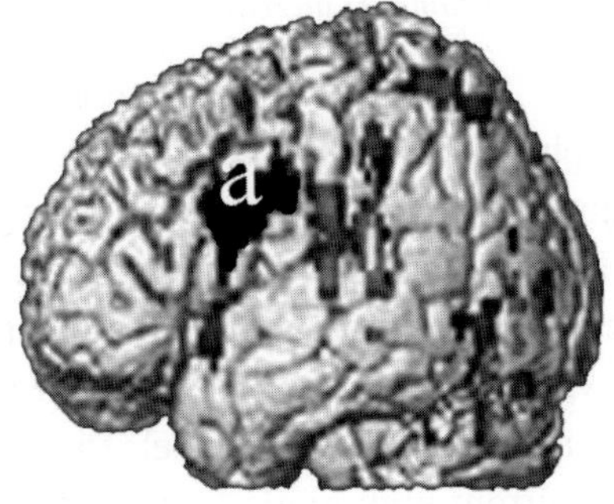

Figure 5-12: fMRI scan of the left cerebral hemisphere demonstrating Broca's area (a).

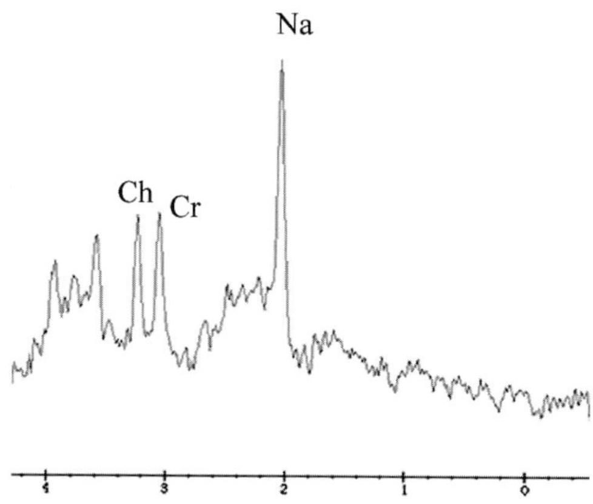

Figure 5-13: Normal MRS (Ch = choline, Cr = creatinine, Na = N-acetyl aspartate).

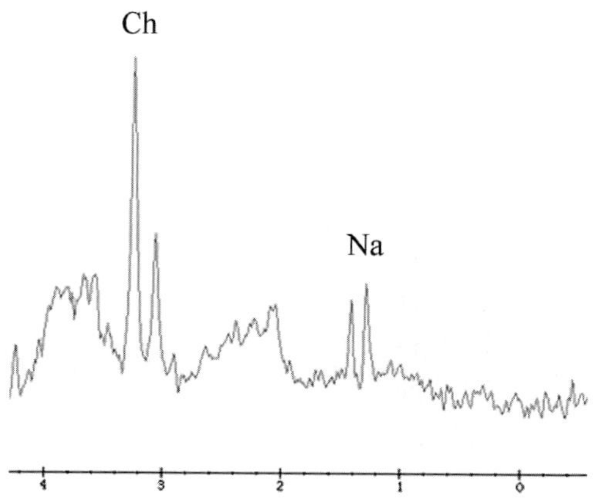

Figure 5-14: MRS-tumour: increased Ch and decreased Na.

necrosis and lymphoma from infective lesions in AIDS. It is a non-invasive alternative to biopsy. However it has limited resolution (detection limited in lesions below 1 cm in size).

4- **Single photon emission tomography (SPECT)**: SPECT also measures: blood flow, sodium-potassium pump activity, and receptor binding. Tracers used in SPECT include: Thallium and HMPAO. It can distinguish recurrent high grade tumours from radiation necrosis and lymphoma from infective lesions in AIDS and therefore it can avoid biopsy. It has poorer resolution and decreased sensitivity relative to PET.

5-1-9 *How to manage gliomas?*

The management of gliomas is dependent on tumour grade, location, KPS of patient and age. The grading system of gliomas is based upon four features: mitotic index, microvascular proliferation, nuclear polymorphism and necrosis. Necrosis is a hallmark of a Grade IV (GBM) and associated with the worst outcome. Grade I is seen almost exclusively in childhood. Grade II is slow-growing and Grade III has two features and classified as malignant. The higher the grade the poorer the outcome. Grading of brain tumours in this way is important for treatment, prognosis, and research. The presumption that GBM could arise "*de novo*" or "progressively" has led the way for multiple factor aetiology of brain tumours. Furthermore, in 2002 a literature review of the epidemiological concepts in primary brain tumours, noted that there was consistently sex and ethnic differences in glioma.[20]

It could be argued that the future of glioma treatment lies not in surgery but within the laboratory. Current management of primary malignant brain tumours at their first presentation is often limited due to their delayed presentation. By the time they present with generalised symptoms from mass effect and increased ICP, the compensation mechanisms of the Monro-Kellie doctrine and cerebral autoregulation had failed. Pre-symptomatic treatment and diagnosis may be possible in the future as scientific advancement in fields of gene therapy and insertion of tumour suppressor genes, retinoblastoma gene transfer, regulated toxin gene therapy, oncolytic viruses, and genetically modified bacteria are a workable reality.

As stated previously, survival rates for GBM are incredibly grim — with one-year survival of 29.3%, two-year survival of 8.7% and five-year survival of 3.3%. The clinical and molecular factors that contribute to long-term survival are still unknown. Current treatment is essentially palliative, and limited. Surgery is the first line of treatment for a number of reasons:

1- Debulking the tumour to decrease ICP and mass effect thus relieving symptoms.

2- Pathological diagnosis for tumour staging, prognosis, treatment options and epidemiological data collection.

3- Decreasing the mitotic index and tumour size helps adjunctive chemo- and radiotherapy.

The surgical management decision between biopsy and resection is a contentious issue. A Cochrane review[21] documented that resection is more risky but relieves symptoms and that there is no evidence to suggest improved survival rates over biopsy. Biopsy itself is a lower risk procedure, but will not reduce symptoms or improve survival. Several studies have shown that resection of 98% of tumour is associated with an increased survival. These studies had sufficient numbers and the extent of resection was confirmed by post-operative MRI scan, while few studies have reported the opposite. The latter studies however, have not had sufficient numbers and were not powered enough or did not evaluate the extent of resection post-operatively. There are clearly times when resection is indicated, such as in acute situations of severe raised ICP, and biopsy is clearly indicated when resection is not possible. The use of fluorescence guided resection (FGR) was reported recently. FGR uses 5-aminolevulinic acid, a non-fluorescent compound in haeme synthesis pathway which leads to the intracellular accumulation of fluorescent porphyrin-IX in malignant gliomas (and other neoplastic tissue). Under blue light in the operating theatre the surgeon is able to visualise fluorescent malignant tissue and therefore be able to perform a more complete resection of the contrast-enhanced tumour — ultimately leading to improved progression-free survival in patients with malignant glioma.[14–16]

Radiotherapy is seen as a useful intervention in the treatment of malignant gliomas (Grades III and IV), with radiation therapy clearly improving survival rates when compared to chemotherapy alone or with supportive care.[22] Radiation after surgical resection in most studies showed a median survival of GBM of 12 months or less.[22] Systemic chemotherapy has been shown to be less beneficial than radiotherapy with a small benefit if any at all.[23] Amongst the most promising agents, temozolamide, a randomised controlled trial comparing radiation alone against radiation with concurrent temazolamide, the temozolamide arm had increased median survival by two months.[24]

Side effects of radiotherapy include hair loss, tiredness, fatigue, drowsiness, headache, nausea, anorexia and skin changes and the risk of radiation necrosis. Side effects of chemotherapy include marrow suppression and its consequences, hair loss, nausea and vomiting and loss of appetite. Moreover, brain tumours themselves affect cognition, behaviour and personality, decrease mobility and loss of independence.[25]

Your personal notes:

....

....

....

....

....

....

....

....

....

....

Problem 5-2:   Raised ICP and secondary brain tumours. How to manage a patient presenting with raised ICP due to secondary brain tumour (SBT)?

Any patient suspected of harbouring intracranial mass lesion (metastases) should have systemic review and systemic examination hunting for primary, chest radiography and staging CT of chest, abdomen and pelvis prior to undertaking cranial biopsy or resection.

Problem based toolkit:

Brain metastases

Symptoms   **Signs**

Investigations   **Treatment**

Prognosis

PCS5-2-1:

A 56-year-old right-handed woman presented with headache, incoordination, nausea, and vomiting of two months duration. She tended to fall to the left. She gradually got worse over the last two months and she suddenly became confused with twitching of the left hand. She had a diagnosis of migraine in 2000, tinnitus in 1998, fibroadenoma of the right breast in 1994, and atopic eczema in 1993. She had left leg varicose vein ligation in 1987, and hiatus hernia in 1979. She had no history of hypertension, diabetes mellitus or seizures. She was on Citalopram 20 mg once daily, Cyclizine 50 mg, and Propranolol 80 mg. She had no known drug allergies and systemic enquiry revealed no additional symptoms. Her father died at the age of 96 of MI and mother died with bronchiectasis, whilst her sister died of ovarian cancer aged 41 years. She was married, never smoked and drank socially. She was fully conscious (GCS 15), speech was normal, and her MMSE was 29/30. Her right pupil was 3 mm reactive and left pupil 4 mm and reactive. Both disc margins were blurred. Rest of cranial nerve examination was normal. Examination of the limbs revealed left side spastic hemiparesis with increased tone, weakness of 4, brisk reflexes and upgoing planter response. Sensation was normal. The rest of general and systemic examination was normal with body temperature of 37.2°C, BP 137/79 mmHg, pulse 68 bpm, RR 16 rpm, and O_2 saturation of 96% on air.

Differential diagnosis:

The features of headache, nausea and vomiting with features of raised ICP are suggestive of a mass lesion such as a tumour. The short history of two months points towards malignancy. The absence of systemic symptoms and signs does not rule out metastases in the brain. The absence of systemic upset such as fever, and tachycardia does not rule out infection. The sudden deterioration and twitching in the left hand suggests a partial complex seizure originating near the motor cortex on the right which is also supported by the mild spastic right hemiparesis. Therefore the differential is;

1- Brain metastases.
2- Malignant glioma.
3- Brain abscess.

Investigations:

CT scan brain demonstrated an ill-defined mass, 4 × 3.5 cm with irregular ring enhancement in the right fronto-temporal region with extensive surrounding oedema and significant mass effect with uncal and subfalcine herniation and midline shift to the left by 18 mm. The temporal horn of the right lateral ventricle was also dilated indicating the beginning of secondary contralateral hydrocephalus (Figure 5-15).

An MRI scan confirmed that there was only one lesion as described above. Her blood tests included: 12.4 g/dl Hb, 131 mmol/l Na, 2.37 mmol/l Ca, 4.1 mmol/l K, 10.6 WCC, 275 Platelet count, 4.7 mmol/l Urea, and 7.3 mmol/l Glucose. Chest X-ray and chest-abdomen and pelvic CT were all negative.

Management Options:

She was given a loading dose of Dexamethasone 8 mg PO followed by 4 mg QID with proton-pump inhibitor. She improved significantly on steroids and the option of surgical excision followed by external beam radiotherapy or biopsy followed by stereotactic radiosurgery was discussed.

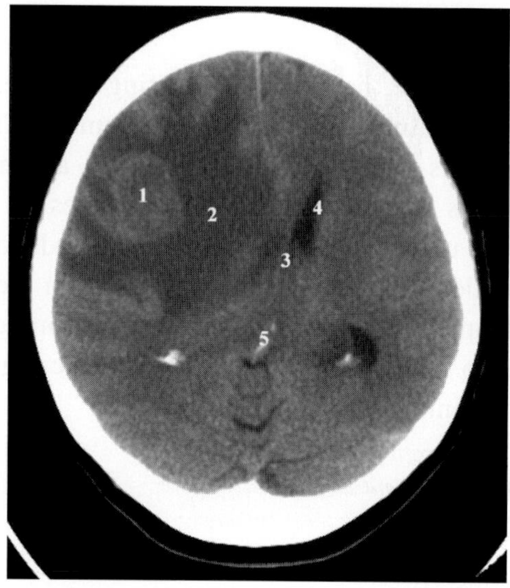

*Figure 5-15: CT of the brain demonstrating a rounded lesion (1) surrounded by exten-
sive oedema (2), producing shift of the midline (3) and pineal body (5) to the left and
contralateral ventricular dilatation (4). This appearance is consistent with cerebral
metastasis (lesion is in the grey-white matter interface and the amount of oedema is
greater than the size of the lesion.)*

Outcome:

She underwent successful resection of her tumour aided by image guided
technology and she made an excellent post-operative recovery followed
by external beam radiotherapy. The histological diagnosis was consistent
with metastatic lesion from lung cancer.

5-2-2 What is the differential of a single intrinsic cerebral lesion?

The differential diagnosis of a patient presenting with a possible cerebral
metastases is brain abscess as the scan appearances are almost the same.
However, a patient with brain abscess may have in addition a source of
infection (dental, mastoid, middle-ear, endocarditis, sinusitis, etc.) and
systemic symptoms such as pyrexia, whilst a patient with brain metastasis
may have a systemic primary in the lung (Figure 5-15), breast (Figure 5-16),

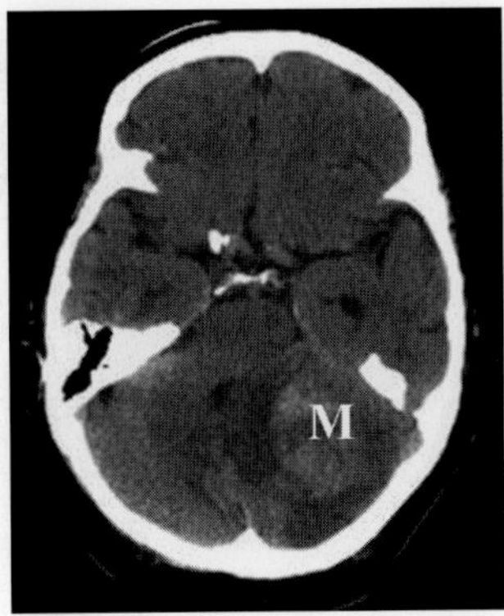

Figure 5-16: *CT demonstrating slightly hyperdense lesion (M) in the left cerebellar hemisphere causing fourth ventricle deviation and oedema. Patient presented with symptoms of raised ICP and ataxia. Pathology confirmed breast cancer as a source of the metastasis.*

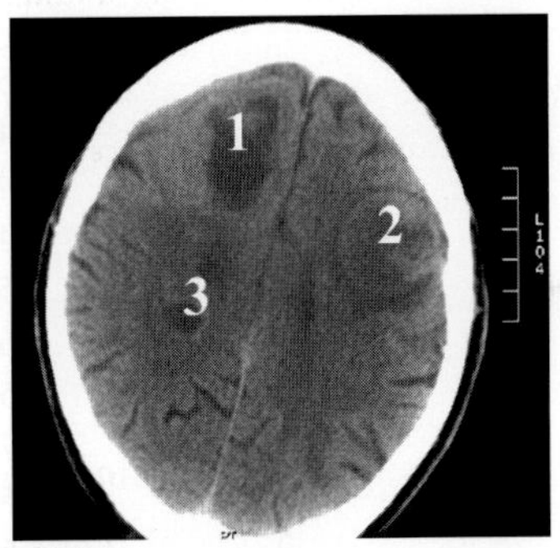

Figure 5-17: *CT showing multiple intracerebral lesions (1–3) in a 65-year-old woman who had bowel cancer resected 18 months ago.*

colon (Figure 5-17), renal, or skin (Figure 5-18). Table 5-3 summarises sources of brain metastases.

5-2-3 *What is the epidemiology and presentation of brain metastases?*

Brain metastases are more common than primary brain tumours and 10–40% of patients with systemic cancer develop brain metastases. Forty

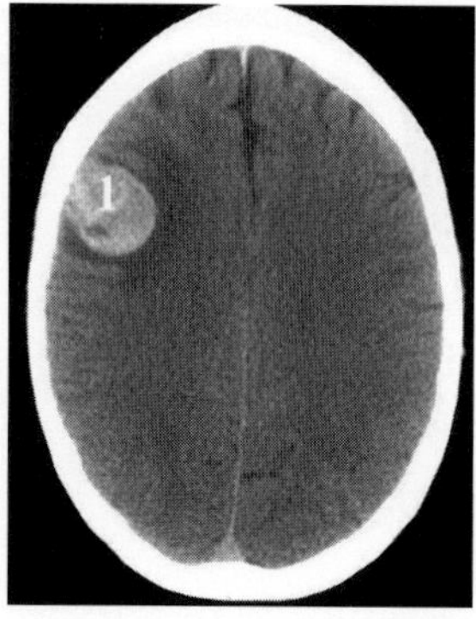

Figure 5-18: Metastatic malignant melanoma (1) on CT presented with haemorrhage in a 45-year-old patient.

Table 5-3: Sources of cerebral metastases[26]

Metastasis source	% of total	Single %	Multiple %
Non-small cell lung cancer	24	50	50
Breast cancer	17	49	51
Small cell lung cancer	15	43	57
Malignant melanoma	11	49	51
Renal cell cancer	6	56	44
Bowel cancer	6	67	33
Uterine cancer	5	53	47
Unknown source	5	70	30
Ovarian cancer	2	57	43
Bladder cancer	2	64	36
Prostate cancer	2	82	18
Testicular cancer	2	55	45
Total metastases	100	53	47

to fifty per cent of patients present with headaches, 10–20% with seizures, 5–10% with stroke-like symptoms, and some present with cognitive decline. On examination 35% will have altered level of consciousness, 44% hemiparesis, 9% hemisensory disturbance, 9% papilloedema, and 13% gait ataxia.[26] Single metastasis occurs in 53%, most commonly from colon, breast, lung and kidney, whilst multiple in 47% most commonly from malignant melanoma and small cell cancer of lung. Brain metastases have poor prognosis: the overall one-year survival is about 10%, if untreated the median survival is one month, with steroids two months, with external beam radiotherapy three to six months, and with surgical excision followed by radiotherapy ten to 16 months. The prognosis is much better in patients who had good KPS (70 or better), controlled primary, absence of other metastases and age under 65 years.[27] The goals of treatment include relief of symptoms, and improvement and extension of good quality of life.

5-2-4 *How to manage brain metastases?*

1) Symptomatic treatment

   — Analgesia (Dihydrocodeine) for headache.
   — Steroids: dexamethazone to reduce oedema.
   — Metoclopramide for nausea and vomiting.

2) Treatment of underlying cancer including hunting for the primary by performing chest X-ray (Figure 5-19), CT chest, abdomen and pelvis (Figures 5-20 and 5-21).
3) Surgical excision when there is good prospect of extending good quality of life or relieving symptoms.

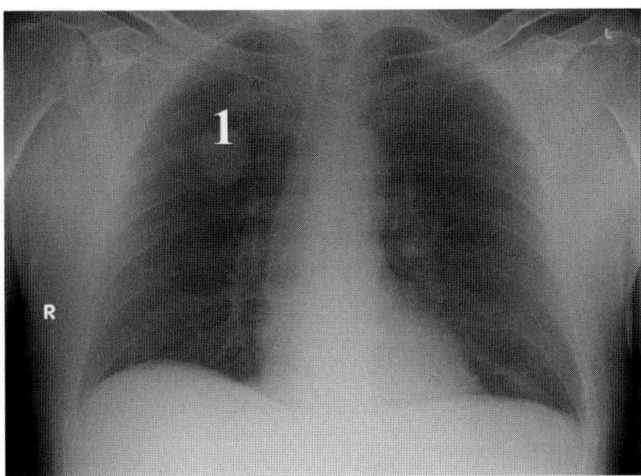

Figure 5-19: Chest X-ray in a man suspected to have brain metastasis confirming a source in the lung (1).

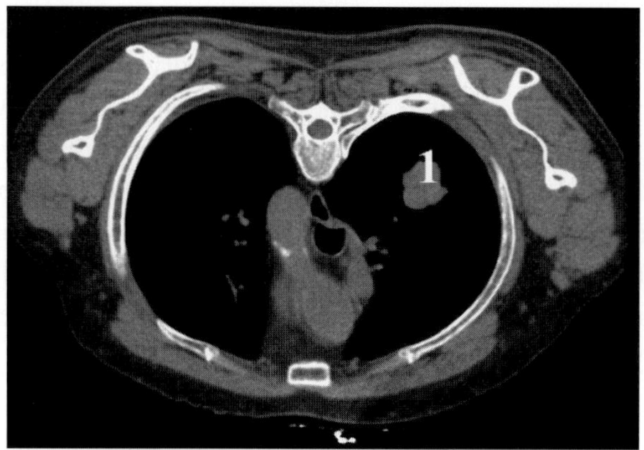

Figure 5-20: CT chest demonstrating primary lung cancer (1).

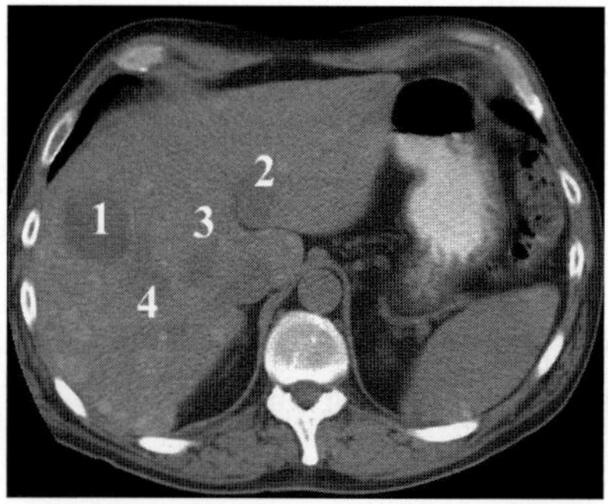

Figure 5-21: CT abdomen demonstrating multiple liver metastases in a patient with malignant melanoma and cerebral metastasis.

4) Radiotherapy following surgery or stereotactic radiosurgery for tumours 3 cm or less in diameter.

5) Supportive care for poor prognosis patients and in the presence of widespread systemic disease.

Problem 5-3:   Raised ICP, brain abscess and CNS infections. How to manage a patient presenting with raised ICP due to CNS infection?

Any patient suspected of harbouring CNS infection requires immediate admission, investigations and antibiotic treatment to prevent death and serious morbidity.

Problem based tool box:	
Brain abscess	Antibiotics
CSF fistulae	CSF leaks
Empyema	Encephalitis
Meningitis	Tuberculosis

PCS5-3-1:

A 34-year-old male, right-handed, shop fitter, presented with short history of headache and nausea. The headaches were acute and sharp all over for the last 24 hours and are made worse on bending. The nausea was of similar onset and duration, was constant and associated with vomiting three times. Three days earlier he had been complaining of earache. He had sore throat and fever associated with dysphagia five days earlier. By the time he presented to hospital, he was on Paracetamol (PO) 1 g, four times daily, Ibuprofen (PO) 400 mg, three times daily, Dihydrocodeine (PO) 50 mg, every four to six hours, Metoclopramide (PO) 10 mg, every eight hours, as required for nausea. He had no allergies. He was married with two children, smoked 15 cigarettes per day and drank alcohol occasionally. He was fully conscious (GCS 15), his temperature was 38.1°C, pulse was 86/min, regular, respiration was 15/min, BP 118/68 mmHg and was not anaemic, jaundiced or cyanosed. Cranial nerve examination was normal, and he had no abnormal focal neurological signs. Rest of examination was normal.

Differential diagnosis:

A patient presenting with acute headache associated with nausea and vomiting with preceding history of infection (sore throat or ear infection in this case scenario) should be suspected of harbouring CNS infection till proved otherwise, the differential diagnosis would be;

1- Cerebral abscess.
2- Bacterial meningitis.
3- Viral encephalitis.
4- Other types of meningitis.

Investigations:

Full blood count		Urea and electrolytes		Others
Hb	13.4	Na	142	CRP 92*
MCV	98.7	K	4.8	
WCC	16.4*	Urea	4.0	
Platelet	421	Creatinine	79	

** Raised.*

Blood culture: No growth after five days for both aerobic and anaerobic microbes.

Left middle ear aspirate culture: No growth after two days of incubation.

CT scan: There was low attenuation lesion in left temporal lobe with ring enhancement. This is likely to be a temporal lobe abscess. There was evidence of bilateral otitis media with extension of infection into the left temporal lobe. There was extensive surrounding oedema.

Management:

- Symptomatic treatment: analgesia (Dihydrocodeine) for headache, Paracetamol for pyrexia and Metoclopramide for nausea and vomiting.
- Treatment of underlying cause (otitis media): antibiotics (Ceftriaxone and Metronidazole) and drainage of middle ear effusion and insertion of grommet.
- Antibiotics for cerebral abscess: empirical therapy (Ceftriaxone and Metronidazole).
- Surgery: burr hole aspiration of the abscess.
- Steroid for reducing oedema once antibiotics have been started IV.

Patient's outcome: After drainage of the abscess and mastoidectomy, he improved gradually and fully recovered.

5-3-2 *What is the epidemiology of CNS infections?*

The central nervous system (CNS) is vulnerable to infection and different organisms cause meningitis, encephalitis and brain abscess. Knowledge and prompt recognition of CNS infections are crucial because many of these conditions are likely to result in death or severe morbidity if not diagnosed and treated promptly. The reasons are that the CNS is protected from the body immune system (the body defence mechanisms against infections) by the blood brain barrier (BBB). Therefore when bugs gain access to the CNS there are no defence mechanisms to counteract their attack. The advent of antibiotics and improved treatment of ear and sinus infections has led to a reduction in intracranial abscess formation but the incidence is still about two to three per million per year. However, cerebral abscess is still common in the developing world. The combined effect of improved diagnostic imaging techniques (hence the earlier discovery of cerebral abscesses) and antibiotic treatments have improved the prognosis of patients with cerebral abscess. Mortality rates have decreased from 40–50% in the 50s to less than 5% recently. Cerebral abscess may occur at any age, with no age or sex predilection.

5-3-3 *What are the causes and sources of CNS infections?*

The mode of spread of CNS infections can be divided into haematogenous spread and local direct spread.

1- Brain infection via haematogenous spread usually originates from a known septic site or occult focus such as skin pustule particularly in the danger zone of the face (the face area around the mouth and nose because its venous drainage goes directly into the cavernous sinus), chronic pulmonary infection (e.g. bronchiectasis), diverticulitis, osteomyelitis and bacterial endocarditis. Congenital septal defects of the heart with right to left shunt are a risk factor for developing multiple brain abscesses because the blood does not filter through the capillary beds within the lungs before reaching the brain. Therefore, it is important to notice any other focus of infection during history taking and examination of a patient suspected to have cerebral abscess.

2- Local spread occurs as a result of infection of adjacent structures such as frontal sinusitis, otitis media, mastoiditis or infected dental caries. The spread of infection can be due to direct penetration of the dura or indirectly via the extension of an infected thrombus or embolus along a vein (emissary veins).

3- Direct implantation of infection occurs following craniocerebral trauma (e.g. compound depressed skull fracture and basal skull fracture) or following cranial surgery.

The best way to predict the causative organism(s) is by looking at the primary source of infection. Middle ear infection is often caused by mixed organisms such as *Strep. milleri, Bacteroides fragilis, E. coli, Proteus* and *Strep. pneumonia.* Infection from sinus or blood is usually by *Strep. pneumonia, Strep milleri* and *Staph aureus.* In circumstances where trauma is the aetiology, *Staph aureus* is the most likely organism responsible for cerebral abscess. In basal skull fractures *Strep. pneumonia* is the most common. Following surgery *Staph aureus* is often seen. Opportunistic infections of the brain are also common in the immuno-compromised patients including *Toxoplasma, Aspergillus, Candida, Nocardia* and *Listeria.*

5-3-4 *What types of CNS infections occur?*

1- Cerebral abscess:

Cerebral abscess is a localised bacterial infection of the brain. The most common sites are: the temporal lobe or the cerebellar hemisphere when the source of infection is located in the ear and the frontal lobe for infections arising from the frontal sinus or teeth (Figure 5-22), parietal lobe or scattered in the brain commonly in the left hemipshere (the left carotid originates from the aortic arch directly) in case of haematogenous spread (Figure 5-23). Diagnosis is made on neuroimaging and the underlying organism is cultured from blood or abscess aspirate. Lumbar puncture (L/P) is absolutely contraindicated.

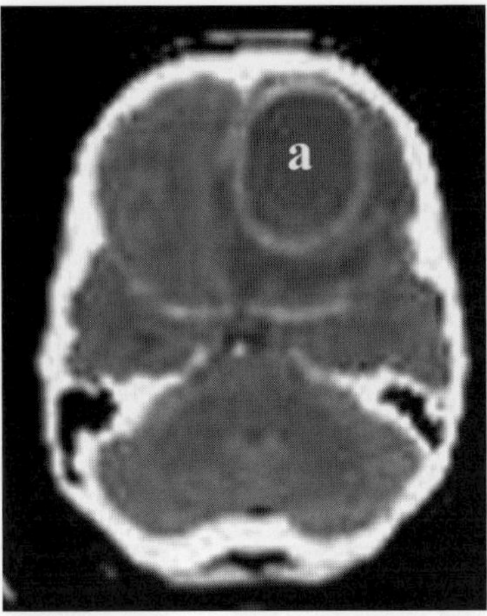

Figure 5-22: CT with contrast showing ring enhancing lesion (a) in the left frontal lobe (brain abscess).

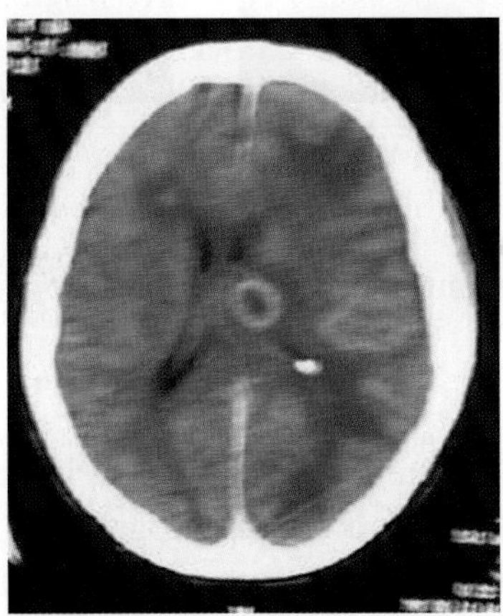

Figure 5-23: CT scan demonstrating multiple intracerebral enhancing lesions with oedema (a case of multiple intracranial abscesses).

It is sometimes difficult to distinguish between single or multiple intracranial brain abscesses and single or multiple malignant brain tumours on neuroimaging alone. Table 5-4 compares the two types of pathologies. It is important to distinguish the two pathologies as their treatment and management is different. Abscesses require intravenous antibiotics and

Table 5-4: Differences between brain abscess and malignant brain tumour

Diagnosis	Brain abscess(es)	Malignant brain tumour (s)
Location (epicentre)	Grey-white matter interface	Grey-white matter interface for metastases and subcortical white matter for high grade glioma (HGG)
Enhancement	Smooth ring-shaped	Irregular ring-shaped with large solid part
Surrounding oedema	Large	Large in metastases, less in HGG
Systemic symptoms	Often present	Often absent: no fever, or leucocytosis
Primary source	Infection	Primary cancer in metastases
C-reactive protein	Very high	Normal or slightly elevated
Compare image		

drainage whilst malignant brain tumours require steroids, biopsy, resection or radiotherapy.

2- Meningitis:

Bacterial meningitis is a life-threatening acute infection of the meninges and subarachnoid space with a rapidly progressive course. Its pathology begins with the multiplication of pathogenic organisms within the subarachnoid space after penetrating the BBB thus making it difficult for host defence mechanisms to reach the infection. An inflammatory process is initiated and neutrophils migrate into the subarachnoid space producing a purulent exudate which gathers in the basal cisterns at the base of the brain before spreading throughout the subarachnoid space. Although the underlying brain is not directly infected by the bacteria it becomes congested, oedematous and ischaemic; at this stage only the pia matter protects the brain from abscess formation. The inflammatory exudates may also affect vascular structures in the subarachnoid space resulting in arteritis or venous thrombophlebitis causing infarction. The pus can in some cases obstruct the flow of CSF in the ventricles and subarachnoid space causing hydrocephalus.

5-3-5 *What are the causes and epidemiology of bacterial meningitis?*

Although only few bacterial organisms are responsible for most cases of bacterial meningitis there is a wide range of causal organisms which vary with age. Worldwide, the three major bacteria accounting for 80% of meningitis are *Haemophylis influenzae* (Hi), *Nisseria meningitidis* (Nm) and *Streptococcus pneumonia* (Sp). Nearly all cases of Hi meningitis occur in children under the age of five years with most presenting between four months and two years of age. It is also more common in boys than girls. It is thought to be rare in those under two months due to the placental transfer of maternal antibodies during pregnancy. Meningitis in an individual older than six years caused by Hi is suggestive of an underlying pathology or immunodeficiency such as otitis media, sinusitis, epiglotitis, diabetes or alcoholism. Meningitis resulting from Nm is primarily a disease of children and young adults with fewer than 10% of cases occurring in over 45 years and is also more prevalent in boys and men. Adults over 24 years of age, who develop Nm, commonly have underlying conditions such as congestive cardiac failure or HIV. Whilst Sp meningitis can affect all ages, Sp is the commonest cause of bacterial meningitis in adults with the highest number of cases reported at the extremes of age. Certain factors have a strong predisposition to causing Sp meningitis: pneumonia present in 15% to 25% of patients and acute otitis media occurring in 30%. In addition, alcoholism and liver cirrhosis are associated features in approximately 20% to 30% of patients that develop Sp meningitis. The circumstances in which meningitis develops can also be indicative of particular bacteria. Meningitis, that develops after a penetrating injury or neurosurgical operation is usually caused by staphylococcal, streptococcal or Gram-negative organisms. However, meningitis following a closed head trauma accompanied by a skull fracture or CSF leak is more commonly due to Sp. Post-traumatic meningitis may occur after basal skull fractures and CSF leaks (Figure 5-24).[28] In particular fractures of the middle third of the face (Le Forte) predispose to

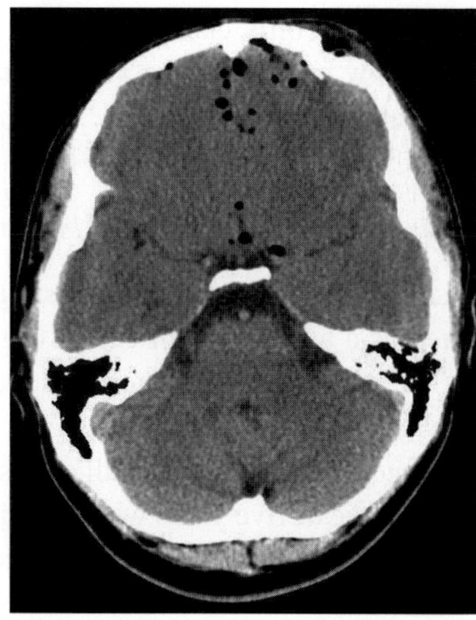

Figure 5-24: Compound depressed skull fracture with skin and dural breach associated with intracranial air (dark bubbles in the subarachnoid space).

CSF rhinorrhoea, or otorrhoea and subsequent meningitis. Depressed skull fractures (Figure 5-24) associated with dural breach predispose to intracranial infection and require antibiotic treatment and surgical toilet of the overlying wound within six hours.

Basal skull fractures with or without CSF leaks (Figure 5-25) are managed with vigilant neurological observation without antibiotic prophylaxis[29] to avoid replacing the normal bacterial flora with more resistant microbes.

5-3-6 *What are the symptoms and signs of meningitis?*

The classic triad of symptoms in bacterial meningitis are high fever, headache and neck stiffness. The fever is generic to systemic infections but the meningitic symptoms of a severe frontal/occipital headache, a stiff "board-like" neck on gentle flexion, photophobia, vomiting and associated neurological signs are all suggestive of meningitis. Often patients may have recently suffered from an upper respiratory tract or ear infection preceding the onset of meningitis. During the initial stages of the illness

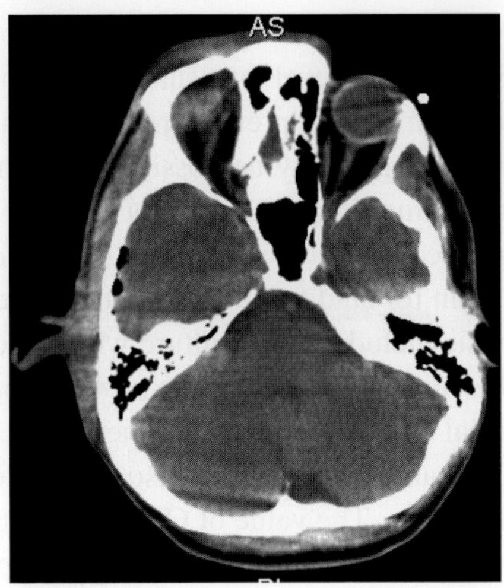

Figure 5-25: Right temporal basal skull fracture, note the bubble of air epidurally.

patients will usually be alert but as many as 90% will go on to experience an impaired conscious level. Without prompt treatment further deterioration of consciousness may result due to hydrocephalus, septic effects on the underlying brain parenchyma or septic thrombosis of cerebral arteries and veins which can cause secondary infarction. Focal or generalised seizures occur in 30% of meningitis, cranial nerve signs in 15% and focal neurological signs such as hemiparesis, dysphasia and hemianopia in 10%. Kernig's sign in which the lumbar roots are stretched by hip flexion producing pain, may also be present suggesting inflammation of the meninges.

5-3-7 *How to investigate a patient with suspected meningitis?*

Patients in which bacterial meningitis is suspected can undergo investigations to confirm the diagnosis. CT brain is essential before CSF examination to rule out mass lesions. CSF is then obtained via lumbar puncture (L/P) to identify the causal organism. In an individual with meningitis the CSF may appear cloudy because of the raised white cell count usually in excess of 500 cells/mm^3. In bacterial meningitis polymorphonuclear leucocytes contributes 80–90% of the white blood cells found in the CSF unlike viral meningitis where neutrophils are far more abundant. The CSF protein level is usually substantially high and a reduced glucose concentration is present in 58% of bacterial meningitis. Identification of the pathogen may be possible through Gram stain in up to 90% of bacterial meningitis when common bacteria are involved. CSF should also undergo specific tests to check for *Mycobacterium tuberculosis* (Ziehl-Neelsen stain for acid fast bacilli). Other investigations that are useful in the diagnosis include blood culture which succeeds in isolating an organism in 80% of *Haemophilus influenzae* but only in 50% of the time in pneumococcal and meningococcal meningitis. Imaging such as chest X-ray and CT scan of sinuses can also be employed to detect the original source of infection. The value of CT scanning in a suspected bacterial meningitis patient is primarily to exclude other possible pathology in the CNS but can be used to detect complications such as signs of raised ICP and causes of focal neurological deficits. Treatment of bacterial meningitis includes immediate high dose intravenous antibiotics until all bacteria have been eradicated from the CSF. In addition, if a patient initially presents in a critical condition or deteriorating intensive care support therapy may be required until the individual improves — this is particularly true in meningococcal meningitis.

Post-traumatic CSF leaks that did not resolve spontaneously within a few days, recurs, or complicated by meningitis require further investigations to localise the underlying CSF fistula. This can be achieved in most cases by fine cuts CT scan (Figure 5-26) or MRI cisternography (Figure 5-27).[30,31] Subsequent repair of the fistula is essential to prevent recurrent meningitis using an endoscope transnasally and dural patch or intradurally using the microscope, The choice of surgical repair is dependent on the location, size and accessibility of the dural defect.[32–34]

A number of tests were developed to distinguish between CSF leak, other body fluids and blood. For example blood mixed with CSF will produce a dark red centre and lighter halo around it while blood alone will produce a spot of red without a halo, all body fluids may contain glucose and protein and estimation of glucose and protein in the fluid leak is not reliable to confirm CSF leak.[35] B2-tranferrin is a byproduct of B1-transferrin and only produced in the CSF and aqueous humour of the eye and therefore

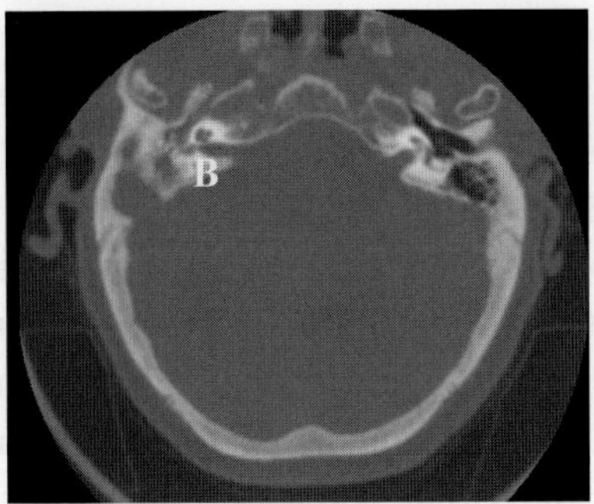

Figure 5-26: Fine cut CT of a patient with paradoxical rhinorrhoea (CSF leaking from the middle cranial fossa into the middle ear, via the Eustachian tube into the nostril) demonstrating a bone defect in the right temporal bone and opacification of the right middle ear and mastoid air cells (B).

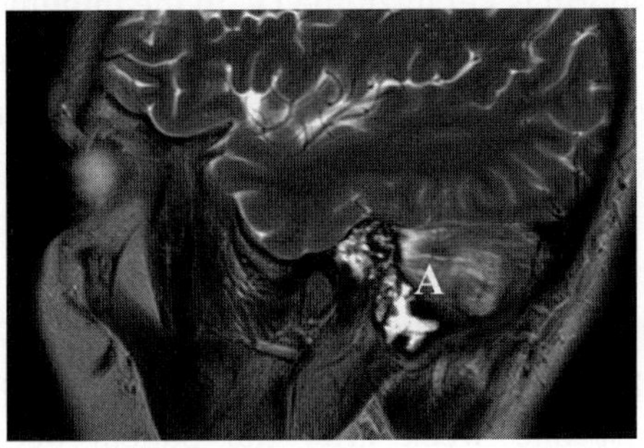

Figure 5-27: MRI cisternography demonstrating CSF in the left mastoid air cells (A) in a patient with paradoxical rhinorrhoea.

can be used to reliably confirm the presence or absence of CSF in the fluid leak.[35]

5-3-8 *How to treat bacterial meningitis?*

Effective antibiotic treatment relies on achieving an adequate concentration of the antibiotic within the CSF to have a bactericidal effect. Several factors contribute to this concentration: the ability of the antibiotic to penetrate the BBB, the bactericidal activity of the antibiotic once it reaches the infected CSF, and the antibiotic's rate of metabolism and clearance from the CSF. The capacity for an antibiotic to penetrate the BBB is dependent on its molecule size and structure but most importantly its lipid solubility. As the BBB behaves like a lipid bilayer the greater the lipid solubility of the antibiotic the greater its ability to penetrate into the CSF. The physiological condition of the BBB can affect its permeability to antibiotics, e.g. it is dramatically increased when the meninges are inflamed. Selection of an antibiotic will also depend on the most likely causative organism, the age of the patient and the original source of the infection. If there is no obvious site of infection and taking into account the patient's age initial antibiotic therapy prior to identification of the pathogen should involve: in neonates (under three months) — ampicillin, aminoglycoside and cephalosporin; in children (under five years) — ampicillin and cephalosporin; and in adults — penicillin G or cephalosporin. The most effective cephalosporin is kefatazidine IV. In the immunocompromised — ampicillin and cephalosporin. Following organism identification the antibiotic therapy may have to change accordingly to ensure the greatest sensitivity and penetration into the CSF. In general Haemophilus infection reponds best to chloramphenicol with cefotaxime to which ampicillin or further cephalosporins can be added. Benzylpenicillin is effective in pneumococcal and meningococcal meningitis with Chloramphenicol and cephalosporins a possible alternative. Antibiotic treatment should be continued for at least one week after the patient becomes afebrile in Haemophilus and Meningococcus infection and ten to 14 days following Pneumococcus meningitis. Recent research has also indicated that children treated with antibiotics and steroids such as dexamethasone improves illness outcome but that benefit in adults was not as significant.

5-3-9 *What is the prognosis of meningitis?*

Prompt diagnosis and treatment with an appropriate antibiotic(s) is normally enough to ensure recovery and protect against the potentially fatal complications of bacterial meningitis. As mentioned previously major complications include cerebral oedema, seizures, hydrocephalus, subdural effusion (particularly in children) and more rarely subdural empyema or brain abscess. Mortality rates from bacterial meningitis vary depending on the causal organism. Haemophilus meningitis occurring in younger children carries a good outcome with death in less than 5%. However, pneumococcal meningitis commonly presenting in adults has a worse prognosis with a mortality rate of 20%. Meningococcal meningitis has a variable outcome; a sudden onset with systemic involvement has a poor prognosis where as a gradual onset has an improved prognosis. Overall mortality occurs in 10%. Bacterial meningitis is just one of numerous ways CNS infection may present. Unlike viral meningitis which is usually self-limiting and fungal infection which tends to present in immunocompromised individuals, bacterial meningitis is a potentially life-threatening illness affecting all age groups with serious complications.

5-3-10 *How to manage subdural empyema?*

3- Subdural empyema:

Subdural empyema depicts pus in the subdural space. The aetiology and pathogenesis is similar to bacterial meningitis. It can follow surgery (Figure 5-28) or spontaneously secondary to haematogenous spread (Figure 5-29).

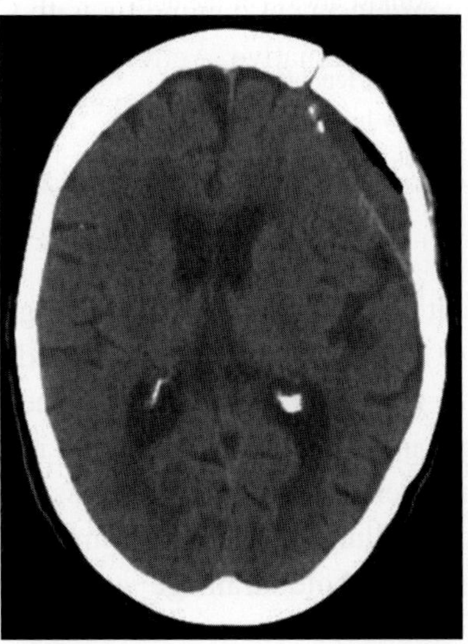

Figure 5-28: Post-craniotomy subdural empyema.

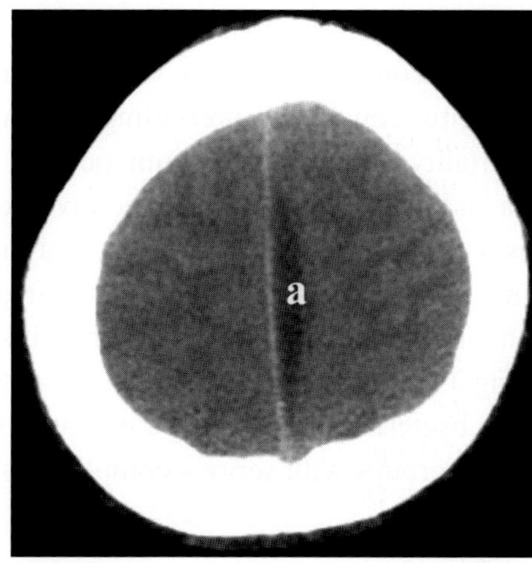

Figure 5-29: Interhemispheric subdural empyema (a).

Table 5-5: Distinguishing features of chronic subdural haematoma and empyema

Diagnosis	Subdural empyema	Chronic subdural haematoma
Location	Lateral/interhemispheric	Lateral or bilateral
Enhancement	Almost always of the dura	Uncommon/rare
Cerebral oedema	Common	Rare
Systemic symptoms	Fever, leucocytosis	None
C-reactive protein	Very high	Normal
Source of infection	Yes	No

It may be difficult to distinguish on neuroimaging between subdural empyema, hypodense subdural haematoma or subdural hygroma as both can follow surgery or trauma. Table 5-5 lists some of the distinguishing features but if you are in doubt treat as infection in the same way as you would treat a ring enhancing lesion as an abscess.

The treatment of subdural empyema is immediate antibiotics intravenously and either burr hole drainage and washout or craniotomy depending on the consistency of the pus and how easily it comes out.

5-3-11 *How to manage encephalitis?*

4- Encephalitis:

Encephalitis is an inflammatory condition of the brain, usually caused by a viral infection, although it can also be bacterial in origin. Cases can range from mild to severe and can lead to serious neurological consequences if missed or the diagnosis was delayed, e.g. in herpes simplex encephalitis (HSE). Mild cases present as flu-like symptoms, whilst serious cases can cause severe headache, sudden fever, drowsiness, loss of consciousness, vomiting, confusion, seizures and coma. Mild cases, respond to rest, fluids and a pain reliever, whilst severe cases, might need to be hospitalised and even ventilated. The incidence of HSE is rare (0.2 per 100,000) but is important to detect and treat. West Nile encephalitis (WNE) is rare and also requires early detection and treatment. HSE is treated with acyclovir. CT and MRI are essential diagnostic tests to be performed prior to CSF examination in these patients primarily to rule out space occupying lesions. MRI in particular often demonstrates high signal on T2-weighted images in the medial temporal structures, subfrontal cortex and the insula. CSF is examined for increased lymphocytes and protein and polymerase chain reaction (PCR). A PCR for DNA Herpes Simplex Virus (HSV) is 100% specific and 75–98% sensitive within the first 25–45 hours. Types 1 and 2 HSV cross-react, but no cross-reactivity with other herpes viruses occurs. Viral serology may also help as complement fixation antibodies are useful in identifying arbovirus. Cross-reactivity exists among one subgroup of arboviruses, the flaviviruses (e.g. St. Louis encephalitis, WNE), and with antibodies raised in persons inoculated with the yellow fever vaccine. EEG may also help in identifying HSE as the EEG may show characteristic paroxysmal lateral epileptiform discharges (PLEDs) (Figure 5-30) are often observed, even before neuroradiographic changes and are found in 80% of cases.

5- Tunberculoma:

Tuberculosis (TB) is uncommon in the west and much reduced in developing countries because of active vaccination programmes. However, due

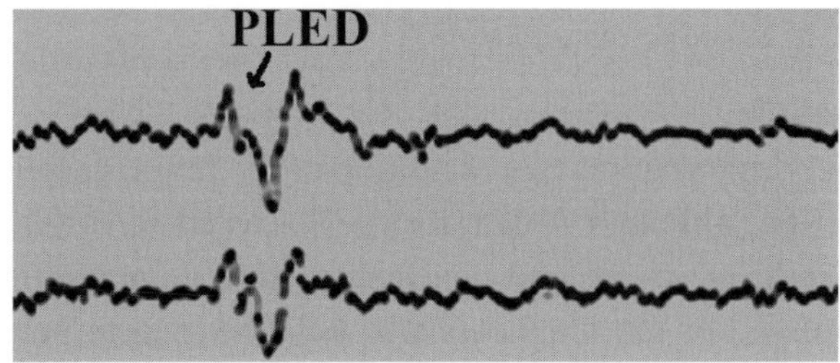

Figure 5-30: EEG demonstrating PLED from the temporal lobe in a patient with HSE.

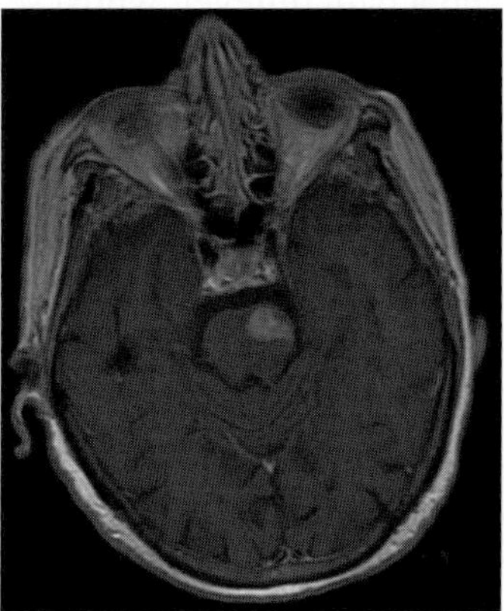

Figure 5-31: Tuberculoma in a young man from the Indian subcontinent.

to worldwide travel and globalisation TB can pop in any country around the world and vigilance is important to clinch the diagnosis and provide appropriate treatment. Tuberculomas are at the top of the list of differential diagnosis of any space occupying lesion in the Indian subcontinent (Figure 5-31).

Problem 5-4:   Raised ICP and hydrocephalus. How to manage a patient presenting with raised ICP due to hydrocephalus?

In patients presenting with symptoms, signs and imaging features suggestive of hydrocephalus, look for a cause as hydrocephalus alone is not sufficient diagnosis.

Problem based toolkit:

Aqueduct stenosis

Hydrocephalus

Normal pressure hydrocephalus

Obstructive hydrocephalus

Shunts and CSF diversions

PCS5-4-1:

A 74-year-old right-handed male presented with deteriorating memory and mobility for nine months. He used to walk one mile a day but unable to mobilise independently at all and rapidly declined in the last three weeks. His decline in memory was stepwise rather than gradual with poor recall and difficulty concentrating. His wife reported increased fatigue and somnolence over the same time period. Recently he was in low spirits. He had an MI and stable angina. He had CABG 1986, hypertension, colonic carcinoma resection three years ago, and diverticular disease. He was alert with good eye contact, normal affect, and MMSE 17/30.

Differential diagnosis:

Vascular dementia, normal pressure hydrocephalus (NPH), Parkinson's disease (PD) with dementia, Alzheimer's disease, and Dementia with Lewy bodies are the main differential in this patient. His blood biochemistry and blood counts showed: Na 131($\downarrow$), K 4.9 (normal), Urea 4.4 (normal), Creatinine 73 (normal), Hb 14.0 (normal), WBC 11.8 (slightly elevated), and PLT 272 (normal). MRI scan demonstrated dilated ventricles with some cerebral atrophy (Figure 5-32).

Because of the MRI appearances and the history NPH was thought to be possible than probable and DaTSCAN was performed to rule out PD. The scan revealed symmetrical and normal pattern of tracer uptake in the basal ganglia bilaterally. No evidence of a pre-synaptic dopamine

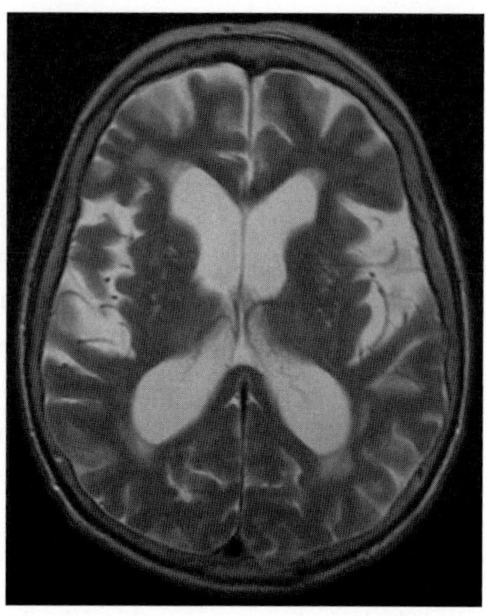

Figure 5-32: NPH presented with dementia and ataxia in a 74-year-old.

receptor deficiency ruling out PD. His cognitive assessment at this point demonstrated Adenbroke's Cognitive Examination (ACE) 47/100, MMSE 15/30, Attention and Orientation 8/18, Memory 9/26, Fluency 1/14, Language 24/26 and Visuospatial 5/16. He had lumbar puncture (L/P): opening CSF pressure was 150 $mmHO_2$ (normal 70–180), WCC none, RBC 8 and no organisms seen, glucose 3.9 mmol/L, protein 422 mg/L (normal 150–450). All CSF parameters were normal. He had CSF drainage of 20 ml on three consecutive days. His cognitive assessments after this showed: ACE 56/100 (better), MMSE 17/30 ((better), Attention and Orientation 9/18 ((better), Memory 11/26 (better), Fluency 4/14 (better), Language 26/26 (better), and Visuospatial 6/16 (better).

He had a shunt inserted and improved following the shunt gradually.

PCS5-4-2:

A 46-year-old right-handed woman presented with a severe circumferential headache that was worse first thing in the morning, and associated with double vision. The symptoms had been ongoing for six days and were present throughout the day. The headache was a dull ache rated 7/10 on VAS. There was little relief with pain medication, and there was no associated aura. The double vision was worse when looking to the left. The patient had been nauseous but had not vomited. There was no associated loss of consciousness or seizures. The patient had complained of being off balance, although this was present for many years and she required the use of a walking stick. She had posterior fossa surgery to remove a dermoid cyst 13 years ago and had a ventriculoperitoneal shunt placed 11 years ago. She was fully conscious with GCS of 15, MMSE 30/30 and had difficulty with upward gaze and partial left sixth nerve palsy.

Differential diagnosis:

A history of headache of insidious onset associated with diplopia of sixth nerve paresis indicates raised ICP. The history of previous PCF surgery and shunt and loss of upward gaze would indicate hydrocephalus due to blocked shunt. The shunt valve could be checked to find out if the reservoir was filling and emptying.

Investigations:

Urea and electrolytes, full blood count, blood glucose, and C-reactive protein were normal. CT head demonstrated obstructive hydrocephalus indicating shunt blockage.

Management options:

This patient needed shunt revision as a matter of urgency. One can buy time by measures to decrease ICP, e.g. aspiration of the shunt reservoir and draining 10–20 ml. However, this will only work if the ventricular catheter was patented.

5-4-3 *How to classify hydrocephalus (differential diagnosis)?*

Hydrocephalus can be divided into congenital and acquired. Congenital is present from birth and can be a manifestation of something else, e.g. aqueduct stenosis. Acquired hydrocephalus is caused by another pathology, e.g. tumour, bleed, or infection. To learn the different types of hydrocephalus you need to understand CSF pathways first.

CSF circulates throughout the central nervous system. It protects the brain and spinal cord as a shock absorber, and metabolically supports neurones and glial cells by delivering nutrients derived from the blood, as well as maintaining homeostasis by detoxifying the environment by removing the cellular waste products. Sixty to seventy per cent of CSF is produced in the ventricles, by choroid plexuses in the lateral and fourth ventricles. It is secreted by a combination of diffusion, pinocytosis and active transfer. The choroid plexus consists of tufts of capillaries with thin fenestrated endothelial cells, covered by modified ependymal cells with bulbous microvilli. The remainder of the CSF is produced by ependymal cells found around blood vessels and along ventricular walls. CSF then circulates from the lateral ventricle (LV) via the interventricular foramina [foramena of Monro (FM)] into the III ventricle (3V) then into the fourth ventricle (4V) via cerebral aqueduct [aqueduct of Sylvius (AS)]. CSF then exits 4V into the subarachnoid space (SAS) through two lateral apertures [foramina of Luschka (FL)], and one median aperture [foramen of Magendie (FM)]. Most of the CSF passes through FM and enters the cisterna magna (CM), which is located between the medulla and cerebellum. Remaining CSF exits through the FL to enter the subarachnoid space in the region of the cerebellopontine angle (CPA). From CM and CPA, the majority of CSF flows superiorly up through the perimesencephalic cistern (PNC) and around the cerebral hemispheres. A small proportion of CSF exiting the fourth ventricle flows inferiorly down into the thecal sac surrounding the spinal cord (Figure 5-33).

CSF is reabsorbed back into the venous sinuses, principally at the superior sagittal sinus (SSS) via numerous arachnoid villi (AV), which consist of invaginations of arachnoid matter through the dural wall and into the lumen of the sinus. AV act as one-way valves between the subarachnoid space and the dural sinuses. Reabsorption occurs at AV because of greater hydrostatic pressure in the subarachnoid space. About half a litre of CSF is produced every 24 hours and any blockage or disturbance of CSF circulation can lead to rapid increase of ICP. From

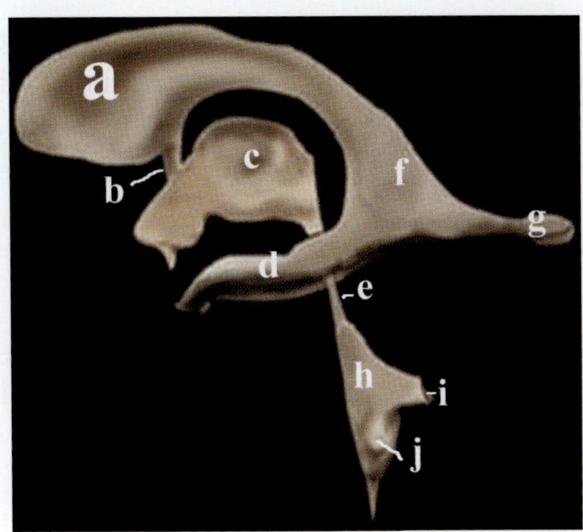

Figure 5-33: CSF circulation. a = Frontal horn of the lateral ventricle, b = FM, c = 3V, e = ADS, f = trigone of the lateral ventricle (LV), g = occipital horn of LV, d = temporal horn of LV, h = 4V, i = FM, and j = FL.

clinical management point of view hydrocephalus could be divided into the following.

1- Communicating hydrocephalus (CHC):

CHC means that there is no obstruction of CSF circulation between the ventricular system and the SAS. This can be further divided into two categories:

a. *Normal pressure hydrocephalus (NPH):*

As the name implies the ICP is within normal limits. It is often seen in the elderly and presents with a triad of symptoms: memory deficit, ataxia and urinary incontinence. Diagnosis is made on clinical grounds and imaging features (Figure 5-32).

The management of NPH is complex and sometimes difficult to distinguish from vascular dementia associated with cerebral atrophy. Up to 10% of those diagnosed with dementia are believed to actually have NPH. In the US alone it is estimated that 750,000 suffer from NPH, and fewer than 20% are appropriately diagnosed and treated. NPH is often mistaken for Alzheimer's disease, Parkinson's disease, or merely accepted as part of old age. There is a greater difficulty in determining whether a patient with NPH is an appropriate candidate for CSF diversion or drainage because no single diagnostic study had emerged as highly reliable.[36]

5-4-4 *How to diagnose normal pressure hydrocephalus?*

Guidelines in diagnosis and treatment of NPH have been developed and are based on the presence or absence of symptoms and signs of NPH as follows:

I. Probable NPH:

Probable NPH patients should fulfil the following criteria: The NPH symptoms are insidious in onset, take origin after the age of 40 years, have a duration of three months or greater, are not attributable to other documented neurological, psychiatric or general medical conditions, and are progressive in nature. Gait disturbance is a mandatory symptom for patients to be categorised as probable NPH. In addition, an impairment of either urinary function or cognition must be present. All three classic symptoms need not be present. Gait disturbance may manifest itself in a variety of ways. At least two of the following signs of gait must be observed for probable NPH: decreased step height, decreased step length, decreased cadence/speed of stride, increased trunk sway during ambulation, widened standing base, toes turned outward on ambulation, spontaneous or provoked retropulsion, and *en bloc* turning (requiring three or more steps for a 180-degree turn). Urinary impairment in probable NPH should include one of the following symptoms not attributable to primary urologic disorders or other causes: episodic or persistent urinary incontinence, urinary urgency as defined by frequent perception of a pressing need to void, urinary frequency as defined by greater than six voiding episodes in an average 12-hour period despite normal fluid intake, and nocturia as defined by the need to urinate more than two times in an average night. Cognition impairment in probable NPH patients must involve at least two of the following that cannot be fully attributable to other conditions: psychomotor slowing (increased response latency), difficulty dividing or maintaining attention, memory lapses (especially short-term), executive dysfunction (e.g. impairment in multi-step procedures, working memory, formulation of abstractions/similarities, insight), and behavioural or personality changes.

II. Possible NPH:

If patients do not meet all of the above criteria but are still suspected to have NPH, certain exceptions are permissible for a designation of possible NPH. The clinical presentation and history may include any of the following six exceptions: subacute or indeterminate mode of onset, onset at any age following childhood, have less than a three-month or indeterminate duration, if symptoms remotely follow events such as mild head trauma, intracerebral haemorrhage, childhood and adolescent meningitis, or other conditions that the clinician judges unlikely to be immediately causally related, if symptoms co-exist with other neurological, psychiatric or general medical disorders that the clinician judges not to be entirely attributable to these conditions, and if symptoms are non-progressive or not clearly progressive. For a "possible NPH" designation, observable gait or balance disturbance is not a mandatory symptom as long as incontinence or cognitive impairment are determined. Similarly, gait disturbance or dementia alone can stand as an acceptable sign of NPH possibility. In brain imaging, evidence of cerebral atrophy of sufficient severity to potentially explain ventricular size is acceptable, as well as the discovery of any structural lesions that might influence ventricular size.

III. Unlikely NPH:

Patients should be classified as unlikely to have NPH if they do not fulfil the criteria for either probable or possible NPH or if they exhibit any of the following eight items: acute presentation of symptoms, recent history of subarachnoid haemorrhage, meningitis, or brain injury, signs of increased intracranial pressure such as papilloedema, no component of the symptom triad (gait, dementia and incontinence), other causes clearly explain findings, no evidence of ventriculomegaly through brain imaging, obstructive hydrocephalus revealed through brain imaging, or congenital hydrocephalus revealed through brain imaging.

5-4-5 *How to treat normal pressure hydrocephalus?*

The best treatment for NPH is still controversial because of the difficulties in diagnosis. However, CSF drainage trial via lumbar puncture (L/P) either through three-day continuous drainage or repeated L/P with assessment of cognition, and gait before and after CSF drainage is reasonable and simple. Those whose symptoms improve have a better chance of response after permanent CSF diversion. CSF diversion using a shunt from either the SAS in the lumbar region (LPS) or ventricle (VPS) to the peritoneum often provides adequate solution. The shunt pressure should be either in the low range or programmable. Immediate complications of shunting include infection, and bleeding. Long term complications include infection or blockage. Only 50–70% of patients respond to shunting and the younger the patient the better the response. The average ICP of NPH is about 150 $mmHO_2$ compared to the normal mean of 122 $mmHO_2$. During prolonged ICP monitoring plateau waves of raised ICP can be observed.

b.   *High pressure CHC:*

This occurs after diffuse SAH, basal meningitis or excessive CSF production: diffuse SAH blocks the arachnoid villi preventing CSF absorption. In the early stages this may respond to repeated L/Ps. In the later stages may require CSF shunt (Figure 5-34). In the acute period while CSF protein and RBC counts are high, repeat LPs will keep CSF pressure down, however, if there was any doubt about the presence of differential pressure between the different intracranial and spinal CSF compartments an external ventricular drain would be recommended to avoid brain shift and herniation. CSF protein had to drop to under 1 g/l before the shunt is inserted.

Basal meningitis blocks the arachnoid villi and prevents CSF absorption because of inflammation. The underling infection needs to be treated and eradicated completely before insertion of a shunt in these patients. In the initial period while the infection is being eradicated repeat L/Ps will keep CSF pressure down, if there was any doubt about the presence of differential pressure between the different intracranial and spinal CSF compartments an external ventricular drain (EVD) would be recommended to avoid brain shift and herniation.

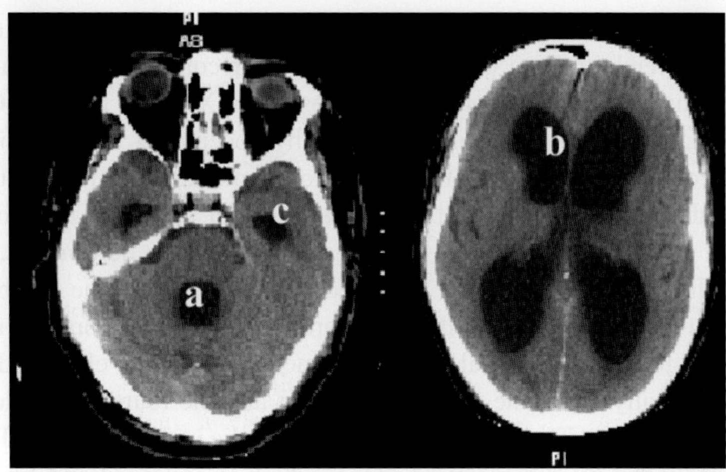

Figure 5-34: CT scan demonstrating CHC after SAH. Note that both the LVs (b) and 4V (a) are dilated. c = Marks the temporal horns that often dilate in acute hydrocephalus.

Increased CSF production is very rare but can occur in secretory choroid plexus papilloma (CPP). The diagnosis would be evident on brain imaging and the treatment is that of the underlying lesion. If the treatment of the underlying CPP did not resolve the hydrocephalus and the CSF protein is low enough, CSF shunt would be the treatment.

2- **Non-communicating hydrocephalus (NCHC):**

This can be divided into:

5-4-6 What is congenital hydrocephalus and Chiari malformations?

a) *Congenital OHC (COHC):*

It affects about one in every 1000 live births and more common when prenatal screening for neural tube defect is not performed. The most common type of NCHC is aqueduct atresia (ADA) and aqueduct stenosis (ADS) followed closely by Arnold Chiari malformation (ACM). ADA occurs *in utero* or post-natally, and may be caused by clots from intraventricular bleeding, infection, or any pathology that causes gliosis that leads to obliteration of the aqueduct. ADS is narrowing of the aqueduct without gliosis. It tends to be a component of a set of complex malformations which may be inherited in autosomal recessive or X-linked patterns. CMF is often associated with Spina bifida and hydrocephalus. The malformation involves abnormalities of the posterior cranial fossa and its contents. These abnormalities consist of a shallow posterior fossa and a low insertion of the tentorium. As a direct result of these deformities, the cerebellum and brainstem are crowded together, forcing the cerebellar vermis, tonsils and the medulla down through an enlarged foramen magnum into the cervical spinal canal. The medulla becomes elongated and folded dorsally while the cerebral aqueduct and the fourth ventricle are forced to collapse. The FL and FM are forced to lie in the spinal canal, and are surrounded by subarachnoid space, which is collapsed and fibrotic. The blockage of CSF pathway from these lesions causes hydrocephalus.

- *ADA and ADS:*

It leads to obstruction of the aqueduct of Sylvius. This manifests in infancy and is recognised by enlarging head circumference, bulging tense anterior fontanel or sunset sign where the infant's sclera is visible superior to the cornea due to defects in upward gaze because of pressure on the tectal plate of the midbrain (Figure 5-35). The treatment is by creating an opening in the floor of the 3V (third ventriculostomy), this would avoid the long term risks of permanent shunt placement. However, if this procedure failed a shunt would be necessary. Patients who had a shunt inserted at childhood need to be kept under surveillance for elective extension of the peritoneal catheter during growth spurt if the child was shunt dependent.

The best way to recognise ADS is finding that LV and 3V are dilated while 4V is normal (Figure 5-35). However, MRI scan using sagittal plane would be the best way to visualise the aqueduct directly (Figure 5-36).

- *4V exit obstruction:*

This is caused by obstruction of the 4V foramena (FM and FL). This would lead to balloon dilatation of the roof of the 4V and can be mistaken for large cisterna magna. This condition is known as Dandy Walker Syndrome (DWS). The treatment is CSF diversion.

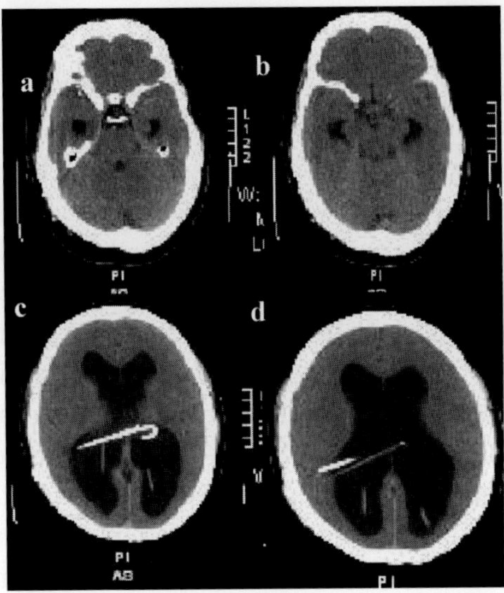

Figure 5-35: Congenital hydrocephalus shunted at birth and required several shunt revisions over the years note: LV and 3V dilated, 4V is normal and previous shunt catheters in the LV.

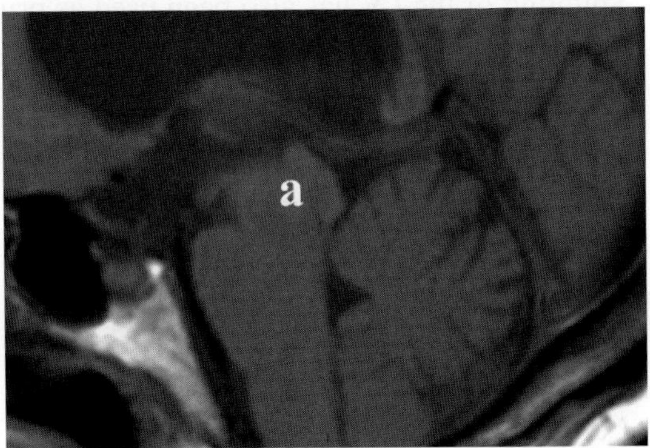

Figure 5-36: Sagittal MRI showing aqueduct atresia (a).

b) *Acquired OHC (AOHC):*

This is a common finding in clinical practice as obstruction from tumours, blood clot, abscess or giant aneurysms can block the CSF pathways in several locations, particularly the FM, 3V, aqueduct and 4V.

5-4-7 *What is colloid cyst and how to manage it?*

- *AOHC at the FM may be caused by colloid cyst:*

Colloid cysts are uncommon and may present with features of chronic hydrocephalus, or drop attacks. The mechanisms of chronic hydrocephalic symptoms: cognitive decline, dementia and ataxia, are as those described under NPH. Drop attacks occur when the cyst obstructs the FM leading to acute rise in ICP. Acute rise in ICP leads to sudden loss of consciousness and collapse. Once the patient drops on the ground the cyst dislodges from the FM causing the CSF to drain normally and the patient regains consciousness as quickly as he had lost it. The differential diagnosis in patients with drop attacks would include colloid cyst, Stoke Adam's Syndrome due to complete heart block or rapidly developing generalised seizures that spread so fast in the two hemispheres of the brain across the corpus callosum. An example of colloid cyst is shown in Figure 5-37. The treatment of symptomatic colloid cysts is surgical removal transcortically, transcallosally or endoscopically. Some surgeons aspirate colloid cysts stereotactically but the thick capsule and the cyst mobility makes it less than ideal target, particularly if the contents of the cyst spills into the ventricles causing chemical meningitis and hydrocephalus. Shunting of the LV has also been used as primary treatment particularly in the elderly and as a rescue procedure after resection.

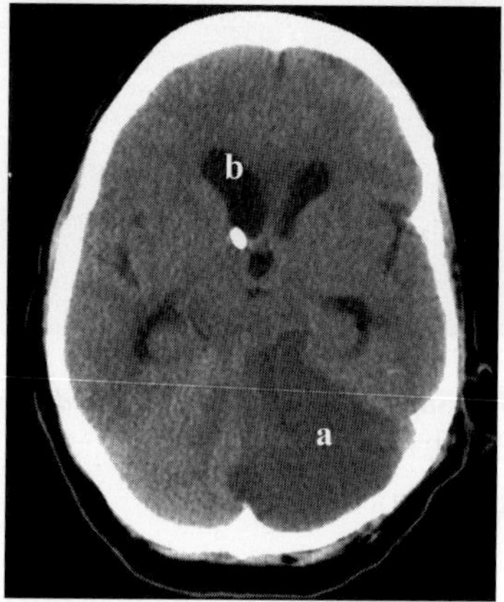

Figure 5-37: A 35-year-old male presented with drop attacks and headaches. MRI scan demonstrating a cyst (a) in the FM.

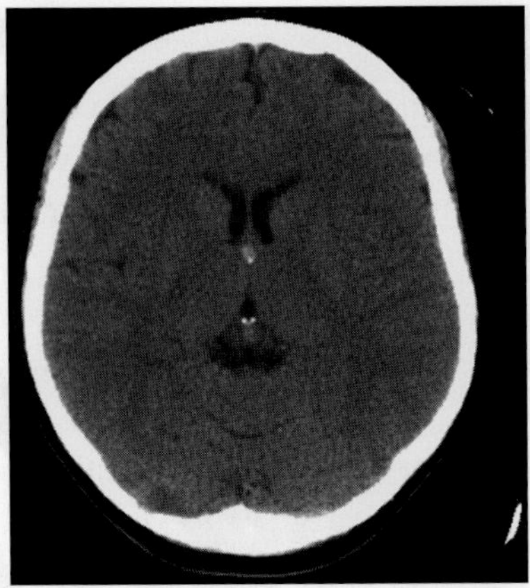

Figure 5-38: *CT showing hyperdense colloid cyst in a 35-year-old woman presented with headaches and drop attacks. She had this removed with excellent results.*

The commonest location of colloid cysts is in the anterior third of the 3V and they appear as high signal on T1 and T2 and hyperdense on CT (Figure 5-38). Isodense cysts are not uncommon and may be missed on CT scan, therefore great care should be taken not to perform L/P in these patients without thorough examination of the MRI scan. Colloid cysts can be removed without problems, but be mindful as potential complications of surgery in particular injury to the fornix leading to complete loss of recent memory is a real risk.

- *AOHC at the anterior third of 3V:*

This could be due to colloid cyst as discussed above, invasive pituitary adenoma (Figure 5-39), craniopharyngioma (Figure 5-40), or a giant anterior communicating artery aneurysm. The treatment of these patients is directed at treating the cause with peri-operative external ventricular drainage (EVD) and Ventriculoperitoneal shunt (VPS) as a rescue procedure to treat persistent hydrocephalus.

- *AOHC due to obstruction of post-3V:*

This could be due to pineal body tumours or cysts (Figure 5-41) or basilar tip aneurysm (BTA) (Figure 5-42). Blood clot in 3V (Figure 5-43) may

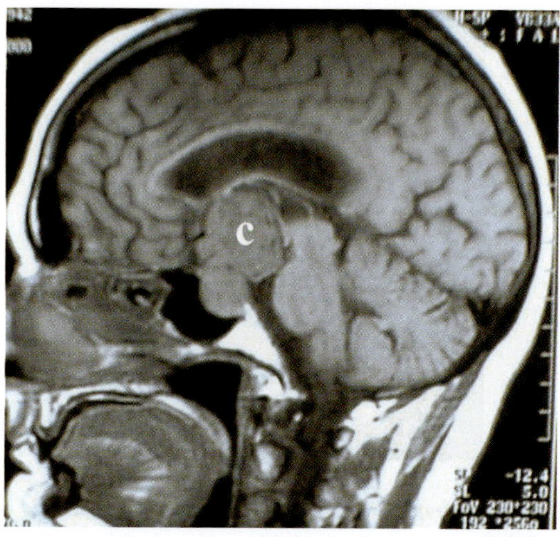

Figure 5-39: OHC due to invasion of 3V with pituitary adenoma (c). This patient was a 46-year-old male who presented with bitemporal visual defects in addition to hydrocephalus. He underwent transsphenoidal resection of non-functioning pituitary adenoma.

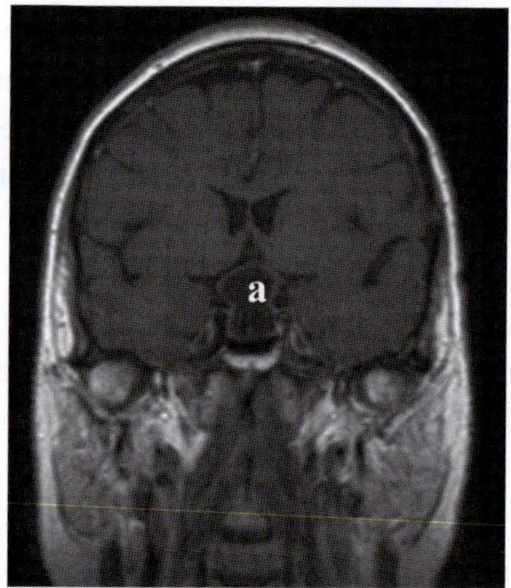

Figure 5-40: AOHC due to craniopharyngioma. This 30-year-old patient presented with fatigue and tiredness with bitemporal visual field defects. He underwent transsphenoidal drainage of the cyst.

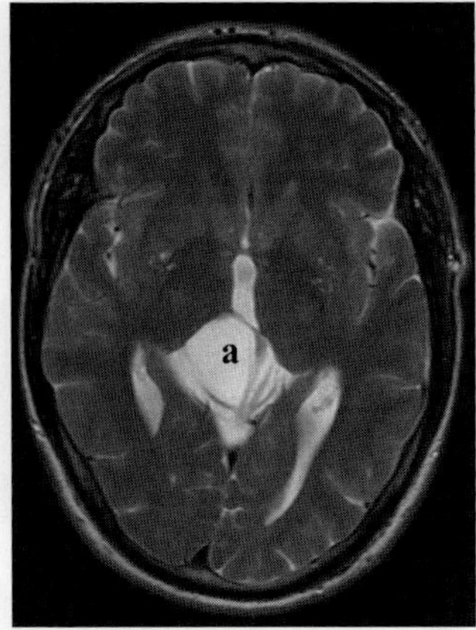

Figure 5-41: *AOHC due to pineal cyst (a) in a 27-year-old man presented with chronic headaches. This was drained endoscopically without the need for a shunt.*

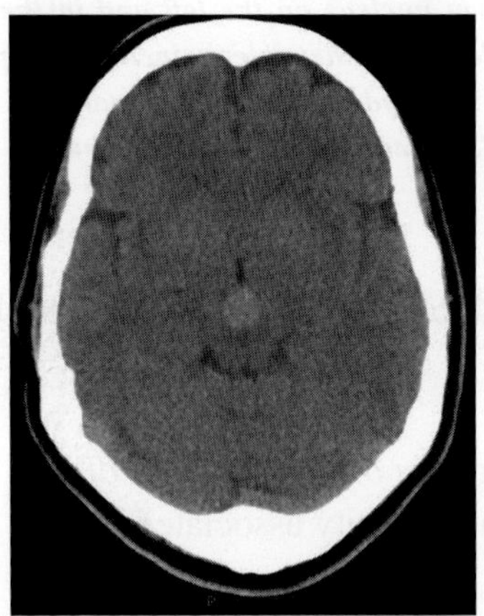

Figure 5-42: *BTAA (hyperdense lesion in the middle of the CT scan image) blocking the post-3V and may lead to hydrocephalus.*

also lead to AOHC in some patients if the clot did not resolve in time or the ADS is blocked.

- *AOHC due to blockage of ADS:*

The aqueduct of Sylvius is vulnerable and can be blocked by blood clot as shown in the previous example but can also be blocked by tumour or any

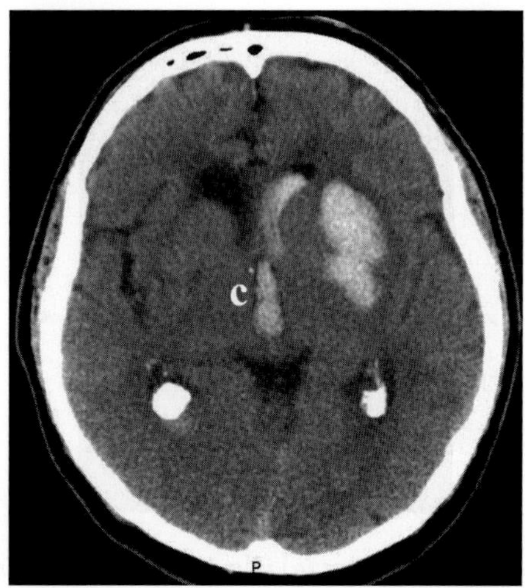

Figure 5-43: AOHC due to blood clot in 3V (hyperdense lesion c). Note that the clot extended from the lentiform nucleus on the left and in the left LV. This 60-year-old patient presented with sudden right hemiplegia including right UMN of VII nerve and patient was hypertensive. The hydrocephalus was managed by EVD till the CSF was clear and the clot resolved. Patient did not require a shunt.

mass lesion in the midbrain, e.g. haemorrhage, midbrain glioma, abscess or cyst (Figure 5-44).

- *AOHC due to blockage or compression of 4V:*

This is a common clinical entity associated with:

1. Intrinsic cerebellar tumours [glioma, medulloblastoma (Figure 5-45), ependymomas, haemangioblastoma, juvenile astrocytomas or metastases].
2. Extrinsic tumours such as giant CPA schwannoma, meningioma (Figure 5-46), clival meningioma, or epidemoid cyst.
3. Cerebellar haematoma or infarct (Figure 5-47).
4. Clot in the 4V (Figure 5-48).

All the aforementioned lesions can present with hydrocephalus in addition to their cardinal symptoms and signs.

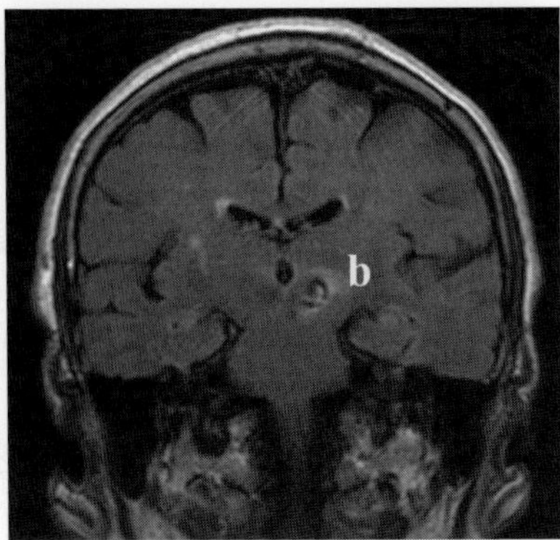

Figure 5-44: Cavernoma of the cerebral peduncle that bled and led to AOHC in a 55-year-old woman. This was associated with drowsiness, hemiparesis, and ipsilateral third nerve palsy.

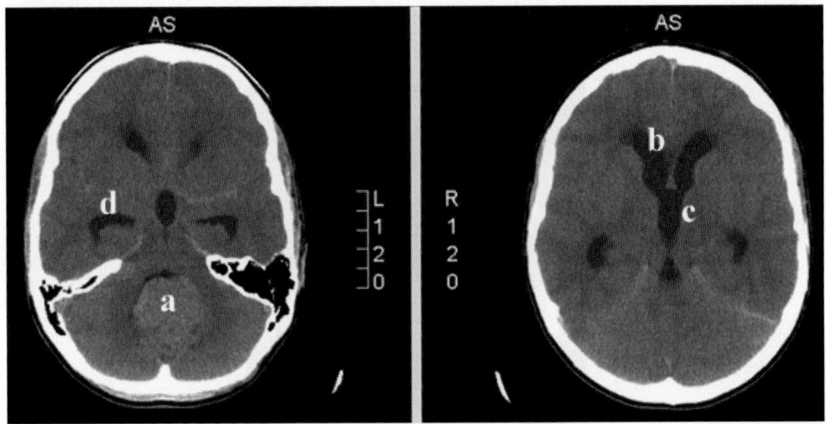

Figure 5-45: Medulloblastoma (a) of 4V in a child leading to AOHC (b) dilated LV, (c) dilated 3V, (d) dilated temporal horn. The tumour was excised via posterior fossa approach without the need for EVD or a shunt. Shunts need to be avoided in these patients to prevent tumour seeding into the peritoneum.

5-4-8 *How does hydrocephalus exert its effects?*

Normal ICP is 80–100 mmH$_2$O in newborns and <180 mmH$_2$O in children and adults compared to venous pressure in the sinuses. As CSF is produced at a rate of 500 ml/day and the total volume of the CSF in the ventricles

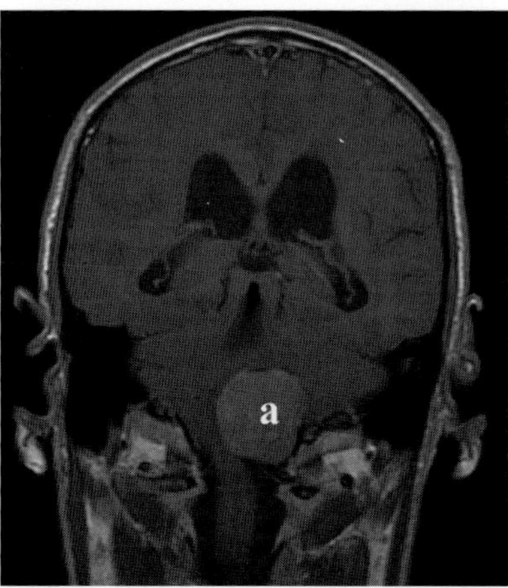

Figure 5-46: CPA meningioma (a) causing obstruction and shift of the 4V and hydrocephalus. This 60-year-old man presented with dysphonia and swallowing difficulties. He had this tumour removed without EVD or shunt. He made an excellent recovery.

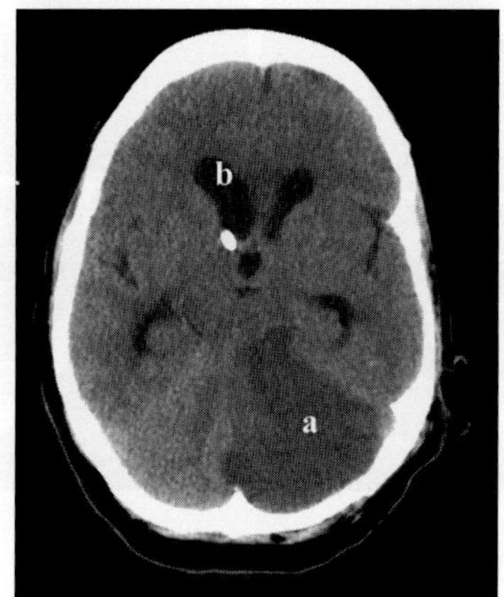

Figure 5-47: Cerebellar infarct (a) in a 70-year-old woman leading to hydrocephalus (b) required an EVD. Some of these patients benefit from sub-occipital decompression.

and subarachnoid space is around 135–150 ml, this creates a turnover of about 3.7 times a day and a pressure gradient leading to CSF reabsorption. This reabsorption is facilitated by the aforementioned hydrostatic pressure gradient and the difference in osmotic pressure between CSF and venous

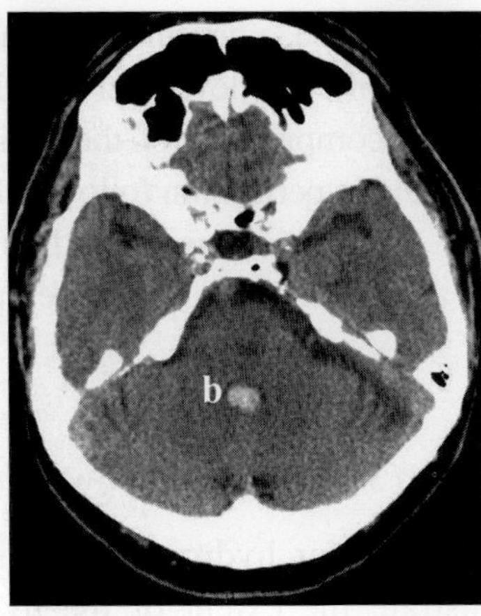

Figure 5-48: Clot in 4V (b) leading to hydrocephalus and requiring an EVD.

blood. The CSF osmotic pressure is lower than plasma because of the lower protein and glucose content of the CSF. Hydrocephalus exerts its effects by increasing ICP. According to the Monro-Kellie hypothesis the cranial cavity is a ridged incompressible box, with a fixed volume. Its contents; brain tissue (80%/1400 ml), CSF (10%/150 ml), and blood (10%/150 ml) create a state of volume equilibrium, such that any increase in the volume of one of the cranial contents must be compensated by a decrease in the volume of another otherwise the ICP will rise.[37] To maintain constant ICP, there are a number of mechanisms which are able to compensate for small increases in ICP. These mechanisms include movement of CSF into the thecal sac, increased reuptake of CSF, and compression of venous sinuses. Once compensatory mechanisms are overcome, any increase in CSF volume will increase the ICP dramatically.[38] Increased ICP may cause brain tissue ischaemia and uncal hernation where the temporal lobe herniates beneath the tentorium and cerebellar tonsils herniation where the cerebellar tonsils are forced through the foramen magnum. Both are clinical emergencies as they can compress the brainstem and lead to death. Hence obstructive hydrocephalus is a neurosurgical emergency even when the patient is apparently fully conscious. Symptoms of acute hydrocephalus vary with age, the rate of disease progression, and underlying cause of the hydrocephalus. In adults and older children the most common presentation is raised ICP; headaches, nausea, vomiting and papilloedema. Impaired upward gaze and impaired conscious level and visual disturbances are also common symptoms due to compression of the brainstem. A late sign of raised ICP is bradycardia and hypertension followed by pupillary dilatation and coma. In infants the signs are enlarged head circumference, dysjunction of sutures, bulging and tense anterior fontanel, prominent scalp veins and sunset sign.

5-4-9 *How to investigate a suspected patient with hydrocephalus?*

The investigation of choice for hydrocephalus is MRI scan because MRI scan can demonstrate the extent of the hydrocephalus and the underlying cause such as PCF lesions and brain stem lesions. While CT scan can diagnose hydrocephalus quite well, its resolution is not good enough for aqueduct and PCF pathology. The key diagnostic signs on brain imaging include; prominence of the temporal horns of LV (Figures 5-35, 5-45 and 5-47). The temporal horns are barely visible in normal brain without hydrocephalus. The ratio between the width of the frontal horn and the biparietal diameter (Evans ratio) would be > 0.4 if hydrocephalus is present and periventricular oedema due to seeping of CSF into the brain parenchyma (Figures 5-43 and 5-45). By comparing and contrasting the dilatation of ventricles, it is possible to identify the obstruction location. Generalised dilatation of all ventricles suggests communicating hydrocephalus (Figure 5-34), while the dilatation of frontal horns of lateral ventricles and third ventricle ("Mickey mouse" ventricles) indicates a non-communicating (Figures 5-35, 5-45 and 5-47). Ultrasound might be useful in neonates before fontanel closure.

5-4-10 *How to manage hydrocephalus?*

The basic principles of hydrocephalus management are:

1- To treat the underlying causes (Figure 5-49).
2- Third ventricolostomy for aqueduct obstruction.

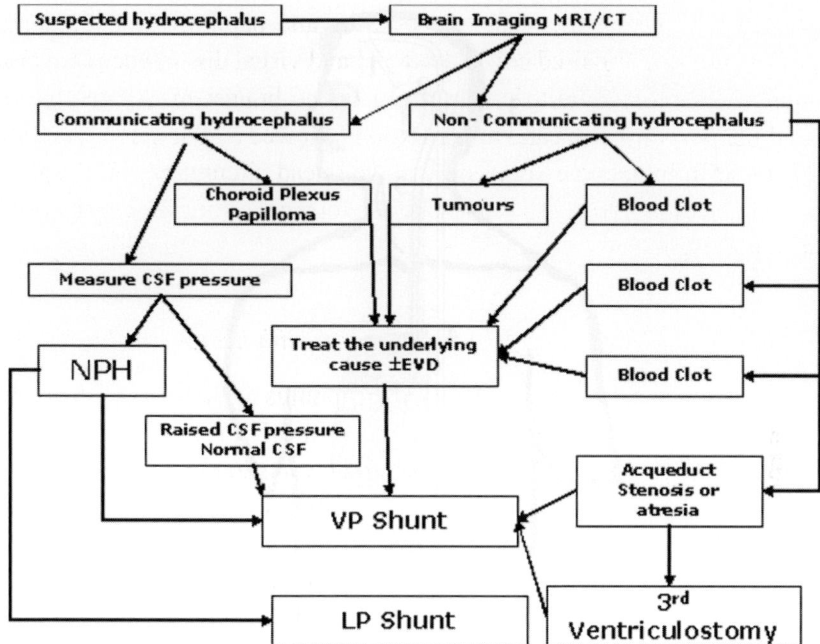

Figure 5-49: Paradigm of managing a patient with suspected hydrocephalus.

3- Ventriculo-peritoneal shunt (VPS).

The choice of shunt is dependent on the patient's age, type of hydro-cephalus and surgical preferences. Each shunt consists of:

1- Ventricular catheter inserted into the LV to drain CSF (Figure 5-50). The ventricular catheter is often connected to a small subcutaneous reservoir to facilitate management of shunt malfunction by measuring the CSF pressure within the reservoir (Figure 5-51).
2- Regulating valve (low, medium or high pressure or programmable valves) that regulates CSF pressure to the predetermined pressure.
3- Distal catheter that carries excess CSF to its final location for re-absorption.

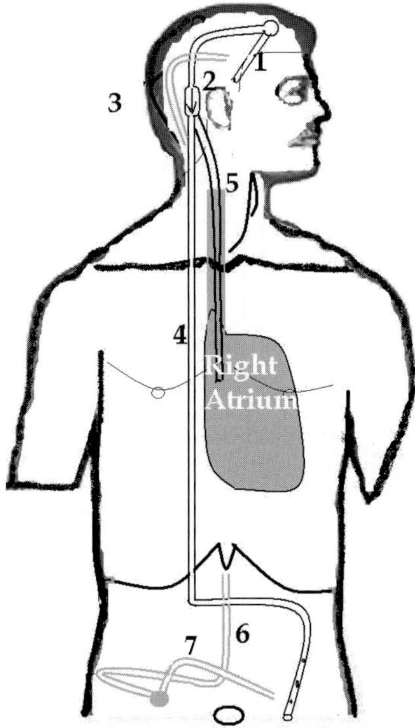

Figure 5-50: Shunt types: 1 = ventricular catheter, 2 = valve, 3 = Torkildson's shunt, 4 = peritoneal catheter in VPS, 5 = atrial catheter in VAS, 6 = intrathecal catheter for LPS, 7 = peritoneal catheter in LPS.

5-4-11 *What are the types of shunts?*

Shunts are divided according to the location of the distal catheter placement into:

a- VPS: Ventriculoperitoneal shunt draining the ventricle to the peritoneum. VPS is the most commonly used shunt at the moment.

b- VAS: Ventriculo-atrial shunt draining the CSF into the right atrium. VAS had gone out of fashion because of venous thrombosis and bacterial endocarditis risks.

c- LPS: Drains CSF from the lumbar thecal sac into the peritoneum, it should only be used in communicating hydrocephalus.

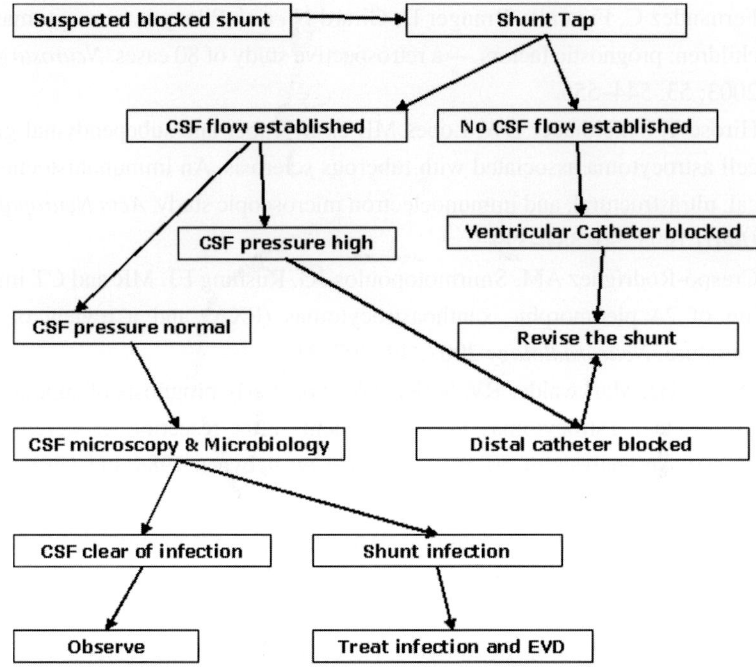

Figure 5-51: Management chart of suspected shunt malfunction.

d- Torkildson's shunt is a simple tube draining CSF from the occipital horn of LV to cisterna magna bypassing the aqueduct. It had gone out of fashion when modern CSF valves came into being.

References

1. Stupp R. Malignant gliomas: ESMO clinical recommendations for diagnosis, treatment and follow up. *Ann Oncol* 2007; 18(Suppl 2): 60–70.

2. Lassman AB, DeAngelis LM. Brain metastases. *Neurol Clin* 2003; 21: 1–23.

3. D'Ambrosio AL, Agazzi S. Prognosis in patients presenting with brain metastasis from an undiagnosed primary tumour. *Neurosurg Focus* 2007; 15: 22(3): E7.

4. Kleihues P, Burger PC, Scheithauer BW. Histological classification of CNS tumours. In: Sobin LH, editor. *Histological Typing of Tumours of the Central Nervous System*, 2nd Edn. Berlin: Springer-Verlag, 1993: pp. 1–105.

5. Fernandez C, Figarella-Branger D, Girard N *et al.* Pilocytic astrocytomas in children: prognostic factors — a retrospective study of 80 cases. *Neurosurgery* 2003; 53: 544–555.

6. Hirose T, Scheithauer BW, Lopes MB *et al.* Tuber and subependymal giant cell astrocytoma associated with tuberous sclerosis. An immunohistochemical, ultrastructural, and immunoelectron microscopic study. *Acta Neuropathol (Berl)* 1995; 90: 387–399.

7. Crespo-Rodríguez AM, Smirniotopoulos JG, Rushing EJ. MR and CT imaging of 24 pleomorphic xanthoastrocytomas (PXA) and a review of the literature. *Neuroradiology* 2007; 49: 307–315.

8. Steiger HJ, Markwalder RV, Seiler RW *et al.* Early prognosis of supratentorial grade 2 astrocytomas in adult patients after resection or stereotactic biopsy. An analysis of 50 cases operated on between 1984 and 1988. *Acta Neurochir* 1990; 106: 99–105.

9. Kleihues P, Cavanee WK (editors). World Health Organization classification of tumours. Pathology and genetics-tumours of the nervous system. Lyon: IARC Press, 2000.

10. Devaux BC, O'Fallon JR, Kelly PJ. Resection, biopsy and survival in malignant glial neoplasms, a retrospective study of clinical parameters, therapy and outcome. *J Neurosurg* 1993; 78: 767–775.

11. Obwegeser A, Ortler M, Seiwald M *et al.* Therapy of glioblastoma multiforme, a cumulative experience of 10 years. *Acta Neurochir (Wien)* 1995; 137: 29–33.

12. Van den Bent MJ, Stupp R, Mason W *et al.* Impact of the extent of resection on overall survival in newly-diagnosed glioblastoma after chemo-irradiation with temozolamide: further analysis of EORTC study 26981. *Eur J Cancer Suppl.* 2005; 3: 134.

13. Keles GE, Chang EF, Lamborn KR *et al.* Volumetric extent of resection and residual contrast enhancement on initial surgery as predictors of outcome in adult patients with hemispheric anaplastic astrocytomas. *J Neurosurg* 2006; 105: 34–50.

14. Stummer W, Reulen HJ, Meinel T *et al.* ALA-Glioma Study Group. Extent of resection and survival in glioblastoma multiforme: identification of and adjustment for bias. *Neurosurgery* 2008; 62: 564–576.

15. Stummer W, Oitchimeier U, Meinel T *et al.* Fluorescence-guided surgery with 5-aminolevulinic acid for resection of malignant glioma: a randomized controlled multicentre phase III trial. *Lancet Oncol* 2008; 7: 392–401.

16. Eljamel MS, Goodman C, Moseley H. ALA and photofrin fluorescence-guided resection and repetitive PDT in glioblastoma multiforme: a single centre Phase III randomised controlled trial. *Lasers Med Sci* 2008; 23: 561–567.

17. Ashby LS, Ryken TC. Management of malignant glioma: steady progress with multimodal approaches. *Neurosurg Focus* 2006; 20(4): E3.

18. Westphal M, Ram Z, Riddle V *et al.* Executive Committee of the Gliadel Study Group. Gliadel wafer in initial surgery for malignant glioma: long-term follow-up of a multicenter controlled trial. *Acta Neurochir (Wien)* 2006; 148: 269–275.

19. Eljamel MS, Jeffreys RV. Mucous-secreting choroid plexus adenoma — case report and review of the literature. *Neuropediatrics* 1990; 21: 55–56.

20. Wrensch M, Minn Y, Chew T *et al.* Epidemiology of primary brain tumors: current concepts and review of the literature. *Neuro-Oncology* 2002; 4(4): 278–299.

21. Hart MG, Grant R, Metcalfe SE. Biopsy versus resection for high grade glioma. *Cochrane Database Syst Rev* 2000; (2): CD002034. DOI: 10.1002/14651858.CD002034.

22. Walker MD, Alexander E Jr, Hunt WE *et al.* Evaluation of BCNU and/or radiotherapy in the treatment of anaplastic gliomas. *J Neurosurg* 1978; 49: 333–343.

23. Gilbert MA. New treatments for malignant gliomas: careful evaluation and cautious optimism required. *Ann Intern Med* 2006; 144: 337–343.

24. Stupp R, Mason WP, van den Bent MJ *et al.* Radiotherapy plus concomitant and adjuvant temozolomide for glioblastoma. *N Engl J Med* 2005; 352: 987–996.

25. Krex D, Klink B, Hartmann C *et al.* Long-term survival with glioblastoma multiforme. *Brain* 2007; 130: 2596–2606.

26. Klos K, O'Neill B. Brain metastases. *Neurologist* 2004; 10: 31–46.

27. Gaspar L, Scott C, Rotman M, Asbell S *et al.* Recursive partitioning analysis (RPA) of prognostic factors in three Radiation Therapy Oncology Group (RTOG) brain metastases trials. *Int J Radiat Oncol Biol Phys* 1997; 37: 745–751.

28. Eljamel MS. Fractures of the middle third of the face and CSF fistulae. *Br J Neurosurg* 1994; 8(7): 289–294.

29. Eljamel MS. Antibiotic prophylaxis in CSF fistulae. *Br J Neurosurg* 1993; 7(5): 501–506.

30. Eljamel MS, Pidgeon CN. Localisation of inactive cerebrospinal fluid fitulas. *J Neurosurg* 1995; 83(5): 795–798.

31. Eljamel MS, Pidgeon CN, Toland J *et al*. MRI-cisternography in CSF fistulae localisation. *Br J Neurosurg* 1994; 8(4): 433–437.

32. Eljamel MS, Foy PM. Non-traumatic CSF fistulae: clinical history and management. *Br J Neurosurg* 1991; 5(3): 275–279.

33. Eljamel MS, Foy PM. Acute cerebrospinal fluid fistulae, the risk of intracranial infections. *Br J Neurosurg* 1990; 4(5): 381–385.

34. Eljamel MS, Foy PM. Post-traumatic CSF fistulae, the case for surgical repair. *Br J Neurosurg* 1990; 4(6): 479–483.

35. Eljamel MS, Waring DJ. The paragon immunofixation for CSF identification. *Biomed Sci* 1993; 4(2): 43–45.

36. Tsakanikas D, Relkin N. Normal pressure hydrocephalus. *Semin Neurol* 2007; 27: 58–65.

37. Mokri B. The Monro-Kellie hypothesis: applications in CSF volume depletion. *Neurology* 2001; 56: 1746–1748.

38. Steiner LA, Andrews PJ. Monitoring the injured brain: ICP and CBF. *Br J Anaesth* 2006; 97: 26–38.

Your personal notes:

....

....

....

....

....

....

....

....

....

....

Chapter 6: Visual Symptoms (Meningiomas, Pituitary Adenomas)

Problem 6-1:   Visual failure and intracranial meningiomas. How to manage a patient presenting with compressive optic neuropathy?

Any patient presenting with gradual slowly progressive unilateral visual failure should be investigated to exclude compressive optic neuropathy.

Problem based tool box:
Compressive optic neuropathy
Foster Kennedy Syndrome
Intracranial meningiomas
Multiple meningiomas and
  NFII

PCS6-1-1:

A 35-year-old female, right-handed, presented with two years history gradual slowly progressive visual failure in the left eye. More recently she noted headache. The headaches were right-sided and were getting worse. The headaches improved on becoming pregnant but in the last three weeks her vision deteriorated further in the left eye. She had no diplopia and she was not on any medications. On examination her visual acuity was reduced in the left eye to 6/60 and had lost colour vision. The left optic disc was pale and the right was normal.

Differential diagnosis:

A patient presenting with gradual slowly progressive visual failure in one eye associated with optic disc pallor means compressive optic neuropathy (CON) till proven otherwise. The causes of CON include:

- Medial sphenoid wing meningiomas.
- Optic nerve meningiomas.

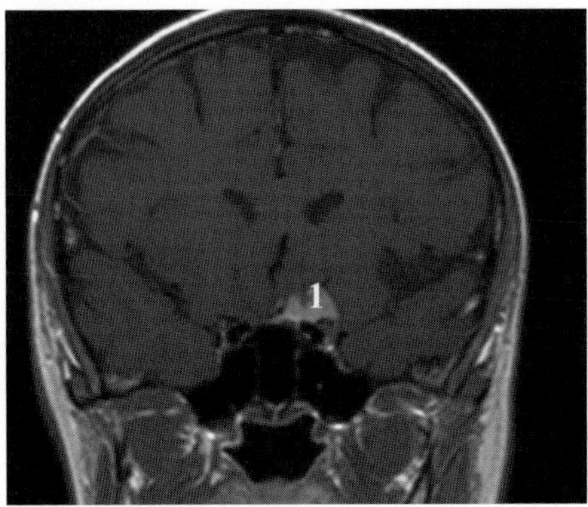

Figure 6-1: T1 MRI with contrast demonstrating intracranial meningioma around the left optic foramen (1) compressing the left optic nerve.

- Ophthalmic artery aneurysm.
- Any other lesion compressing the optic nerve: tumour or granuloma.

Investigations:

This patient needed urgent brain imaging in the form of an MRI. Because she was pregnant CT scan was avoided at this stage. The MRI scan demonstrated a lesion around the left optic foramen compressing the left optic nerve. The lesion was iso-intense on T1-weighted MRI and enhanced well on gadolinium. This appearance was consistent with optic nerve meningioma. The lesion was also closely related to the left intracranial carotid artery and the apex of the left orbit. It had not crossed the midline and there was no oedema or midline shift (Figure 6-1).

PCS6-1-2:

A right-handed 49-year-old female presented with visual disturbance for several months. She had also developed amenorrhea in 1986 and was subsequently diagnosed with hyperprolactinoma. This was treated with Bromocriptine and later with Cabergoline. The patient had no history of angina, MI, hypertension, asthma, TIA, diabetes, epilepsy, rheumatic fever, jaundice/hepatitis or peptic ulcer disease. Her temperature was

36.4°C, pulse was 57 bpm, BP was 138/72 and the rest of the general examination was normal. Cranial nerve examination revealed no problem with sense of smell, bitemporal visual field defect, normal visual acuity and colour vision, normal extra-ocular movements and pupillary responses, facial sensation and functions were normal, and the rest of the physical examination was normal.

Differential diagnosis:

A patient presenting with gradual slowly progressive bitemporal visual failure should be investigated for optic chiasm compression (OCC). The causes of OCC include:

1- Giant pituitary adenoma.
2- Suprasellar meningioma.
3- Optic nerve glioma.
4- Other rare lesions.

Investigations:

This patient needed urgent brain imaging in the form of an MRI or CT. MRI would be preferred because it provides much better detail. The MRI scan demonstrated a lesion in the suprasellar region consistent with meningioma (Figure 6-2).

6-1-3 *What is the epidemiology of meningiomas?*

Meningiomas are tumours of the lepto-meninges of the brain and spinal cord. Meningiomas account for 13–26% of all primary intracranial neoplasms and approximately 25% of all spinal tumours. Meningiomas are thought to originate from the arachnoidal cap cells, which form the outermost layer of the arachnoid mater and have a role in the absorption of CSF. Consequently, meningiomas occur most frequently around the dural venous sinuses where the arachnoid granulations are located. Most meningiomas are benign, and present themselves due to compression and shift of the adjacent brain tissue. As these tumours gradually enlarge, they lead

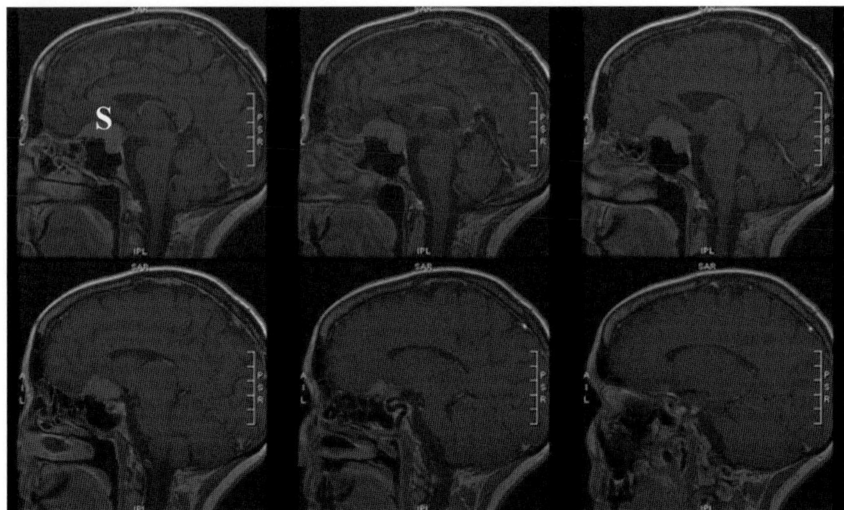

Figure 6-2: Sagittal T1 MRI with contrast demonstrating suprasellar lesion (S) with wide dural base that enhances well, consistent with suprasellar meningioma.

to a slowly progressive pattern of focal neurological deficit, seizures or raised intracranial pressure. With recent advances in neuro-imaging more and more of incidental asymptomatic meningiomas are discovered. Autopsy studies have estimated that as many as 2–3% of the population have an incidental asymptomatic meningioma. Females are twice as commonly affected compared to males.[1] Meningiomas are increasing with age, usually occurring after the seventh decade of life.

6-1-4 *What are the causes of meningiomas?*

Whilst most meningiomas are idiopathic and have unknown aetiology, there are several recognised risk factors for the development of these tumours, including genetic factors[2] such as neurofibromatosis type 2 (NFII) and exposure to ionising radiation. NFII is an autosomal dominant multi-system genetic disorder, with an incidence of one per 37,000 per year. The disease is characterised by the presence of multiple meningiomas[3,4] as well as vestibular schwannomas (Figure 6-3), spinal cord schwannomas, gliomas and juvenile cataracts.

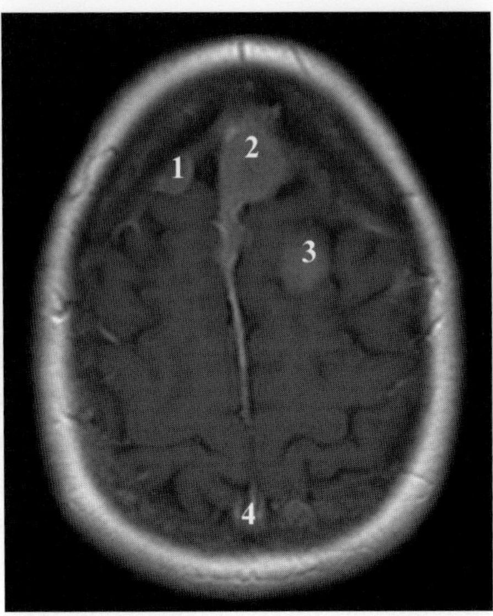

Figure 6-3: A case of multiple meningiomas (1,2,3,4) and vestibular schwannoma in a 30-year-old woman who presented with right sensori-neural hearing loss.

Approximately 40% of children presenting with meningiomas suffer from NFII, and this genetic syndrome must be ruled out in any child known to have such a tumour. NFII results from mutations in the NFII gene located on the long arm of chromosome 22. This gene produces a protein known as merlin (schwannomin), which serves as a tumour-suppressor gene and protects against the formation of various tumours within the central and peripheral nervous systems. Of interest, up to 60% of all idiopathic meningiomas also show mutations in the *NFII* gene. Of the remaining 40% without mutations in *NFII*, there is often evidence for additional mechanisms of merlin inactivation, such as calpain-mediated proteolysis of merlin. It is also well established that the risk of developing meningiomas is increased following exposure to ionising radiation.[5] Local low dose irradiation with 8 Gy, used for the treatment of tinea capitis in the 1950s, has been found to carry a 2.3% lifetime risk for the development of meningiomas. An association has also been found between the development of meningiomas and previous radiotherapy to the skull for the treatment of intracerebral tumours. In the Hiroshima and Nagasaki tumour registries, 88 meningiomas were discovered within 80,160 atomic bomb survivors, and there is even evidence that very small doses of radiation, such as those used in dental radiography, could lead to an increased risk of meningioma development. A less well established risk factor for the development of meningiomas is previous head trauma. The possible mechanism for this relationship is the local alteration of the BBB due to the head injury, associated with a large influx of cytokines, histamine and bradykinin into the extravascular space. Some studies have shown that patients with meningiomas have a higher incidence of head trauma than controls, usually with a long delay between trauma and presentation. However, the significance of this link is questionable, with meningiomas having a higher incidence in females despite males suffering from head trauma two to three times more frequently.[6] Another aetiological factor which has been related to an increased risk of meningioma development is the presence of high levels of sex hormones. Approximately two-thirds of all meningiomas express progesterone receptors on their cell membranes. Expression of oestrogen and androgen receptors by meningiomas is also commonly demonstrated. The precise role of sex hormones in the development of meningiomas is as yet unclear. However, it is now becoming obvious that progesterone must at least be a factor in the growth of some meningiomas. This follows the observation that reversible aggravation of symptoms caused by meningiomas occurs during both the luteal phase of the menstrual cycle and pregnancy, when levels of circulating progesterone are increased. In addition, there has also been some success with *in vitro* inhibition of meningioma cell lines using progesterone receptor (PR) antagonists. Another interesting discovery is that the level of PR expression of a meningioma approximates roughly with both tumour proliferation and histological grade, with higher expression equating to a more benign growth.[7] A study in Sweden identified a significant correlation between patient meningioma diagnosis and familial history by using data from the Swedish Family-Cancer Database and a family history of meningiomas increases the risk by 2.5.[8]

6-1-5 *How do meningiomas look like and where are they located?*

Macroscopically, meningiomas appear smooth and lobular, with a fine vascular pattern on their surface. They most commonly exhibit a globular

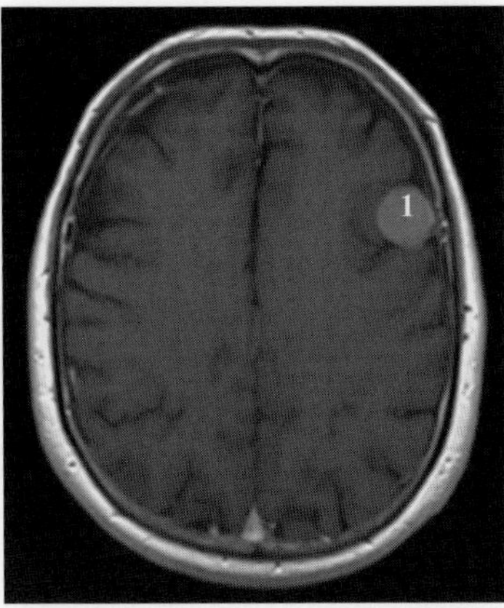

Figure 6-4: Globular meningioma on the left frontal region (1) seen on MRI T1-weighted with gadolinium presenting with seizures or found incidentally.

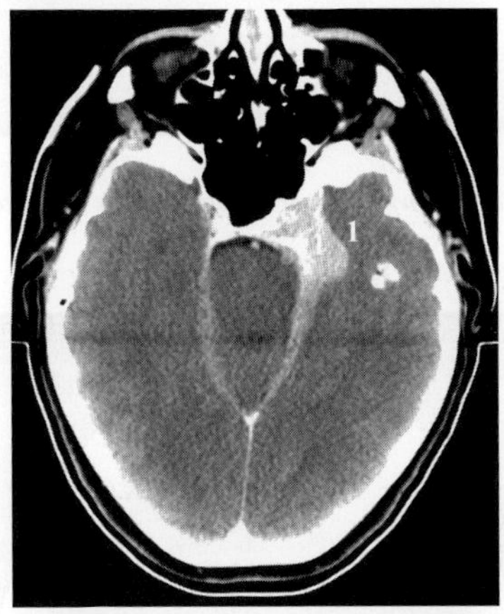

Figure 6-5: Meningioma of the lateral wall of the left cavernous sinus (1) taking the shape of en plaque on CT with contrast presenting with diplopia due to partial third nerve palsy.

shape (Figure 6-4), although this may differ depending on the location of the tumour within the cranium. For example, meningiomas arising from the optic sheath often have a characteristic tubular form, while those lying next to the sphenoid ridge may grow in a flat and diffuse pattern over the dura, termed meningioma en plaque (Figure 6-5).

The most common sites of intracranial meningiomas are parasagittal near the falx cerebri (Figures 6-6 and 6-7), convexity (Figure 6-8) and near the sphenoid ridge (Figures 6-9 and 6-10). However meningiomas can occur at other locations as demonstrated in Table 6-1.

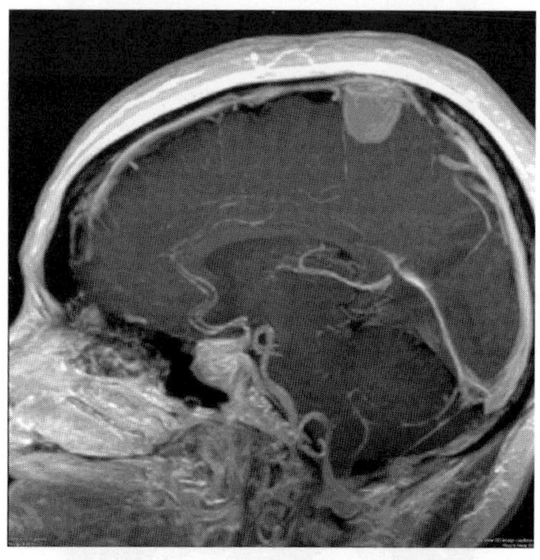

Figure 6-6: Parasagittal meningioma presenting with seizures or found incidentally.

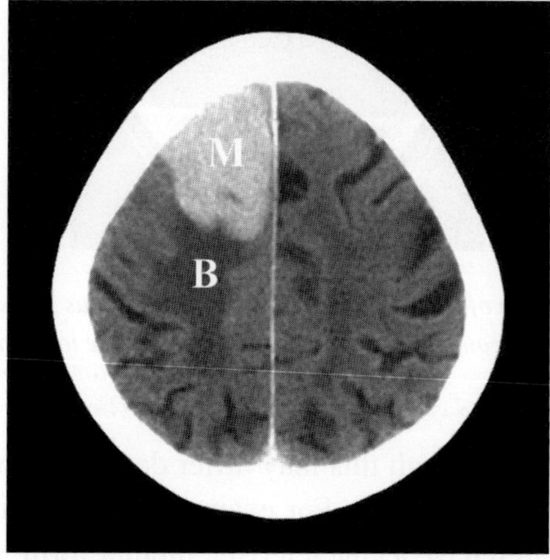

Figure 6-7: CT scan with contrast demonstrating large frontal parasagittal meningioma (M) and surrounding oedema (B) presented with raised intracranial pressure.

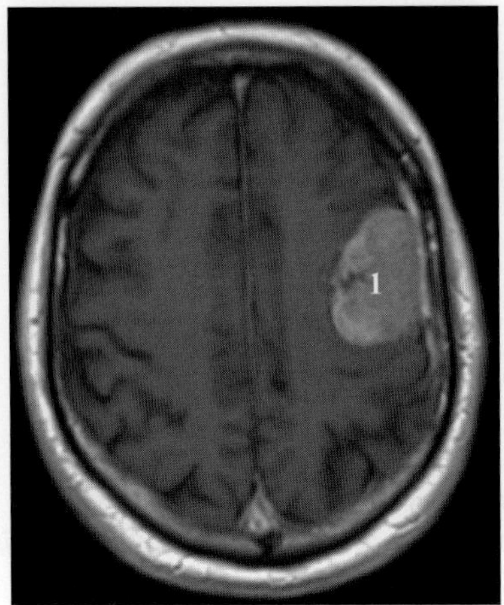

Figure 6-8: MRI scan T1 with gadolinium demonstrating left temporal convexity meningioma presented with seizures and focal neurological deficit (dysphasia).

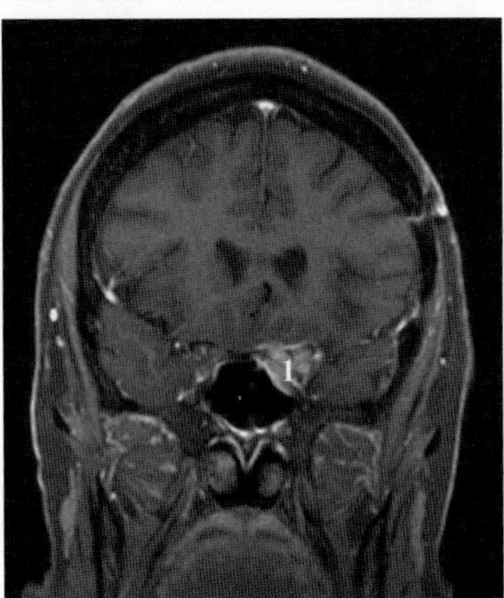

Figure 6-9: MRI scan T1 with gadolinium demonstrating medial sphenoid wing meningioma close to the optic nerve. This may present with unilateral visual failure or ipsilateral optic atrophy and contralateral papilloedema (Foster-Kennedy Syndrome).

6-1-6 *What are the pathological classifications of meningiomas?*

Meningiomas are graded according to the WHO classification into three categories: benign (WHO grade I), atypical (WHO grade II) or anaplastic

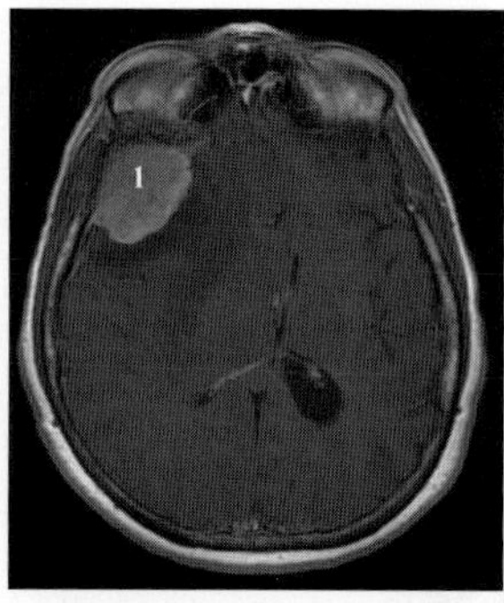

Figure 6-10: MRI scan T1 with gadolinium demonstrating lateral sphenoid wing meningioma (1) surrounded with oedema and midline shift. This patient presented with raised intracranial pressure.

Table 6-1: Locations of meningiomas

Location	Incidence	Location	Incidence
Parafalcine	25% (Figure 6-6)	Convexity	19% (Figure 6-8)
Sphenoid ridge	17% (Figure 6-9)	Suprasellar	9% (Figure 6-2)
Posterior fossa	8% (Figure 6-11)	Olfactory groove	8% (Figure 6-12)
Cavernous sinus	4% (Figure 6-5)	Peritorcular	3% (Figure 6-13)
Tentorial	3% (Figure 6-14)	Lateral ventricle	1.5% (Figure 6-15)
Foramen magnum	1.5% (Figure 6-16)	Optic nerve	1.5%
Clivus	1% (Figure 6-17)		

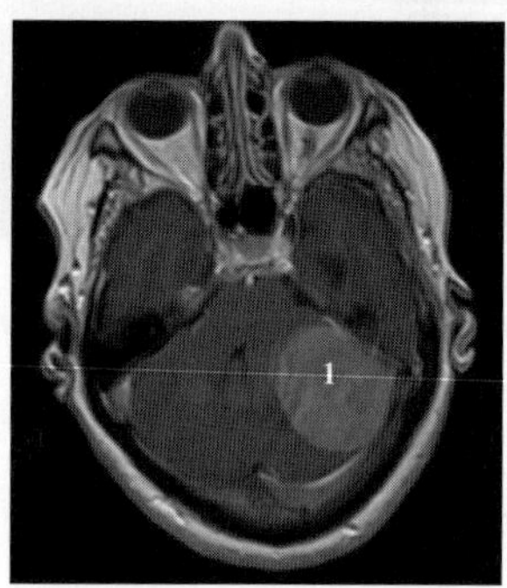

Figure 6-11: MRI scan T1 with gadolinium demonstrating large meningioma (1) in the left posterior cranial fossa causing midline shift and compression of the fourth ventricle presented with raised intracranial pressure due to hydrocephalus.

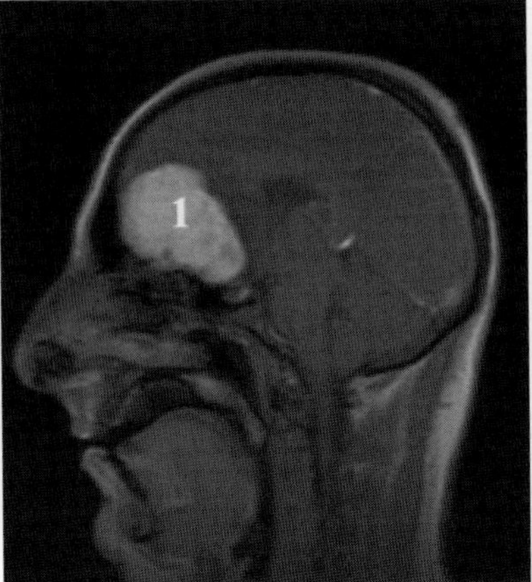

Figure 6-12: MRI scan T2 demonstrating a large mass in the anterior cranial fossa (olfactory groove meningioma 1) causing raised intracranial pressure and anosmia in a 45-year-old woman. These tumours can extend into the nose.

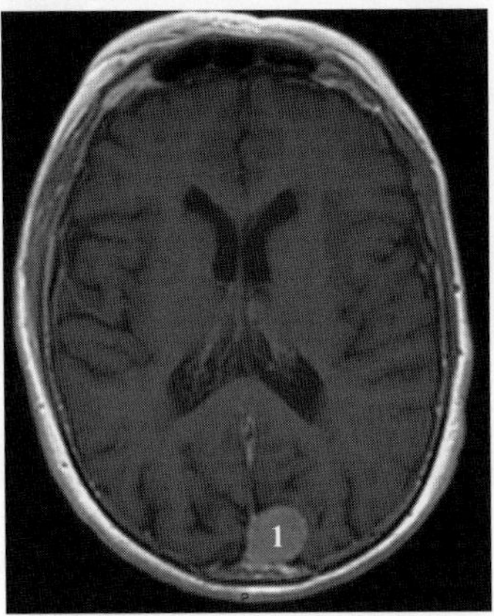

Figure 6-13: MRI scan T1-weighted with gadolinium demonstrating a small meningioma near the torcula (1).

(WHO grade III). Table 6-2 summarises the WHO classification of meningiomas.

WHO grade II is characterised by mitotic index greater or equal to four mitoses per ten high-power fields (HPF), and at least three of the following five parameters: increased cellularity, high nuclear/cytoplasmatic

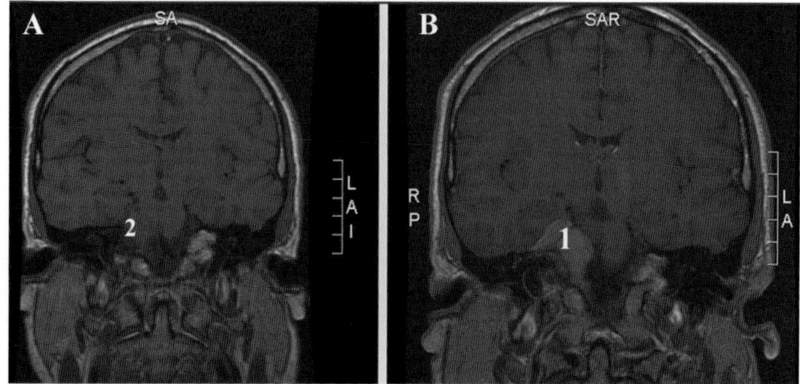

Figure 6-14: MRI scan T1 with gadolinium demonstrating a lesion at the tentorium before gadolinium (2) and after gadolinium (1).

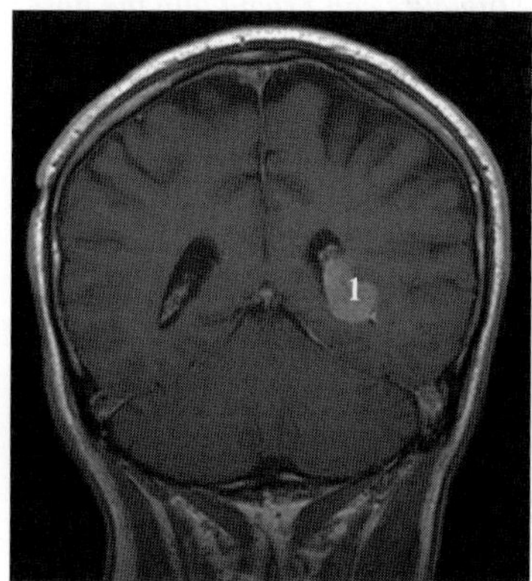

Figure 6-15: MRI scan T1 with gadolinium demonstrating intraventricular meningioma (1) in the trigone of the left lateral ventricle.

ratio (small cells), prominent nucleoli, uninterrupted patternless or sheet-like growth, foci of spontaneous necrosis, or brain invasion. WHO grade III on the other hand is characterised by mitotic index greater or equal to 20 mitoses per ten HPF, and anaplasia (sarcoma, carcinoma, or melanoma-like histology). Eighty per cent of meningiomas are benign, WHO grade I and approximately 15–20% are atypical and the remaining 1–5% are considered anaplastic.

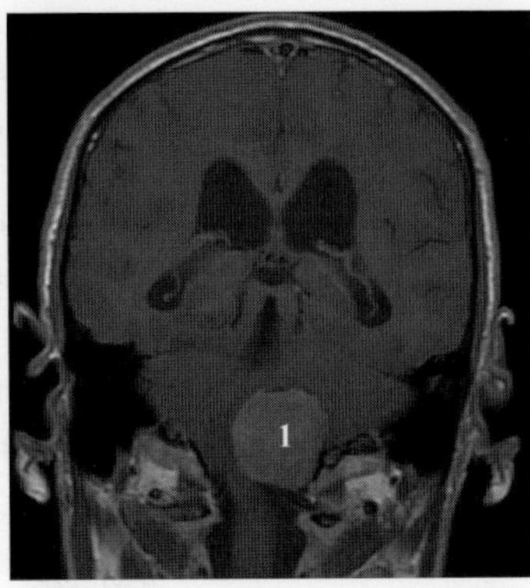

Figure 6-16: MRI scan demonstrating a meningioma at the foramen magnum.

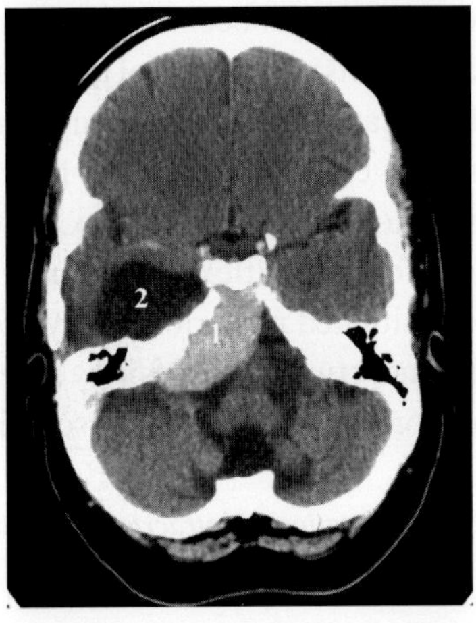

Figure 6-17: CT scan with contrast demonstrating clival meningioma (1).

Table 6-2: WHO classification of meningiomas

Grade	Tumour types
I	Syncytial, Transitional, Fiberous, Psammomatous, Angiomatous, Microcystic, Secretory, Clear cell, Choroid, Lymphoplasmocyte-rich, Xanthomatous, Myxoid, Osseous and Cartilagenous.
II	Atypical meningioma.
III	Anaplastic meningioma (malignant).

6-1-7 *How do meningiomas present?*

Meningiomas may present in several ways (Table 6-3):

1- Seizures: Epileptic seizures in a previously healthy individual are a common phenomenon with meningiomas, and approximately a quarter of all patients will present in this way. These seizures often have a focal component, closely related to the location of the tumour. The pathophysiology of tumour-induced epilepsy remains a poorly understood topic, although focal cortical hypoxia, direct mass effect, perilesional oedema and altered levels of excitatory amino acids are thought to contribute.

2- Raised ICP: In the remainder of patients, the onset is more insidious with pressure effects such as headache and vomiting often developing before focal neurological signs become evident.

3- Focal neurological deficits: When focal signs do occur, they can be used to predict the location of the tumour. For example; parasagittal/parafalcine tumours close to the vertex may affect the "foot" and "leg" area of the motor or sensory cortex, with partial seizures or weakness affecting foot dorsiflexion, then knee and hip flexion. Parasagittal tumours situated posteriorly may present with a homonymous hemianopia and tumours arising anteriorly may produce impairment of memory, intellect and personality if they grow to a

Table 6-3: Presentation of intracranial meningiomas

History	%	Physical signs	%
Headaches	36	Paresis	30
Personality change	22	No signs	26
Weakness	19	Memory impairment	15
Generalised seizures	19	Cranial nerve signs	12
Visual disturbance	16	Visual field deficit	10
Focal seizures	15	Paraesthesia	9
Imbalance	15	Speech impairment	9
Speech difficulty	10	Papilloedema	8
Decreased conscious	7	Reduced visual activity	6
Numbness	6	Reduced conscious	5
Vertigo	1	Nystagmus	3

large enough size. Medial sphenoidal wing and parasellar meningiomas may compress the optic nerve and produce visual impairment, often with a central scotoma or other field defect. Suprasellar meningiomas often present early, once compression of the optic chiasm has led to a visual field defect, usually a bitemporal hemianopia. Optic nerve sheath tumours may produce a progressive unilateral visual loss. Olfactory groove meningiomas, may destroy the olfactory bulb or tract causing unilateral anosmia. This can often pass unnoticed by patients, until tumour expansion leads to a bilateral defect of smell.

4- Asymptomatic: With the ever-increasing availability and image quality of CT and MRI, the diagnosis of meningioma is usually quite straightforward. These tumours appear as well defined extra-axial masses, which displace the adjacent brain.

6-1-8 *How do meningiomas appear on neuroimaging?*

Meningiomas tend to be hyperdense compared with normal brain on CT (Figure 6-18), and following intravenous contrast injection, there is strong uniform enhancement of the lesion (Figure 6-7). MRI is the preferred investigation to show the dural origin of the tumour. Meningiomas usually appear isointense (Figure 6-14) or slightly hypointense to brain on T1-weighted MR imaging and hyperintense on T2-weighted imaging (Figure 6-19). Meningiomas show strong uniform enhancement after intravenous injection of a paramagnetic contrast such as gadolinium (Figure 6-12). On cerebral angiography meningiomas demonstrate a "tumour blush".

Meningiomas may cause midline shift, oedema, calcification or cystic formation (Table 6-4).

6-1-9 *How to manage symptomatic meningiomas?*

The primary management of symptomatic meningioma is surgical excision of the tumour including its dural (Simpson grade 1). A total excision may not be possible in some locations, particularly when important neural or vascular structures are enveloped by the tumour. Gross total excision with diathermy of the dural origin (Simpson grade 2) without dural diathermy (Simpson grade 3) or subtotal excision

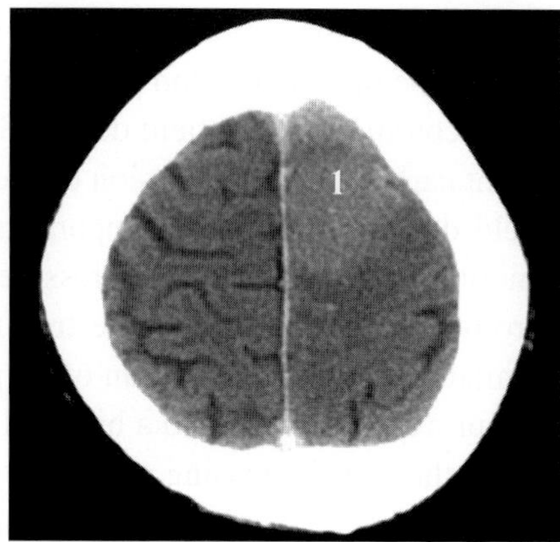

Figure 6-18: CT scan demonstrating hyperdense lesion in the left frontal region (1).

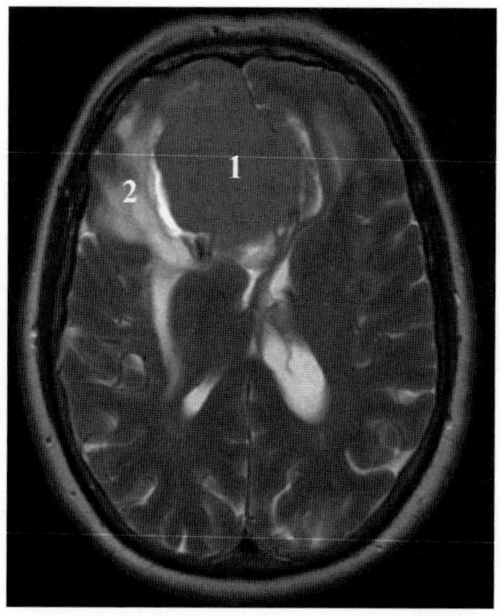

Figure 6-19: T2-weighted MRI scan demonstrating a large bifrontal lesion (1) slightly hyperintense with surrounding oedema (2) and brain shift.

(Simpson grade 4) may therefore lead to post-surgical recurrence. Rates of recurrence are directly related to the extent of surgical excision. Based on this system, recurrence rates at five years were estimated at 9% for Simpson's grade 1 excision, 19% for a grade 2 and 29% for a

Table 6-4: Neuro-imaging characteristics of meningiomas

Features	%	Features	%
Midline shift	78	Homogenous enhancement	72
No oedema	48	Mixed enhancement	23
Mild oedema	31	Severe oedema	16
Hyperostosis (Figure 6-20)	18	Calcification	27
Fringing or dural tail*	1	Mushroom appearance*	0

*These appearances are more common in WHO grade III meningiomas.

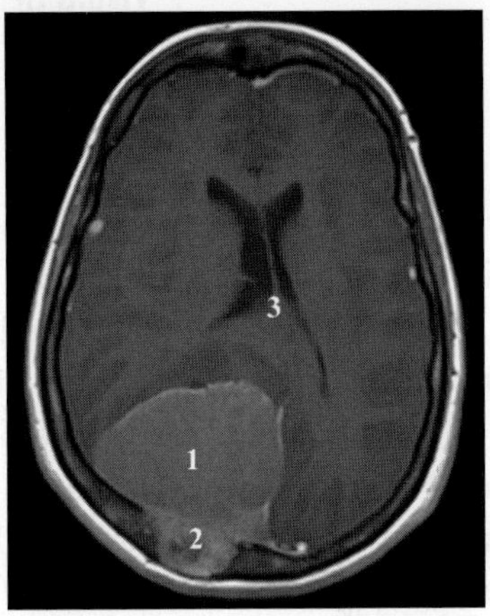

Figure 6-20: MRI scan demonstrating bone invasion (2) of meningioma (1) in the right occipital region.

grade 3. Simpson grade 5 is merely tumour biopsy. Pre-operative steroid therapy is desirable to prevent intra- and post-operative brain swelling. Emobilisation of meningiomas before surgery is rapidly gaining support to minimise intra-operative blood loss. Stereotactic radiotherapy is also commonly employed in the management of meningiomas, either as an adjuvant to surgery for example in skull base or cavernous sinus meningiomas or as a primary treatment in patients who refuse or unfit for surgery.

Problem 6-2:   Visual symptoms and pituitary adenomas. How to manage a patient presenting with visual field defect?

Any patient presenting with progressive bitemporal visual field defect (BTVD) should be treated as pituitary adenoma unless and until proven otherwise.

Problem based toolkit:

Acromegaly Cushing's

  Craniopharyngiomas

Pituitary abscess/adenoma

Pituitary apoplexy

Rathke's cleft cysts

Visual field defects

PCS6-2-1:

A 60-year-old woman presented with six months history of difficulty in reading where the right side of each word was missing. Vision has remained unchanged for the past six months. She had a number of falls in the past as a result of her poor vision. Past medical history included coronary angioplasty (1990), bilateral cataract removal, and age-related macular degeneration. Neurological examination showed bitemporal hemianopia and visual acuity of 6/12 bilaterally. Systemic review revealed no additional useful information.

Differential diagnosis:

This patient presented with visual problems of insidious onset of six months duration. She had a history of previous eye problems; macular degeneration and cataracts therefore primary eye disease should be considered as a cause; other local eye diseases that should be considered include retinopathy, retinal detachment, iridocyclitis, glaucoma and optic neuritis. However other extra-ocular causes of visual failure should be considered, particularly intracranial compressive lesions such as meningiomas and pituitary adenomas. The absence of local eye disease to explain the history and the finding of bitemporal visual field defects pointed to a chiasmatic compression most likely from giant pituitary adenoma. The differential diagnosis of bitemporal visual field defects include:

- Pituitary adenoma.
- Pituitary abscess.
- Pituitary metastases.
- Craniopharyngioma.
- Suprasellar meningioma
- Giant aneurysm AComA.
- Hypothalamic glioma.
- Optic chiasm glioma.
- Rathke's cleft cyst.
- Other sellar cysts.

The classical presentation of non-secreting pituitary adenomas is bitemporal hemianopia. Some may present with sudden headache and diplopia similar to SAH (pituitary apoplexy).

Investigations:

Visual field examination: This confirmed the presence of bitemporal VFD (Figure 6-21).

Brain MRI confirmed a pituitary lesion that stretched the optic chiasm. The lesion enhanced with contrast (Figure 6-22).

Endocrine tests confirmed hypopituitrism with slightly elevated prolactin. Her electrolytes, blood glucose, urea and full blood counts were all normal.

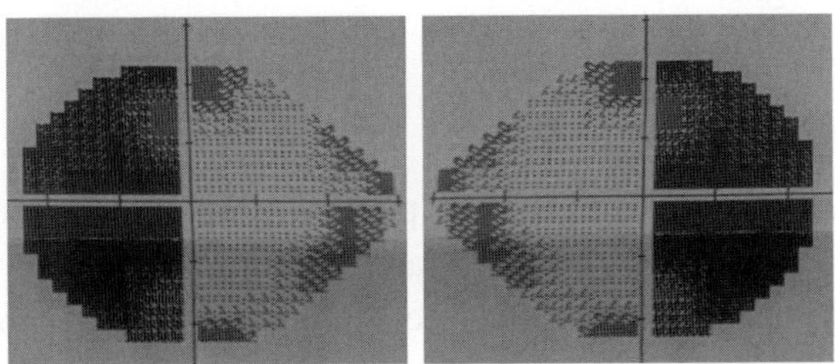

Figure 6-21: Visual field examination showing bitemporal VFD.

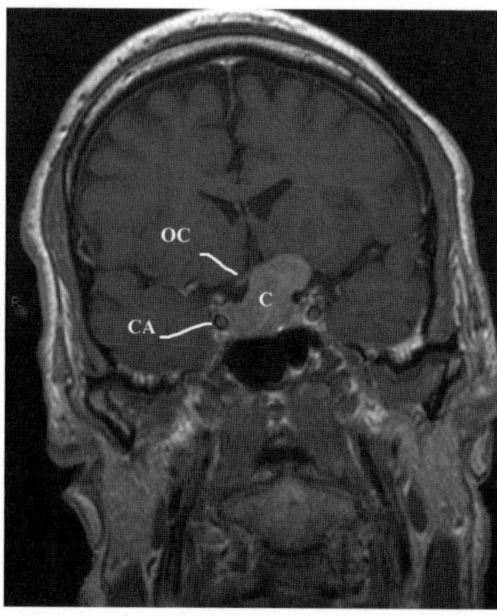

Figure 6-22: MRI demonstrating large pituitary adenoma (C) compressing the optic chiasm (OC), invading the cavernous sinus encircling the internal carotid arteries (CA).

Management: She was pretreated with hydrocortisone 100 mg QID and underwent transsphenoidal excision of the pituitary adenoma.

PCS6-2-2:

A 75-year-old right-handed woman presented with sudden severe headache. On questioning she had visual loss of insidious onset for several months and felt fatigued. No other significant history. Examination revealed that she was fully conscious, with bitemporal visual field defect and no other signs.

Differential diagnosis:

Sudden severe headache raised the possibility of subarachnoid haemorrhage (SAH) and thunderclap headache syndrome, but the presence of visual symptoms and visual field defect in the temporal VF points to optic chiasm compression. Putting the two together a diagnosis of pituitary apoplexy will be most likely.

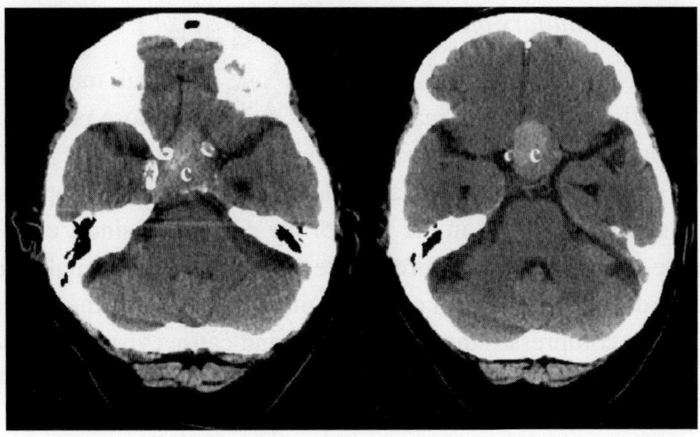

***Figure 6-23:** **Axial CT scan demonstrated a large lesion in the sella turcica (c). The
lesion is hyperdense.***

Investigations:

Full blood counts, urea, electrolytes and blood glucose were all normal.
VF examination demonstrated bitemporal VF defects similar to those
shown in Figure 6-21.

CT brain demonstrated hyperdense lesion in the sella turcica region
consistent with a bleed in a giant pituitary adenoma (Figure 6-23).

The patient was treated with hydrocortisone 100 mg QID and underwent transsphenoidal excision of the adenoma. At surgery there was clear
evidence of haemorrhage.

6-2-3 *What is the epidemiology of pituitary adenomas?*

Pituitary adenomas (PA) are benign tumours of the pituitary gland and represent about 12% of all intracranial tumours.[9,10] They are classified according
to their function into secreting or non-secreting PA. Secreting adenomas tend
to be small (microadenomas) that present with syndromes of hypersecretion
such as Cushing's disease, acromegaly or hyperprolactinaemia. Whereas
non-secreting adenomas tend to present late and by the time they reveal
themselves clinically they have often already compressed the optic chiasm[11–15] or invaded the cavernous sinus and surrounding structures.[15,16]

6-2-4 *How do pituitary adenomas present?*

The clinical presentation of PA can be due to local mass effect or endocrine effects. The local mass effect is due to the close position of the PA to the optic chiasm and cavernous sinuses. Large tumours (greater than 10 mm), otherwise known as macroadenomas can cause compression of adjacent neural structures in the wall of the cavernous sinus, e.g. III cranial nerve causing partial third nerve palsy and periorbital pain and headaches due to enlargement of the pituitary fossa. When the PA expands up the way it compresses the optic chiasm and causes visual field defects. This usually affects the superior temporal quadrants (Figure 6-24) progressing to bitemporal hemianopia (Figure 6-21).

The PA can also compress normal pituitary gland, leading to reduced hormone secretion and eventually panhypopituitarism. Compression of the pituitary stalk leads to slight elevation of prolactin levels.

The endocrine presentation of PA can be due to either hypo- or hypersecretion. As the pituitary gland controls many other glands in the body the symptoms can be variable. However, only one or two of the pituitary hormones are affected at any one time. The cause of hyposecretion, is a result of large PA compressing the pituitary gland. This can cause weight gain, loss of libido, fatigue, secondary amenorrhoea, sterility, glucocorticoid and androgen deficiency, muscle weakness and secondary hypothyroidism. Panhypopituitarism is when all of the pituitary hormones are diminished. Hypersecretion on the other hand presents in different ways dependent upon the hormone secreted in excess: growth hormone-secreting PA causes acromegally in adults and gigantism in children;

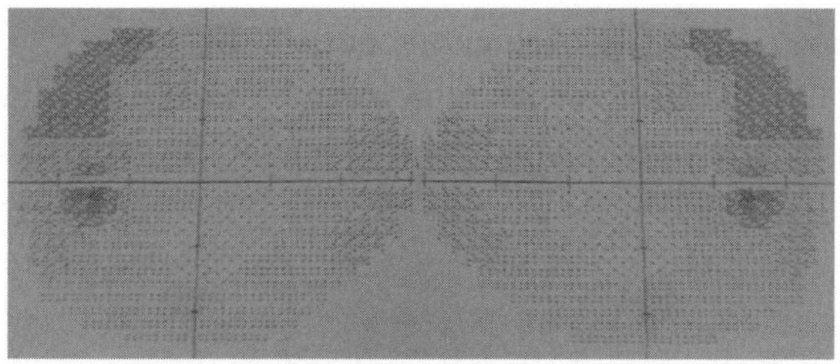

Figure 6-24: Bitemporal upper quadrantanopia.

prolactinomas cause galactorrhoea, impotence and secondary amenorrhoea; and ACTH-secreting PA causes Cushing's disease. TSH and FSH/LH-secreting tumours are very rare. Rarely, pituitary tumours can present with severe sudden headache similar to that of SAH, rapidly progressive visual defects and acute pituitary insufficiency (pituitary apoplexy), where there is infarction followed by haemorrhage into the PA.

6-2-5 *How to investigate a patient with possible PA?*

Investigation of a suspected PA involves visual fields, neuro-imaging and endocrine tests.

1- *Visual flied (VF) assessment*: VFs are assessed in patients with PA because of the aforementioned reasons. VF compromise in any way dictates the type of therapy and the urgency of therapy. Generally if there are significant VF defects, surgery will be necessary to decompress the optic chiasm and preserve vision. The commonest VF defect in PA is bitemporal VF defect, initially affecting the upper quadrants (Figure 6-24) and then bitemporal hemianopia (Figure 6-21). However other types of VF defects can be found if the optic chiasm is pre- or post-fixed (Figure 6-25).

2- *Neuro-imaging*: The scan of choice is an MRI scan for obvious reasons; it details the anatomy well and can show the chiasm and cavernous sinuses (Figures 6-22). CT however, can be useful (Figure 6-23).

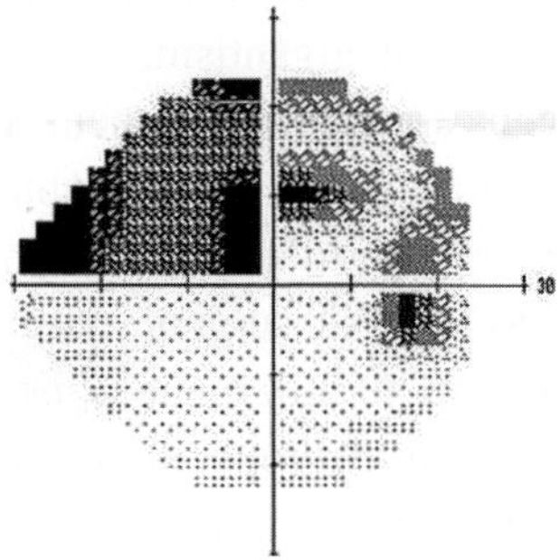

Figure 6-25: VF defect in post-fixed chiasm and large PA affecting the left VF superior temporal and nasal fields.

3- *Endocrine tests*:

a. **Prolactin:** This hormone is kept under control via the pituitary hypothalamic axis where dopamine secreted in the hypothalamus keeps the prolactin level within normal range. Prolactin is elevated by stress, pregnancy, beast feeding and during sleep. This is a physiological response and returns to normal when the physiological stimulus ceases. A number of drugs can elevate prolactin: dopaminergic inhibitors (oestrogen, metoclopramide, verapamil, domperidone, cocaine, and opiates), antipsychotics (phenothiazines, benzamides; sulpiride, butyrophenones; haloperidol, benperidol, risperidone, molindone, quetiapine), antidepressants (selective serotonin reuptake inhibitors (SSRI), tricyclics; chlomipramine, desipramine and mono amine oxidase inhibitors; pargyline, clorgyline), and adrenergic inhibitors (reserpine, methyldopa). Hyperprolactinaemia can occur also due to stalk compression or irritation such as in non-functioning PA, head injuries, and following cranial surgery, in hypothyroidism, and in prolactinomas. Prolactinomas present in females as secondary amenorrhea or irregularity of menstruation, infertility and galactorrhoea in 30–80% of patients. In males they present late with galactorrhoea in < 30%, VF defects, headaches, impotence and hypopituitrism.

b. **Growth hormone (GH):** GH over-secretion causes acromegaly in adults and gigantism in children. GH over-secretion may present in many forms and to different specialists, e.g. it may present to a paediatrician with gigantism, to a general physician with lethargy or sleep apnoea, to a neurologist with sleepiness, headaches, and paraesthesia, to an ophthalmologist with visual failure and field defects, to a dentist with malocclusion of teeth, or clicking jaw, to an ENT surgeon with snoring, sinusitis, large tongue, voice change, to a dermatologist with greasy thick skin, and sweating, to an orthopaedic/rheumatologist with large hands/feet (Figure 6-26), joint pains, or carpal tunnel syndrome, to a cardiologist with hypertension, or heart failure symptoms, to a gastroenterologist with large spleen and liver, to a diabetologist

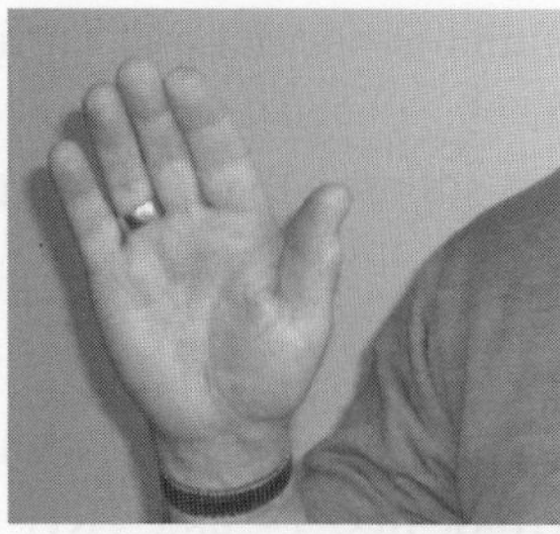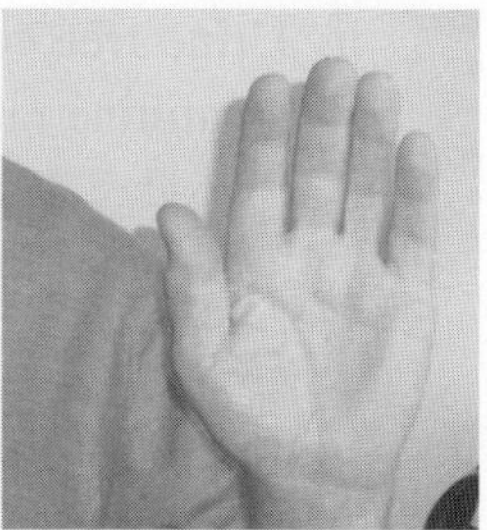

Figure 6-26: Photograph of acromegalic hands with other features listed.

with diabetes mellitus and to a urologist with polyuria, or urine calculi. The diagnosis is made by measuring IGF1 which would be markedly elevated compared to matched age and sex levels. The diagnosis is confirmed by glucose-tolerance-test (GTT). In normal individuals GH suppresses to < 5 mu/l after glucose ingestion whilst in acromegaly the GH is unchanged and shows no suppression or paradoxically rises. GH remains > 5 mu/l after glucose ingestion.

c. **ACTH and cortisol measurements**: Excess ACTH produces Cushing's disease if the source of the excess ACTH is PA or Cushing's syndrome if the source of excess ACTH is outside the pituitary. Excess cortisol leads to protein loss, myopathy and wasting of muscles, osteoporosis and bone fractures, thin skin, striae, and bruising; altered carbohydrate metabolism leading to diabetes mellitus; altered psyche leading to psychosis and depression; mineralocorticoid effects leading to hypertension and oedema, obesity, buffalo hump and round moon face; and excess androgens leading to virilism, hirsutism, acne and oligo/amenorrhoea in women. To distinguish Cushing's from obesity Cushing's is characterised by thin skin, proximal myopathy, frontal balding in women, conjunctival oedema (chemosis) and osteoporosis. To confirm the diagnosis of Cushing's disease dexamethasone suppression tests are performed:

   i. Overnight 1 mg dexamethasone suppression test: If cortisol level was < 50 nmol/l the next morning = normal, not Cushing's.

    ii. Urine free cortisol: Total < 250 units is normal and cortisol/ creatinine ratio of < 25 is normal.

    iii. Two-day 2 mg/day dexamethasone suppression test: Cortisol < 50 nmol/l six hours after last dose indicates that there is no Cushing's.

  d. **Complete pituitary function tests:** Required in patients with PA after treatment, these include — Thyroid: free T4 and TRH test. Gonadotrophins and in females oestradiol and LHRH test; in males testosterone. Adrenal; insulin tolerance test (ITT) and short synacthen test (SST) and glucagon test. GH: IGF1, ITT or glucagon and anti-diuretic hormone (ADH) water deprivation test (WDT).

6-2-6 *What is the differential diagnosis of PA?*

Lesions in the region of the sella are varied in nature:

1- PA is the most common (Figure 6-22).
2- Rathke's cleft cyst: Rathke's cleft cyst is a benign cystic lesion that affects the pituitary gland. It is the most common incidental finding in the pituitary and comprises about 3.7% of all the incidental findings that were greater than 2 mm and they tend to be medially located. Symptomatic Rathke's cleft cyst is relatively uncommon. When these cysts are large enough (Figure 6-26) they may cause headaches, visual disturbances, nausea, decreased energy, vomiting, seizures, pituitary dysfunction, and diabetes insipidus because of mass effect on the pituitary stalk, the third ventricles and the surrounding structures. Haemorrhage occasionally precipitates symptoms. The mean age at presentation is 34 years with female predominance. Relief of symptoms is common with operative management with resolution of symptoms in 78% of cases. The recurrence rate varies from 19–28%. During the third week of gestation an invagination of the floor of the third ventricle (the infundibulum) starts to coalesce to form the pituitary gland and another from the stomodeum (Rathke's pouch). The latter requires sequential induction from the neighbouring diencephalon to attain the morphology required to reach the

infundibulum. Both of these entities are from the ectoderm; Rathke's pouch develops into the anterior and middle lobes, and the infundibulum develops into the posterior lobe and stalk of the pituitary gland. The lumen that connects Rathke's pouch to the oral cavity begins to obliterate around the sixth week of gestation by the development of the sphenoid bone. The lumen of Rathke's pouch is usually obliterated by proliferation of the anterior and posterior walls of the pouch that will become the anterior and middle lobes. The apical extremity of the Rathke's pouch will remain as a small remnant into post-natal life and adulthood as a small cleft between the anterior pituitary (pars distalis) and the posterior pituitary (pars nervosa). The cleft is lined by columnar to cuboidal epithelium that is often ciliated and occasionally associated with mucous-secreting goblet cells. Accumulation of secretory products forms a cyst in this space. It should be noted that some authors have stated that one cannot differentiate a Rathke's cleft cyst from a neuroepithelial cyst, such as a colloid cyst of the third ventricle, based on histology or histochemistry. They propose that some Rathke's cleft cysts have neuroepithelial origin due to pinching off cells from the infundibulum into the cells that make up the dorsal wall of Rathke's pouch. On MRI they have several distinctive features. They are most often intrasellar cysts with or without suprasellar extension. Radiologically, it occurs as a single, well demarcated cyst without calcification (Figure 6-27). The content is homogenous. Depending on the content of the cyst, the MRI signal intensities can vary greatly. The radiological features overlap with that of craniopharyngioma particularly those with extensive cystic changes and without calcification. Histologically, they are lined by a single layer of cuboidal to columnar cells that are often ciliated. Occasional mucous cells may be present. Squamous metaplasia may occur and raises the possibility of a craniopharyngioma. Occasional cells of anterior pituitary gland may be present. In Rathke's cleft cysts that have substantial prior haemorrhage, there may be cholesterol cleft and foreign body giant cell reaction.

3- Arachnoid cyst: Arachnoid cysts in the sella are uncommon and can easily be confused both clinically and radiologically with intrasellar cystic pituitary neoplasms such as Rathke's cleft cysts,

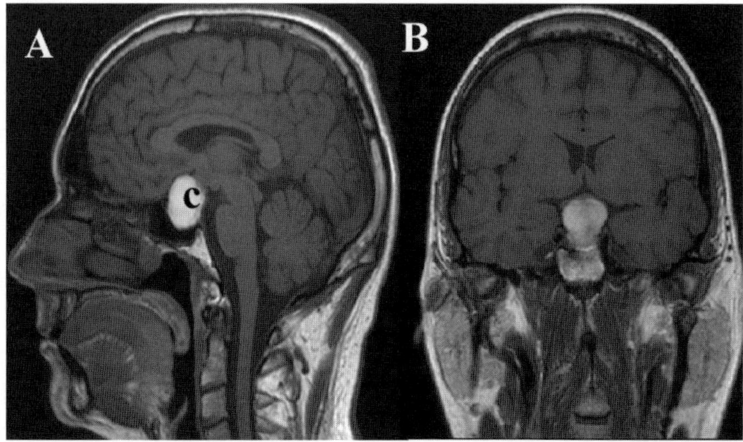

Figure 6-27: MRI scan demonstrating a Rathke's cleft cyst (c) in a 35-year-old man who presented with headaches and diplopia.

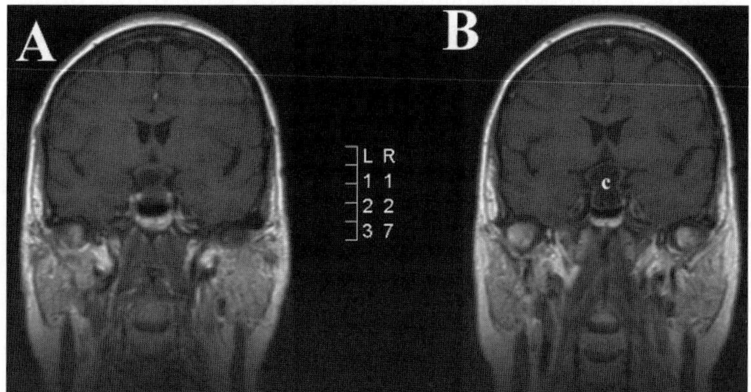

Figure 6-28: Sellar arachnoid cyst (c).

craniopharyngiomas or even empty sella. Adequate diagnosis is quite important because of different treatment modalities and different prognosis. Cystic lesions of the sellar and parasellar regions have a fluid-filled compartment and a connective tissue wall and/or epithelial lining but no communication with the subarachnoid space that distinguishes them from an empty sella (Figure 6-28). These lesions are classified according to the site of origin, tissue of origin and pathological features. They are broadly classified into primary and secondary cysts. The primary lesions arise within the sella and are confined to the pituitary fossa including true intrasellar arachnoid cysts (Figure 6-28), pituitary cysts, Rathke's cleft cysts and other rare types. Secondary non-neoplastic cystic lesions of the sella may arise from the sphenoid sinus or the parasellar region and extend into the fossa, as sphenoid sinus mucocele, arachnoid cysts, or Leptomeningeal cysts. Arachnoid cysts are lined by a single layer of mesothelial cells, surrounded by collagenous layer.

4- Sellar and suprasellar meningioma: Meningiomas constitute about 15% of all intracranial tumours and are the most common primary non-glial lesions. Suprasellar location is the fifth most common site of origin with 5%. Suprasellar meningioma arising from tubereculum sellea clinoid processes and diaphragma sellae may grow downward into the sella turcica. But pure intrasellar meningiomas are well-known lesions. These tumours seem to be exceptional and are thought to arise within the sella turcica and extend superiorly into the chiasmatic cistern, causing visual and endocrine dysfunction by compressing optic pathways and pituitary stalk. CT and MRI demonstrate contrast-enhancing intrasellar or suprasellar lesion (Figure 6-29). Serum prolactin levels may be slightly elevated and visual fields may

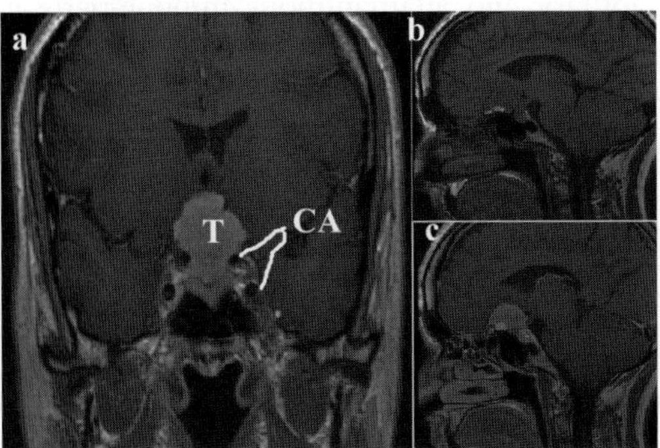

Figure 6-29: a = MRI showing suprasellar meningioma (T), CA = carotid artery. b = Before contrast and c = with contrast. This was a woman who presented with bitemporal VF defects and lethargy.

show bitemporal VF defect similar to that in Figure 6-21. Surgery is the main treatment with the aim of total resection.

5- Pituitary abscess: Pituitary abscess is a rare but potentially life threatening condition if not adequately diagnosed and treated. Since the first description in 1941, over 121 cases have been reported in the literature.[17] Pituitary abscess implies pituitary gland involvement by an infectious process within the sella turcica characterised by the presence of an acute or chronic inflammatory reaction. This process may derive from a localised or generalised infection source (meningitis, sepsis), facilitated or not by a previous existing sellar lesion such as adenoma, craniopharyngioma or Rathke's cleft cyst. Pituitary abscess is treated as an emergency by drainage and IV antibiotics.

6- Craniopharyngioma: Craniopharyngiomas are classified into two histopathologically and clinically distinct subtypes — adamantinous and squamous-papillary variants.[18] The adamantinous type consists of a predominantly cystic lobulated tumour, which is often observed in an intrasellar/suprasellar location in children. These cysts contain various amounts of cholesterol, triglycerides, methaemoglobin, protein, desquamated epithelium, and watery fluid content. Squamous-papillary craniopharyngioma, on the other hand, consists of a predominantly solid or mixed solid-cystic spherical tumour in a suprasellar location in adults. The solid tumour parts have an inhomogeneous but intense enhancement with small necrotic areas and calcifications. The combination of papillary and adamantinous tumour parts within the same neoplasm has been described in 15% of these tumours. Craniopharyngiomas arise anywhere along the migration of Rathke's pouch, which extends from the vomer and the roof of the nasopharynx, through the midline sphenoid bone to the floor of the sella turcica. Thus, craniopharyngiomas can potentially arise in unusual locations such as the nasopharynx,[18] sphenoid bone,[19] third ventricle,[20] and posterior fossa. Craniopharyngiomas are rare, they make up 6–10% of all childhood brain tumours with the majority of children being diagnosed between the ages of five and ten years old. However, they can grow into, and cause problems with, the pituitary and hypothalamus, and the third ventricle, and can damage the optic chiasm. Adverse prognostic factors include; young age at diagnosis, hydrocephalus, hypothalamic invasion, large size and optic chiasm compression. In children, cranio-pharyngiomas present with either raised ICP from hydrocephalus or slowly forming symptoms of pressure on adjacent structures. Raised ICP with hydrocephalus is found in 50%. Visual symptoms and hormonal deficiency, e.g. dwarfism and possibly diabetes insipidus and hypothalamic problems, for example obesity, represent other forms of presentations. MRI scan will be the best investigation to determine the diagnosis, location and extent of craniopharyngioma and provide the roadmap for treatment (Figure 6-30). The appearances of adamantinous and papillary subtypes are not dissimilar (Table 6-5).

CT brain can also be helpful in detecting craniopharyngiomas as they can demonstrate a cystic lesion in the suprasellar region with calcification (Figure 6-31).

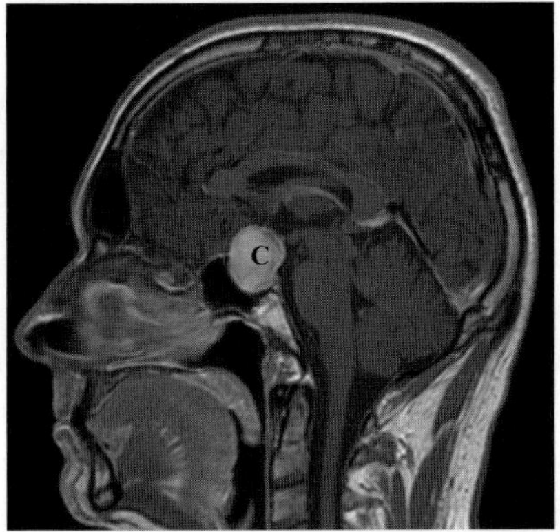

Figure 6-30: MRI of adamantinous craniopharyngioma (C) presenting in an adult with visual failure.

Table 6-5: MRI appearances of craniopharyngiomas

Craniopharyngioma	Adamantinous	Papillary
Site	Often suprasellar	Often third ventricle
Appearance	Predominantly cystic	Predominantly solid
T1 signal	Often hyperintense	Often isointense
T2 signal	Often hyperintense	Often hyperintense
Enhancement	Yes	Yes

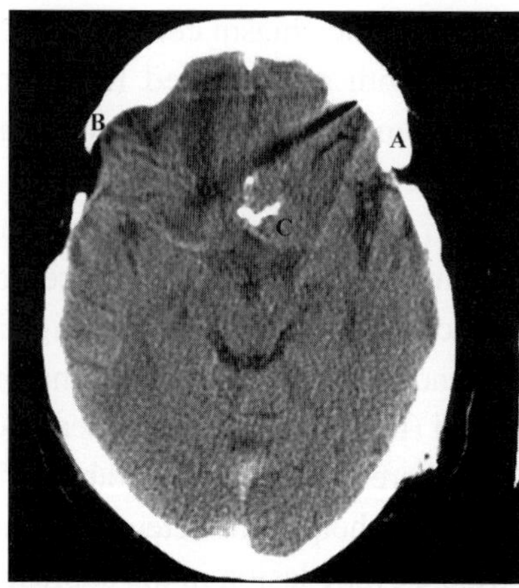

Figure 6-31: CT scan demonstrating calcified remnant of craniopharyngioma (C). Patient had bilateral pterional craniotomy (A and B) and VP shunt.

The main objectives of treatment are: lowering raised ICP, decompression of the optic apparatus, and preservation of pituitary functions. Complete surgical resection should be the aim of surgery followed by radiotherapy if a remnant was left after surgery. Hormonal replacement of any deficient hormones is instituted.

7. Metastases: Metastasis to the pituitary gland is a recognised complication in almost all extracranial cancers such as breast, lung, kidney, gut, thyroid, prostate and other cancers. The incidence of pituitary metastases varies from 0.14% to 28.1% of all brain metastases and is higher in autopsy series.[21] They most frequently originate from lung cancer in males and breast carcinoma in females. Pituitary metastases more commonly affect the posterior lobe and the infundibulum than the anterior lobe. A review of 201 reported cases showed that the frequency of involvement within the pituitary gland was 50.8% in the posterior lobe alone, 33.8% in both lobes, and 15.4% in the anterior lobe alone.[21] The predilection of metastases for the neurohypophysis may reflect the fact that the posterior lobe receives its blood supply directly from the inferior hypophyseal arteries, whereas the anterior lobe is nourished indirectly by portal vessels. On MRI scan pituitary metastases can be differentiated by their intrasellar and suprasellar

dumbbell-shaped appearance that indent the diaphragma sellae, which is morphologically different in pituitary adenoma that usually expands the diaphragma sellae.

8-　Chordoma: Clival chordoma is a locally aggressive and relatively rare tumour of the skull base that is thought to originate from embryonic remnants of the notochord. Chordomas account for 1% of all intracranial tumours and 4% of all primary bone tumours.[22] Chordoma may occur at any age but it is usually seen in adults, with peak prevalence in the fourth decade of life. Chordomas have a 2:1 male predilection. Clival chordomas constitute one-third of all chordomas. Although clival chordomas are generally slow-growing, their intimate relation to critical structures and their extremely high local recurrence rate have often resulted in high mortality. MRI and CT allow precise delineation of chordomas with respect to volume and relation to adjacent neural structures, thereby helping achieve their eradication. Generally, chordomas grow slowly and produce symptoms insidiously. Symptoms of intracranial chordomas vary with lesion location and proximity to critical structures, reflecting the specific sites of extension from the clivus; sellar, parasellar, and retroclival areas and, occasionally, the sphenoid sinus. The most common initial complaint is diplopia related to cranial nerve palsy and headaches. Among cranial nerves, the abducent nerve is the most commonly affected. Headache is usually reported in an occipital or retro-orbital location. The classic appearance of intracranial chordoma on CT is well-circumscribed, expansile soft-tissue mass that arises from the clivus with associated extensive lytic bone destruction. The bulk of the tumour is usually hyperdense relative to the adjacent brain. Intratumoral calcifications appear irregularly on CT and are usually thought to represent sequestra from bone destruction rather than dystrophic calcifications in the tumour itself. On conventional T1-weighted MR images, intracranial chordoma has intermediate to low signal intensity and is easily recognised within the high signal intensity of the fat of the clivus (Figure 6-32).

　　Small foci of hyperintensity can sometimes be visualised in the tumour on T1-weighted images, a finding that represents intratumoral

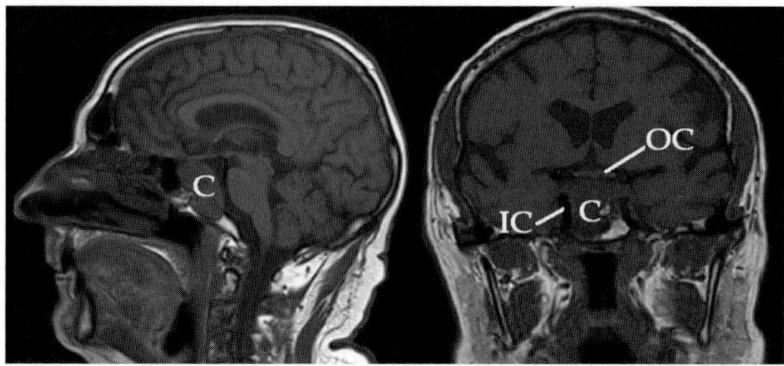

Figure 6-32: MRI scan demonstrating chordoma in a 35-year-old man who presented with diplopia due to sixth nerve palsy.

haemorrhage or a mucus pool. The presence of haemorrhagic foci can be confirmed with gradient-echo imaging that is susceptible to blood, at which the foci appear as dark areas. Classic intracranial chordoma has high signal intensity on T2-weighted images, a finding that likely reflects the high fluid content of vacuolated cellular composition. The intratumoral areas of calcification, haemorrhage, and highly proteinaceous mucus usually demonstrate heterogeneous hypointensity on T2-weighted imaging. Radical total resection with sparing of vital structures is the main treatment followed by radiation is the current therapy. The use of fractionated proton beam radiation therapy permits delivery of tumour doses 15–35% higher than those associated with standard external beam radiotherapy, allowing improved local control and higher survival rates.[22] The recurrence-free five-year survival rate for patients with skull base chordoma who undergo combined treatment with surgery and radiation therapy is 60–70%.

9- Mucocoele: Sphenoid sinus mucocele is rare and often misdiagnosed.[23] Since its first description, less than 150 cases have been reported in the literature. This benign, readily treatable lesion is potentially fatal if misdiagnosed. To make the correct diagnosis preoperatively careful radiological examination and interpretation is essential. The aetiology of paranasal mucoceles is controversial and usually occurs when drainage of a sinus is obstructed by inflammation, fibrosis, trauma, previous surgery or anatomical abnormality.[23] Mucoceles occur most commonly in the frontal and ethmoid sinuses but are quite infrequent in the sphenoid sinus.[24] Out of 63 reported cases, 29 patients (46%) had previous diagnosis of sinusitis, intranasal polyps, nasal mass or nasal discharge. The clinical and radiographic features of sphenoid sinus mucoceles are usually related to sinus expansion and extension of the lesion beyond the confines of the sinus. This usually follows the path of least resistance, namely anteriorly to involve ethmoid air cells and orbits, but occasionally posteriorly into the clivus and superiorly into the sella. Clinically the symptoms and signs are of orbital apex syndrome, superior orbital fissure syndrome and anterior cavernous sinus syndrome. The most common complaint was headache occurring in 55 out of 63 cases (87%). The headache is typically frontal or retro-orbital and tends to be worse towards evening. It may be due to dural stretching if the lesion breaks through the sella turcica. Visual symptoms often alert the patient and his physician to the problem; these occur in 62% with diplopia in 30%. Plain skull X-rays show opacification of the sphenoid sinus and any erosion of the sellar floor. Ballooning of the sella turcica characteristic of pituitary adenoma is unusual with sphenoid sinus mucocele. Very infrequently the petrous apex may be eroded. The sella was eroded in 29 out of 63 cases reviewed (46%). CT and bone window studies are essential for evaluating the cribriform plate, the roof of the ethmoid sinuses, the involvement of the supraorbital ethmoid extension and extension into the superior orbital fissure. Mucoceles appear isodense, hypo- or hyperdense and lack contrast enhancement but may show rim enhancement. MRI is better than CT in delineating sphenoid muco- celes and their relationship to sellar and parasellar anatomy. They have higher protein content, resulting in a shorter T1 and longer T2 that produce high signals on both T1- and T2-weighted images. Surgical drainage is the primary treatment leading to cure in most cases.

10- Giant aneurysms: Aneurysms in the sellar and parasellar regions can arise from the internal carotid artery and the anterior communicating artery (Figure 6-33).

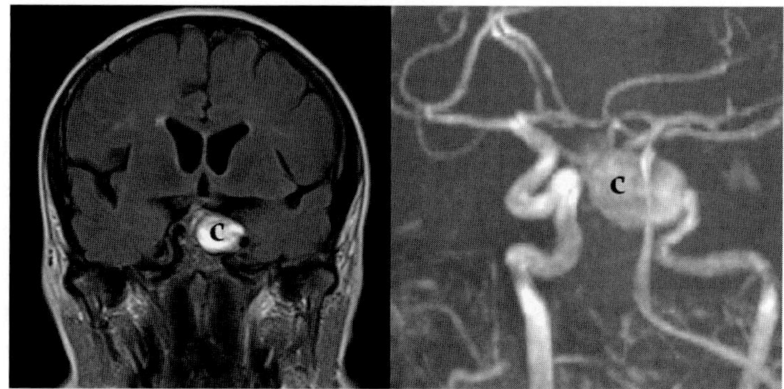

Figure 6-33: Giant aneurysm from the internal carotid artery.

References

1. Claus EB. Epidemiology of intracranial meningiomas. *Neurosurgery* 2005; 57: 1088–1095.

2. Black P. Meningiomas. *Neurosurgery* 1993; 32: 643–658.

3. Eljamel MS. Multiple meningiomas. *J Neurosurg* 1990; 72(5): 834–835.

4. Eljamel MS, Foy PM. Multiple meningiomas and their relation to neurofi-bromatosis. Review of the literature and report of seven cases. *Surg Neurol* 1989; 32(2): 131–136.

5. Musa BS, Pople IK. Intracranial meningiomas following irradiation — a growing problem? *Br J Neurosurg* 1995; 9: 629–637.

6. Brenner AV, Linet MS, Fine HA *et al.* History of allergies among adults with glioma and controls. *Int J Cancer* 2002; 99: 252–259.

7. Hsu DW, Efird JT, Hedley-Whyte ET. Progesterone and oestrogen receptors in meningiomas: prognostic considerations. *J Neurosurg* 1997; 86: 113–120.

8. Hemminki K, Li X, Collins VP. Parental cancer as a risk factor for brain tumours (Sweden). *Cancer Causes Control* 2001; 12: 195–199.

9. Oruckaptan HH, Senmevsim O, Ozcan OE *et al.* Pituitary adenomas: results of 684 surgically treated patients and review of the literature. *Surg Neurol* 2000; 53: 211–219.

10. Yildiz F, Zorlu F, Erbas T *et al.* Radiotherapy in the management of giant pituitary adenomas. *Radiother Oncol* 1999; 52: 233–237.

11. Amar AP, Hinton DR, Krieger MD *et al.* Invasive pituitary adenomas: significance of proliferation parameters. *Pituitary* 1999; 2: 117–122.

12. Anson JA, Segal MN, Baldwin NG *et al*. Resection of giant invasive pituitary tumors through a transfacial approach: technical case report. *Neurosurgery* 1995; 37: 545–546.

13. Ebersold MJ, Quast LM, Laws ER Jr *et al*. Long-term results in transsphenoidal removal of nonfunctioning pituitary adenomas. *J Neurosurg* 1984; 64: 713–719.

14. Majos C, Coll S, Aguilera C *et al*. Imaging of giant pituitary adenomas. *Neuroradiology* 1998; 40: 651–655.

15. Meij BP, Lopes MB, Ellegala DB *et al*. The long-term significance of microscopic dural invasion in 354 patients with pituitary adenomas treated with transsphenoidal surgery. *J Neurosurg* 2002; 96: 195–208.

16. Scheithauer BW, Kovacs KT, Laws ER Jr *et al*. Pathology of invasive pituitary tumors with special reference to functional classification. *J Neurosurg* 1986; 65: 733–744.

17. Vates GE, Berger MS, Wilson CB. Diagnosis and management of pituitary abscess: a review of twenty-four cases. *J Neurosurg* 2001: 95; 233–241.

18. Kanungo N, Just N, Black M, *et al*. Nasopharyngeal craniopharyngioma in an unusual location. *Am J Neuroradiol* 1995; 16: 1372–1374.

19. Graziani N, Donnet A, Bugha TN *et al*. Ectopic basisphenoidal craniopharyngioma: case report and review of the literature. *Neurosurgery* 1994; 34: 346–349.

20. Linden CN, Martinez CR, Gonzalvo AA *et al*. Intrinsic third ventricle craniopharyngioma: CT and MR findings. *J Comput Assist Tomogr* 1989; 13: 362–368.

21. Kucharczyk W, Lenkinski RE, Kucharczyk J *et al*. The effect of phospholipid vesicles on the NMR relaxation of water: an explanation for the MR appearance of the neurohypophysis? *Am J Neuroradiol* 1990; 11: 693–700.

22. Dahlin DC, MacCharty CS. Chordoma: a study of 59 cases. *Cancer* 1952; 5: 1170–1178.

23. Chui MC, Briant TD, Gray T *et al*. Computed tomography of sphenoid sinus mucocele. *J Otolaryngol* 1983; 12: 263–269.

24. Hesselink JR, Weber AL, New PFJ *et al*. Evaluation of mucoceles of the paranasal sinuses with computed tomography. *Radiology* 1979; 133: 397–400.

Your personal notes:

....

....

....

....

....

....

....

....

....

....

Chapter 7: Hearing Loss, Ataxia, Vertigo and Facial Pain (CPA Lesions)

Problem 7-1:   Hearing loss and cerebellopontine angle (CPA) lesions. How to manage a patient presenting with hearing loss?

Any patient presenting with unilateral hearing loss with or without vertigo and tinnitus could have CPA lesion.

Problem based toolkit:

Deafness	**Dizziness**
Tinnitus	**Vertigo**

CPA meningioma

CPA epidermoid cyst

Vestibular schwannoma

PCS7-1-1:

A 68-year-old man presented with slowly worsening left hearing loss first noticed 18 months ago when he did not seem to hear the alarm clock while a sleep on his right side. He tried his phone on both ears and was not able to hear as clearly in the left ear compared to his right. He went to his family practitioner who examined his ears and did not find any earwax or any other external ear problem and observed normal eardrums. He was referred to the local otolaryngology. Examination revealed that his hearing was reduced on the left. Air conduction (AC) was better than bone conduction (BC) in both ears and Weber's test lateralised to the good ear (right). He went on to have pure tone audiogram that confirmed sensory neural deafness on the left and MRI scan that confirmed a CPA lesion consistent with vestibular schwannoma.

7-1-2 What causes unilateral sensory neural deafness?

1- Vestibular schwannoma (VS) (most common 92%).

2- CPA meningiomas (second most common 3–7%).

3- Epidermoid cyst (2–6%).
4- Trigeminal schwannoma.
5- Facial schwannoma.

The main presentation of VS is unilateral sensory neural hearing loss with high frequency and speech discrimination being the most affected. Tinnitus and dizziness are common but true vertigo is rare. As the VS expands into the CPA it stretches the adjacent cranial nerves. The facial nerve is very resistant to stretch and facial weakness is very rare in VS. (If facial weakness is a feature of CPA lesion think of facial schwannoma.) If VS expands superiorly the trigeminal nerve will be affected with reduced corneal reflex or facial numbness. Trigeminal neuralgia is rare in VS. *VS is the diagnosis until proven otherwise by imaging in any patient presenting with unilateral sensory neural hearing loss and reduced ipsilateral corneal reflex or ipsilateral facial numbness.* With further VS enlargement the cerebellum and brain stem will be affected and ataxia or long tract signs may be detected clinically. Downward growth of the VS may result into compression of the lower cranial nerves leading to difficulty in swallowing, aspiration or hoarseness. In very large VS the fourth ventricle can be obstructed leading to hydrocephalus, papilloedema and reduced level of consciousness.

CPA meningioma presents slightly different in that they often present with facial pain similar to trigeminal neuralgia, facial weakness and then hearing loss. Trigeminal schwannoma presents with trigeminal nerve dysfunction such as facial numbness and impaired sensation rather than trigeminal neuralgia. CPA lesions presenting with multiple lower cranial nerve dysfunctions are unlikely to be one of the above lesions and may well be malignant in nature such as metastases.

7-1-3 *What is the epidemiology of VS?*

VS represent about 6% of all intracranial tumours. They are benign, slow-growing tumours, which arise from Schwann-cells in the nerve sheath that surrounds the vestibular nerves. Their growth is slow and difficult to predict in individual patients. The advent of MRI had resulted in the diagnosis of asymptomatic VS in patients who were scanned for other unrelated conditions.[1–3] The incidence of VS is around 13 cases/million/year.[4] However, the incidence was reported to have increased over the last 20 years.[5] This increased incidence is probably a reflection of better diagnostic methods, ageing population and availability of MRI, rather than a true increase in VS incidence. The median age at diagnosis is approximately 50 years.[2] The tumours are unilateral in more than 90%,[6] affecting the right and left sides with equal frequency.

7-1-4 *What are the risk factors for VS?*

The vast majority of VS are sporadic and unilateral in more than 90%.[6] Bilateral vestibular schwannomas are primarily limited to patients with autosomal dominant neurofibromatosis (NFII).[7]

7-1-5 *What is the natural history of VS?*

VS are slow growing tumours. The growth rate of individual VS cannot be predicted accurately. However, many studies had demonstrated that these tumours are slow growing and may shrink in size spontaneously.[8–10] Some authors recommended an initial one year radiological surveillance in all small VS and if they grew in the first year they were treated.[8] Others recommended that surveillance should be abandoned in favour of intervention if the tumour grew by 2 mm in the first year.[9,10]

7-1-6 *What investigations should a patient with unilateral hearing loss have? What is the interpretation of these tests?*

All patients presenting with unilateral hearing loss should have the following examinations:

- Thorough neurological examination.
- Extra-ocular movements.
- Funduscopic examination.
- Facial motor and sensory functions.
- Auroscopy/Weber/Rinne tests.

- Hitselberger's sign (loss of sensation in the ear canal supplied by Arnold's nerve (branch of Vagus nerve to the ear).
- Gag reflex and Sternocliedomastoid and trapezium muscles.
- Pure tone and speech discrimination audiometry (Figure 7-1)
- Impedance audiometry (acoustic reflex and tone decay).
- Auditory brainstem evoked response (ABR) (Figure 7-2).
- Vestibular testing (ENG).
- Neuro-imaging:

    1- MRI: MRI is the investigation of choice in patients suspected to have VS. On a FLAIR (fluid attenuated inversion recovery) or CISS (constructive interference in steady state) sequence where liquid signals are suppressed by inversion-recovery at an adapted TI, VS appear as dark signal (Figure 7-3).

    On T1-weighted MRI sequence VS appears as isointense or slightly hypointense that enhances with gadolinium homogenously

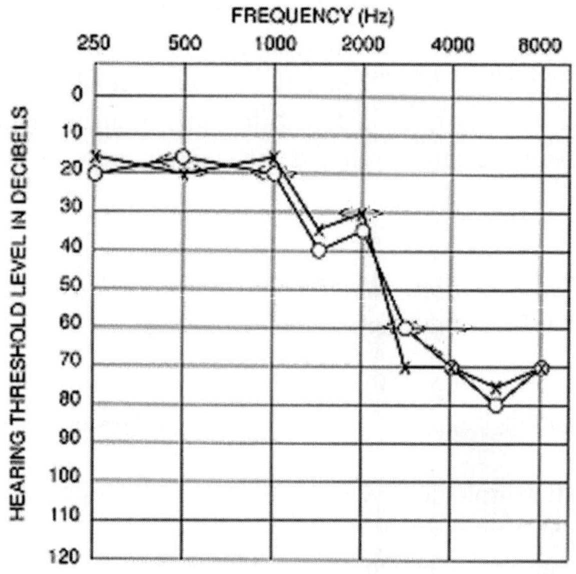

Figure 7-1: Pure tone audiogram. In VS hearing loss usually in the high frequency and if the hearing loss is more than 50 decibels the hearing is not useful.

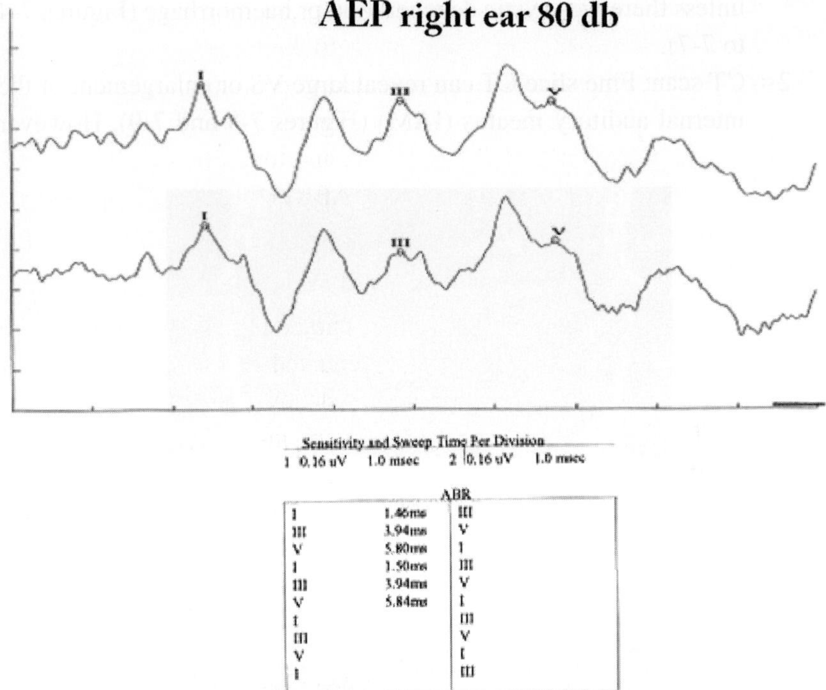

Figure 7-2: AER (AEP): Wave I originates from cochlear nerve, II = dorsal and ventral cochlear nucleus, III = superior olivary complex, IV = nucleus of lateral lemniscus, V = inferior colliculus, VI = medial geniculate body, and VII = auditory radiation (cortex).

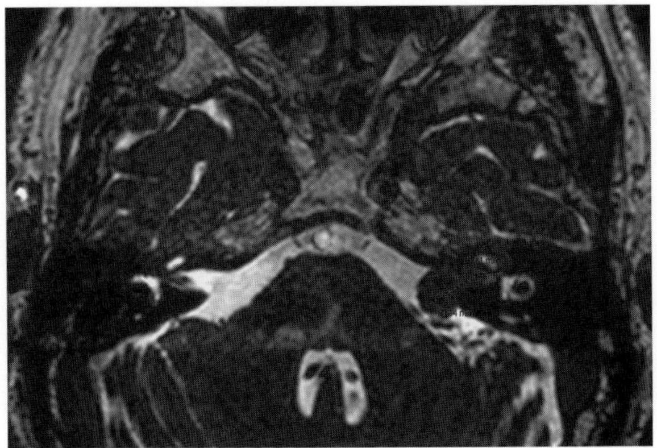

Figure 7-3: Left VS on CISS 3D MRI scan.

unless there was cystic degeneration or haemorrhage (Figures 7-4 to 7-7).

2-   CT scan: Fine slice CT can reveal large VS or enlargement of the internal auditory meatus (IAM) (Figures 7-8 and 7-9). However

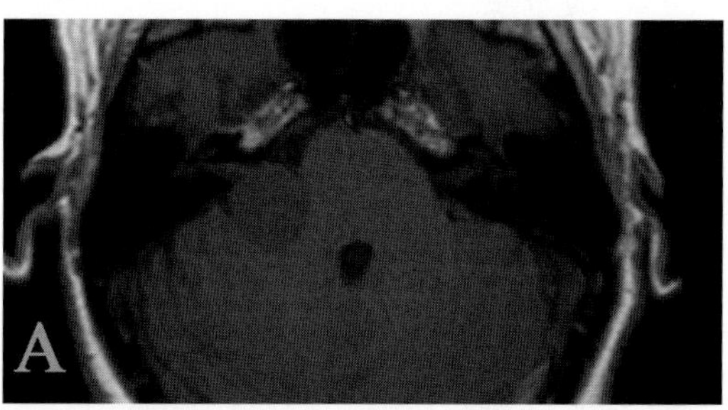

Figure 7-4: Right VS on T1-weighted MRI before contrast (a). The VS is slightly hypointense and globular in shape.

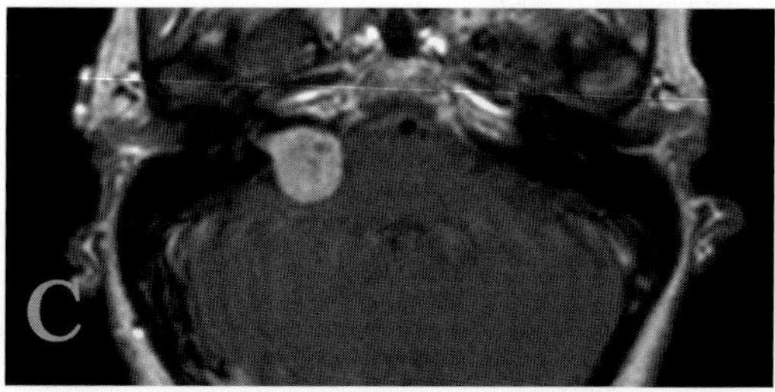

Figure 7-5: Same right VS after IV gadolinium, note VS enhances homogenously.

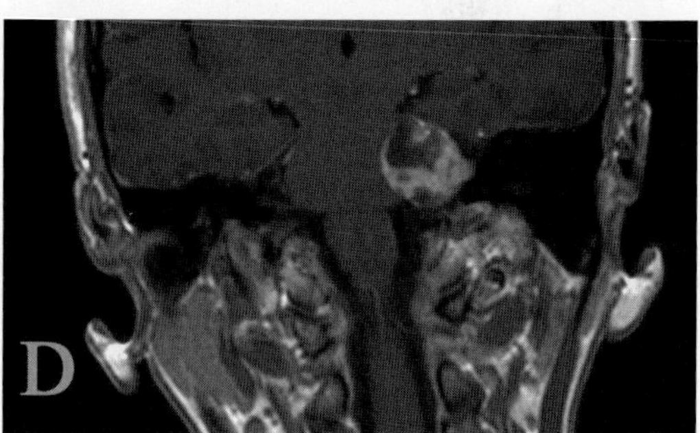

Figure 7-6: VS with gadolinium demonstrating cystic degeneration.

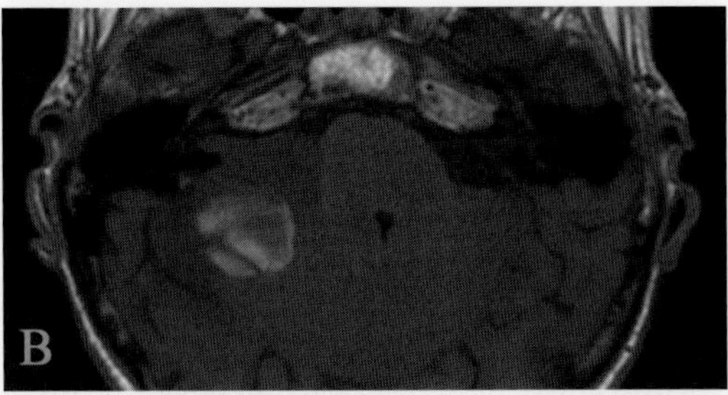

Figure 7-7: Large right VS slightly hypointense with high signal posteriorly due to haemorrhage.

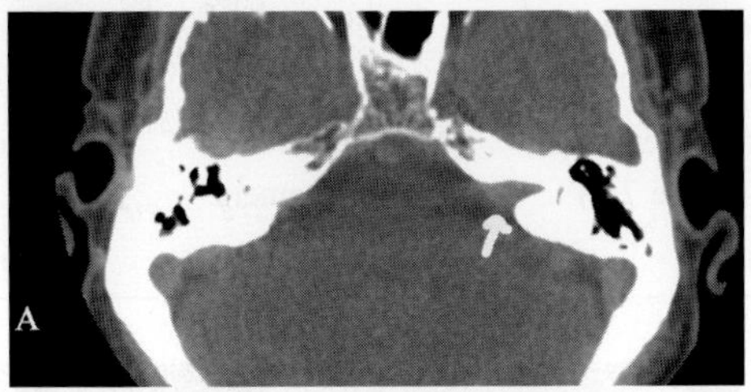

Figure 7-8: CT scan demonstrating enlargement of the left IAM (arrow).

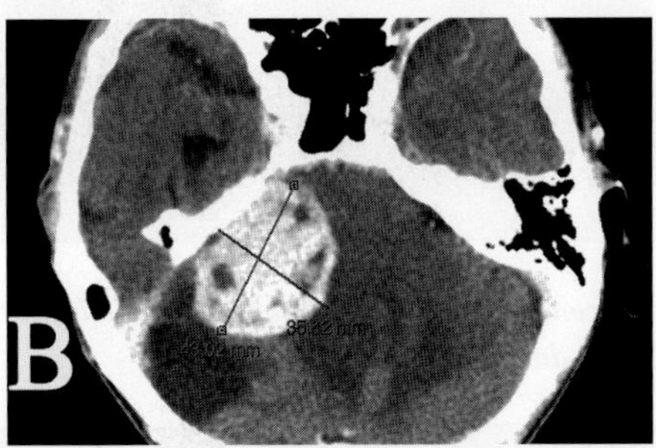

Figure 7-9: CT scan demonstrating large right VS.

the sensitivity of CT is very low and CT nowadays only used to identify the jugular bulb to avoid a high one during surgery.

7-1-7 *How to recognise VS, CPA meningioma and epidermoid of CPA?*

Table 7-1 summarises the difference between VS and CPA meningioma and CPA epidermoid cyst.

Table 7-1: The difference between VS, CPA meningioma and CPA epidermoid

Diagnosis	VS	CPA meningioma	CPA epidermoid
Location	Centred to IAM	Eccentric to IAM	Anterior/posterior to brain stem
Bone changes	Enlarges IAM	Hyperostosis occasionally	Bone erosion
Shape	Spherical or ice cream shaped (Figure 7-4)	Hemispherical or en plaque (Figure 7-10)	Irregular shape and dumbbell (Figure 7-11)
Appearance	Isodense on CT and lower signal on T1 (Figure 7-4)	Hyperdense and more likely to show calcification	Hypodense
Enhancement	Strongly enhance (Figure 7-5)	Moderate enhancement	None
Dural tail	None	Often present	None

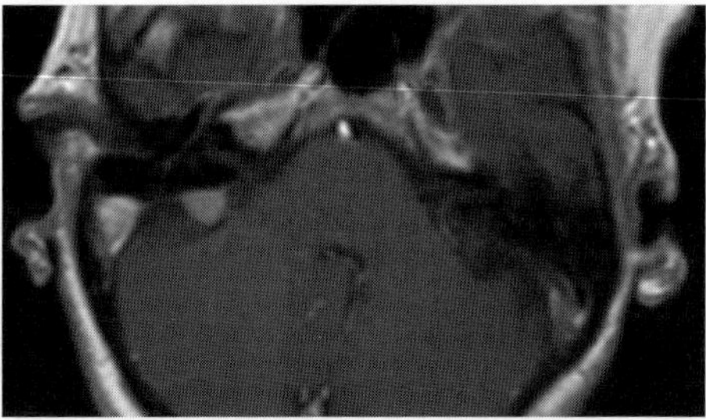

Figure 7-10: MRI with contrast of CPA meningioma, note location eccentric to IAM, hemispherical shape, wide dural base with small tail.

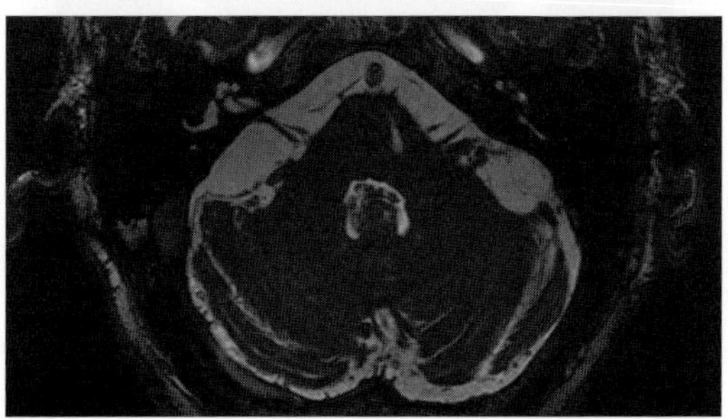

Figure 7-11: MRI scan (CISS) of an epidermoid cyst in the right CPA region.

7-1-8 *How to manage VS?*

The management of VS is close surveillance, microsurgical removal or stereotactic radiosurgery.

1- Conservative radiological surveillance is justified at least in the first 12 months after diagnosis in small VS and has become more popular as many studies have demonstrated that VS are slow growing and may shrink in size spontaneously.[8–10] Surveillance should be abandoned in favour of intervention if the tumour grew by 2 mm in the first year.[9,10] Another group recommended intervention for tumours of 15 mm or bigger and radiological surveillance could be stopped if tumours were unchanged after five years.[11]

2- Microsurgery is recommended in tumours over 3 cm in diameter and in the presence of brain stem compression and hydrocephalus. Surgical approaches of CPA lesions vary depending on the pathologic entity as well as the size and involvement of adjacent structures. While complete excision is planned for most cases, the intimate involvement of surrounding structures may impose unwarranted morbidity if complete excision is attempted. Meningiomas are excised completely more readily than epidermoids, whereas adequate therapy for arachnoid cysts is drainage. Standard approaches to the CPA include the translabyrinthine, suboccipital (retrosigmoid = RS), or middle fossa (MCF) craniotomies. The choice of approach is based on specific location and hearing status. Occasionally, these craniotomies can be combined or performed in addition to an infratemporal fossa dissection for larger tumours. In a large series of 1000 VS, a group of multidisciplinary team achieved total excision in 97.9%, with serviceable hearing in 47%, good eye closure in 79%, facial weakness in 48% and mortality of 1.1%.[12] In small tumours < 3 cm in diameter normal facial function had been preserved in more than 90%, hearing was preserved in 57% and mortality was 0.16%. If one of the goals of surgery was to preserve hearing then the retrosigmoid (RS) or middle cranial fossa (MCF) approaches would be preferred. If the VS was mainly in the CPA, the RS approach would be preferable and for intracanalicular VS the MCF approach would be preferred. Otherwise the translabrynthine approach is preferred by some teams although drilling the pertrous bone can take significantly longer time than the RS approach. The largest reported series of 1000 surgically treated VS at the time of discharge from the hospital, 73% of the patients in this series had satisfactory facial nerve function with complete eye closure; 59% showed good function (House-Brackmann (HB) Grades 1 and 2), and 14% with HB Grade 3 were expected to recover within weeks to months. In cases of nerve discontinuity or loss of the facial nerve stump at the brain stem, it is recommended that reconstruction be performed immediately by transplantation or by nerve reanimation with a donor nerve, respectively. Cochlear nerve deafness can be prevented in increasing numbers by increasing the rates of anatomic (68%) and functional (39%) nerve preservation. The RS approach is the only one that enables hearing preservation regardless of tumour size. Good pre-operative hearing and small tumour sizes are favourable factors. The mortality rate was 1.1% in this study. It may be lowered if patients with severe pre-operative morbidity do not undergo surgery or if they are not transferred from other centres at a last desperate moment but at a time when surgery still offers a realistic lifesaving chance. Cystic schwannomas require special surgical and post-surgical attention, because they are more dangerous to remove with regard to brain stem and facial nerve integrity and are more likely to lead to haemorrhage in the acute and subacute postoperative periods.

3- Stereotactic radiosurgery (SRS): SRS had become a universally accepted treatment option for small VS (< 3 cm in diameter). Ninety-four per cent tumour control rate, 77% normal facial preservation rate and 51% hearing preservation rate was reported with SRS.[13] In view of the natural history of VS not changing or shrinking in size in the majority of cases[8–10] the reported tumour control rate may be misleading. However, the lack of mortality remains attractive to patients and the small risk of malignant transformation may be a persuading factor to other patients to favour other options.

Your personal notes:

....

....

....

....

....

....

....

....

....

....

Problem 7-2:   Facial pain and trigeminal neuralgia. How to manage a patient presenting with facial pain?

Not every patient presenting with facial pain has trigeminal neuralgia (TN). Facial pain can be the only presentation of invasive skull base tumours and you need to keep this in mind. As a result in current medical practice it would be advisable that these patients have at least one MRI scan of the head and the skull base before merely diagnosing TN.

> **Problem based toolkit:**
> **Atypical Trigeminal neuralgia**
> **Classical Trigeminal neuralgia**
> **Facial pain**
> **Microvascular decompression**
> **Percutaneous rhizotomy**

PCS7-2-1:

A 49-year-old female presented with lancinating pain in the right side of her face for two weeks. She was unable to sleep, eat, laugh or talk because of the pain. There were no other features. She had several episodes in the past since 2004. Her pain was sharp and stabbing in nature and scored 10 on VAS (Visual Analogue Scale). There were no relieving factors and no obvious triggers apart from laughing, eating and talking. She was receiving carbamazepine 100 mg tid. The family doctor tried paracetamol, codeine, diazepam, and Ibuprofen without any lasting effect. She had no drug allergies. Neurological and systemic examinations were normal.

7-2-2 What is the differential diagnosis of facial pain?

1-   Classical or idiopathic trigeminal neuralgia (ITN).
2-   Symptomatic or Atypical TN (ATN) which is trigeminal neuralgia with unusual features, e.g. facial numbness.
3-   Tempero-mandibular pain arising from TM Joint.
4-   Jaw claudication as a result of temporal (giant cell) arteritis.
5-   Toothache arising from tooth related infections, e.g. abscess.
6-   Maxillary sinusitis.

When considering an underlying pathology, think of:

i- CPA lesions: Vestibular schwannoma, epidermoid, facial schwannoma and meningioma.

ii- MCF tumours: Trigeminal neuroma, and cavernous sinus meningioma.

iii- Skull base tumours: Meningioma, chordoma, invasive pituitary adenoma, metastasis, and nasopharyngeal carcinoma.

iv- Demyelination.

v- TMJ arthritis.

vi- Temporal giant cell arteritis.

vii- Maxillary conditions: Sinusitis and tumours.

viii- Tooth abscess.

7-2-3 *How to manage a patient with facial pain?*

This patient had already been investigated with MRI scan to rule out an underlying pathology and vascular compression (Figure 7-12). The MRI scan ruled out MS, CPA lesion (Figures 7-13 and 7-14), middle cranial fossa lesions (Figures 7-15 and 7-16) and skull base lesion (Figures 7-17 to 7-19). It was confirmed vascular compression at surgery.

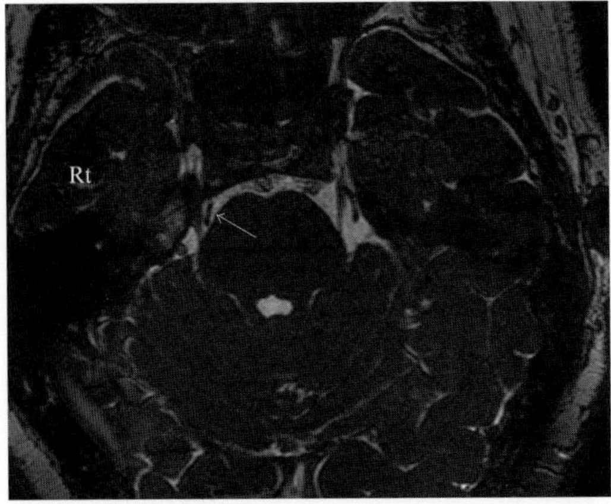

Figure 7-12: MRI inversion recovery (CISS) revealing vascular compression (arrow) of trigeminal nerve presenting with ITN.

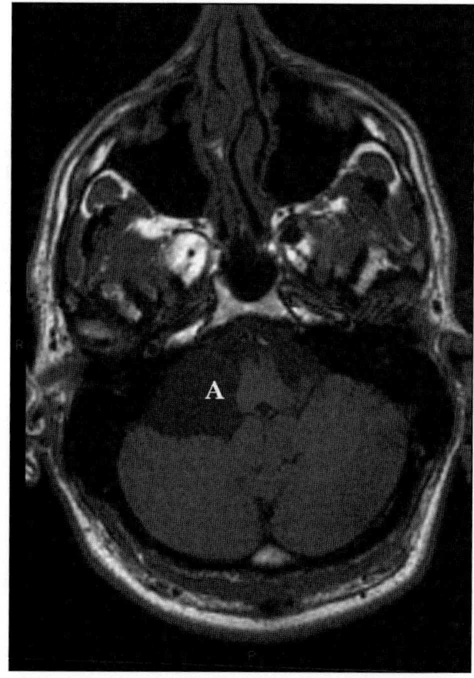

Figure 7-13: MRI (CISS) demonstrating PCF epidermoid cyst (A) in a 31-year-old male presenting with ATN.

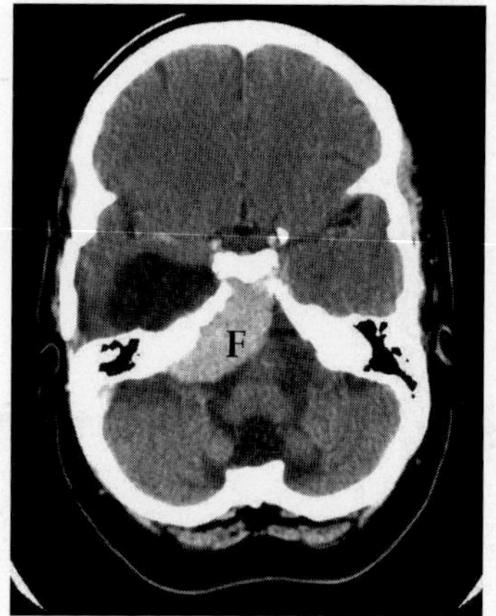

Figure 7-14: CT scan with contrast demonstrating clival meningioma (F) in a 35-year-old presenting with mild hemiparesis and ATN.

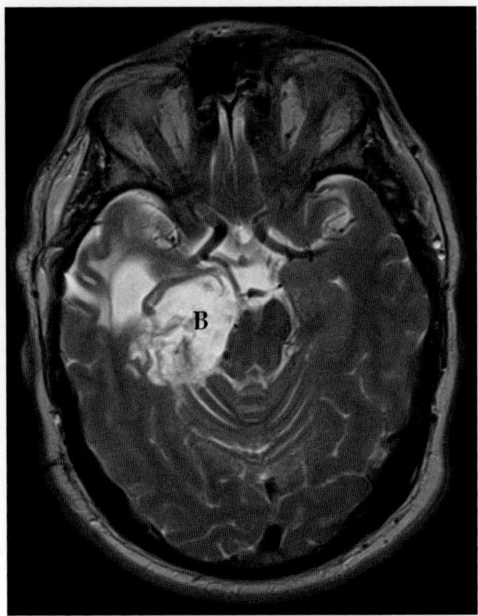

Figure 7-15: MRI (T2) demonstrating MCF epidermoid cyst (B) in a 40-year-old female presenting with ATN.

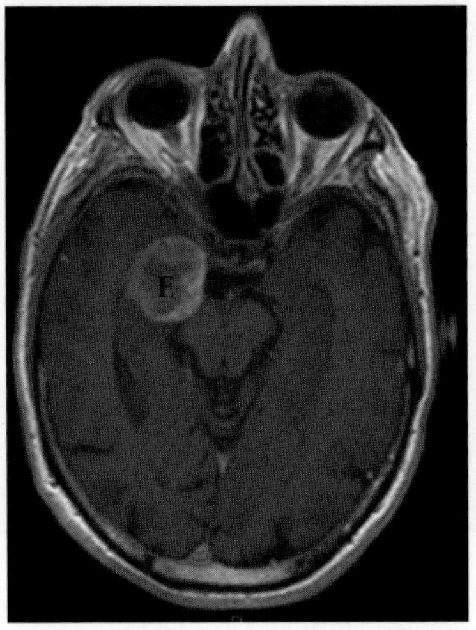

Figure 7-16: MRI (T1 with contrast) demonstrating MCF meningioma (E) in a 65-year-old female presenting with ATN and partial III nerve palsy.

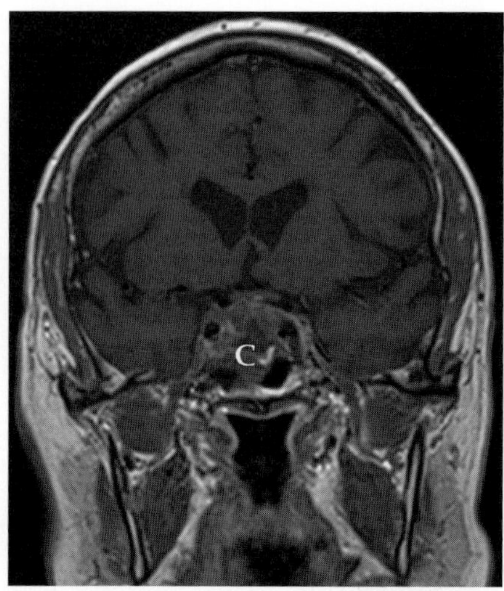

Figure 7-17: MRI with contrast demonstrating skull base invasive chordoma (C) in a 45-year-old man presenting with ATN and partial III nerve palsy.

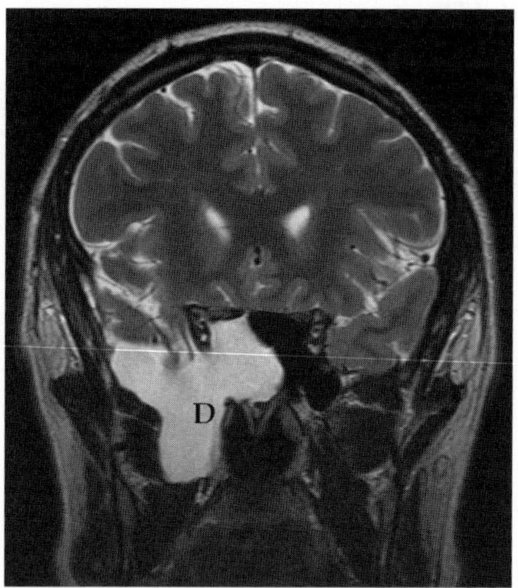

Figure 7-18: MRI (T2) demonstrating fibrous dysplasia of the skull base (D) in a 30-year-old male presenting with ATN and headaches.

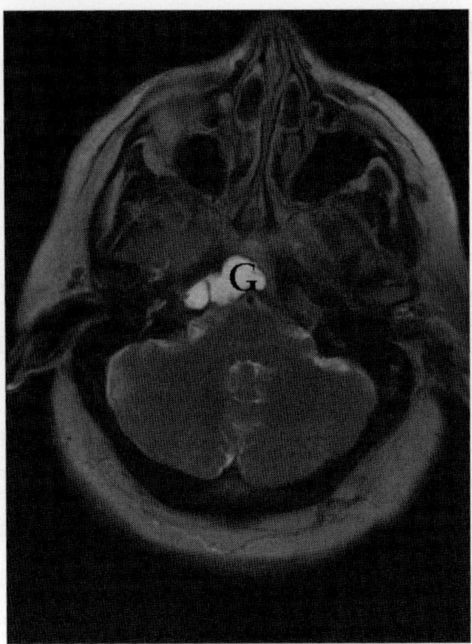

Figure 7-19: MRI (T2) demonstrating cholesterol cyst (G) in the petrous apex in a patient presenting with ATN.

7-2-4 *What is the epidemiology of ITN?*

ITN or tic douloureux is a neuropathic disorder of one or both of the trigeminal nerves. It is relatively rare and affects around four to five per 100,000 of the population and is twice as common in females.[14] Its incidence increases with age and is rare among people below the age of 40 years. It is characterised by sudden, lancinating, severe facial pain that is often described as "stabbing" or "shooting", which lasts for minutes at a time. It remits and relapses and often worsens over time. It is often made worse by chewing, laughing, shaving, and exposure to cold wind.

7-2-5 *What is TN?*

Trigeminal neuralgia (also known as tic douloureux) has been defined by the International Association for the Study of Pain as "sudden, usually unilateral, severe brief stabbing recurrent pains in the distribution of one or more branches of the fifth cranial nerve".[15] Usually the second (V2 maxillary) and third (V3 mandibular) divisions are more affected than the first

(V1 ophthalmic), with only around 3% of cases occurring bilaterally. Other symptoms include tingling or numbness in the face before the development of pain and spasms that can last from a few seconds to minutes each time.

7-2-6 *What are the classification of TN?*

The International Headache Society has classified TN into classical (ITN) and symptomatic trigeminal neuralgia (ATN).[16] Included in ITN are all the cases without an established aetiology such as idiopathic and those with vascular compression. The majority of cases within this group are classified as idiopathic. However there is increasing evidence that 80–90% of these cases are caused by an aberrant loop of artery or vein compressing the trigeminal nerve close to its root entry into the pons.[14] Such evidence includes: an aberrant loop of the artery or vein being found compressing the trigeminal nerve of patients at surgery; demyelination of the trigeminal nerve; after surgery for decompression most patients experience long term relief and improvement of any sensory defects.[17,18] A diagnosis of ATN is made secondary to a number of different causes, including tumours, multiple sclerosis and structural abnormalities of the skull base as described above.[19] Approximately 1–5% of patients suffering from MS will develop trigeminal neuralgia.[17]

7-2-7 *What is the diagnostic criteria and natural history of TN?*

Attacks occur infrequently and can last from several days to weeks at a time, however when these attacks settle the patient can become pain free for months at a time. During severe attacks the patient can experience spasms of pain hundreds of times a day. For the majority of trigeminal cases the diagnosis is clinical. The International Headache Society has put forward the following diagnostic criteria for trigeminal neuralgia:

A- Paroxysmal attacks of pain lasting from a fraction of a second to two minutes, affecting one or more division of the trigeminal nerve and fulfilling criteria B and C.
B- Pain has at least one of the following characteristics:

    a- Intense, sharp, superficial or stabbing.
    b- Precipitated from trigger areas or by trigger factors.

C- Attacks are stereotyped in the individual patient.
D- There is no clinically evident neurological deficit.
E- Not attributed to another disorder.

Trigger factors stated in the above criteria include certain actions or movements such as: chewing, speaking, washing the face, tooth-brushing, cold winds or even touching a specific "trigger spot" on the face. Frequently the pain described in many cases does not exactly fit these criteria, for example, a constant ache between the paroxysms or mild sensory loss in the face. These cases have been named "atypical" or mixed trigeminal neuralgia and are usually more likely to be due to symptomatic disease rather than classical trigeminal neuralgia.

A review in the *European Journal of Neurology*[18] recommended that for patients with non-trigeminal neurological symptoms, routine imaging should be considered to identify ATN. Electrophysiological studies may also prove useful for distinguishing ATN from ITN. Five studies looked at the accuracy of using electrophysiological testing. This was found to be relatively high, especially when using trigeminal reflexes. Of particular note from the review was the lack of evidence to either support or refute the usefulness of MRI in identifying ITN patient.

7-2-8 *How to manage ITN?*

The main aim of treating ITN is to control the pain. Drug therapy is the first line treatment, commonly using anticonvulsants. From the limited evidence available, carbamazepine is the drug of choice[20,21] and proves effective in most patients (and also may confirm the diagnosis). However many patients develop side effects including drowsiness, ataxia, nausea and constipation. If the patient responds and goes into remission, the dosage can be gradually lowered. If carbamazepine was intolerable or ineffective there are a number of second line drugs, although the evidence is weaker for their usage. Oxcarbazepine is found to be better tolerated (fewer side effects) and being a pro-drug of carbamazepine, is often the chosen alternative. Gabapentin is also generally effective in dealing with neuropathic pain; however the evidence is lacking of its specific use in treating trigeminal neuralgia. Other drugs which may benefit when pain control is limited include baclofen, lamotrigine and phenytoin.

If medical therapy does not work then a review of the diagnosis should be made. Surgical options should then be considered if there is persistence of the pain. Surgical interventions for trigeminal neuralgia can be classified according to the principal treatment target, splitting the treatment options into four groups: peripheral techniques targeting portions of the trigeminal nerve distally to the ganglion; percutaneous ganglion techniques targeting specifically the ganglion; gamma knife radiosurgery targeting the trigeminal root and posterior fossa vascular decompression techniques. Peripheral techniques involve blocking or destroying portions of the trigeminal nerve, using substances such as alcohol or phenol. Studies have shown that these techniques only provide temporary relief, with 50% of patients having recurrence of pain after one year. The morbidity of these procedures is low. Percutaneous procedures on the ganglion itself entail penetrating the foramen ovale with a cannula and then controlled compression, chemical or thermocoagulation of the trigeminal ganglion or root.[22] The methods include: thermal (radiofrequency thermocoagulation), chemical (injection of glycerol, which is corrosive to the nerve fibres thus mildly injuring the nerve enough to hinder the pain signals) or mechanical (compression by a balloon inflated into Merkel's cave). Percutaneous techniques have been particularly helpful in treating elderly patients for whom surgery is contraindicated due to co-existing health conditions. These procedures are usually very effective at providing pain relief (around 90%). This figure drops though to 72% after three years for patients who underwent the thermal method.[22] Several side effects have been reported with this group with almost some patients experiencing sensory loss. Around 4–6% developed dysaesthesias/anaesthesia dolorosa (troublesome sensory disturbance) as a result of the destructive technique. Post-operatively around 12% complain of discomfort, which dramatically increases with the balloon technique, with around half of all patients suffering temporary masticator problems.[23] The mortality of these procedures, however, is extremely low. Gamma knife radiosurgery is the only technique which involves aiming a focused beam of radiation at the point where the trigeminal nerve leaves the brain (posterior fossa), in order to destroy it. Initially there was quite a high percentage of patients experiencing complete pain relief but the number falls to around 50% by three years.[23] Also, as the previous group, the complications are 6% suffering from sensory complications. Facial numbness is also reported, although this has been seen to improve with time. Lastly, microvascular decompression allows exploration of the CPA to look for any vessels compressing the nerve. These are then moved out of contact with the nerve and a non-absorbable sponge is inserted to prevent the vessel from returning to its offending position. As with the other groups the initial percentage of patients who are pain-free is around 90%, dropping to 80% after one year. However the figure after five years is the highest with around 73% of patients still pain-free.[22] On average the mortality associated with this procedure is between 0.2–0.5% depending on patient selection. Other major problems related to the surgery include CSF leaks, infarcts and haematomas, with the commonest complication being aseptic meningitis. Other complications to note include hearing loss and transient diplopia, though they are rare.

References

1. Lin D, Hegarty JL, Fischbein NJ *et al*. The prevalence of incidental acoustic neuroma. *Arch Otolaryngol Head Neck Surg* 2005; 131: 241–244.
2. Propp JM, McCarthy BJ, Davis FG *et al*. Descriptive epidemiology of vestibular schwannomas. *Neuro-oncol* 2006; 8: 1–11.
3. Selesnick SH, Jackler RK, Pitts LW. The changing clinical presentation of acoustic tumors in the MRI era. *Laryngoscope* 1993; 103(4): 431–436.
4. Moffat DA, Hardy DO, Baguley DM. Strategy and benefits of acoustic neuroma searching. *J Laryngol Otol* 1989; 103: 51–59.
5. Tos M, Charabi S, Thomsen J. Incidence of vestibular schwannomas. *Laryngoscope* 1999; 109: 736–740.
6. Edwards CG, Schwartzbaum JA, Lonn S *et al*. Exposure to loud noise and risk of acoustic neuroma. *Am J Epidemiol* 2006; 163: 327–333.
7. Eldridge R, Parry D. Vestibular schwannoma (acoustic neuroma). Consensus development conference [see comments]. *Neurosurgery* 1992; 30: 962–964.
8. O'Reilly B, Murray CD, Hadley DM. The conservative management of acoustic neuroma: a review of forty-four patients with magnetic resonance imaging. *Clin Otolaryngol* 1999; 25: 82–86.

9. Smouha EE, Yoo M, Mohr K *et al.* Conservative management of acoustic neuroma: a meta analysis and proposed treatment algorithm. *Laryngoscope* 2005; 115(3): 450–454.

10. Nedzelski JM, Schessel DA, Pfleiderer A *et al.* Conservative management of acoustic neuromas. *Otolaryngol Clin N Am* 1992; 25(3): 691–705.

11. Stangerup SE, Caye-Thomasen P, Tos M *et al.* The natural history of vestibular schwannoma. *Otol Neurotol* 2006; 27(4): 547–552.

12. Samii M, Matthies C. Management of 1000 vestibular schwannomas (acoustic neuromas): surgical management and results with an emphasis on complications and how to avoid them. *Neurosurgery* 1997; 40: 248–262 http://www.c3.hu/~mavideg/ns/samii1-97.html.

13. Kondziolka D, Lunsford LD, McLaughlin MR *et al.* Long-term outcomes after radiosurgery for acoustic neuromas. *N Engl J Med* 1998; 339: 1426–1433.

14. Bennetto L, Patel NK, Fuller G. Trigeminal neuralgia and its management. *Br Med J* 2007; 332: 201–205.

15. Zakrzewska JJM, Linskey ME. Neurosurgical interventions for the treatment of classical trigeminal neuralgia (Protocol). *Cochrane Database Syst Rev* 2008, Issue 3.

16. Headache Classification Subcommittee of the International Headache Society. The International Classification of Headache Disorders, 2nd edition. *Cephalalgia* 2004; 24(Suppl 1): 9–160.

17. Nurmikko TJ, Eldridge PR. Trigeminal neuralgia — pathophysiology, diagnosis and current treatment. *Br J Anaesth* 2001; 87: 117–132.

18. Love S, Coakham HB. Trigeminal neuralgia: pathology and pathogenesis. *Brain* 2001; 124: 2347–2360.

19. Nurmikko TJ, Eldridge PR. Trigeminal neuralgia — pathophysiology, diagnosis and current treatment. *Br J Anaesth* 2001; 87: 117–132.

20. Wiffen P, Collins S, McQuay H *et al.* Anticonvulsant drugs for acute and chronic pain. *Cochrane Database Syst Rev* 2005, Issue 3.

21. Wiffen PJ, McQuay HJ, Edwards JE *et al.* Gabapentin for acute and chronic pain. *Cochrane Database Syst Rev* 2005, Issue 3.

22. Haridas A, Mathewson C, Eljamel S. Long-term results of 405 refractory trigeminal neuralgia surgeries in 256 patients. *Zentralbl Neurochir* 2008; 69(4): 170–174.

23. Gronseth G, Cruccu G, Alksne J *et al.* Practice parameter: the diagnostic evaluation and treatment of trigeminal neuralgia (an evidence-based review): report of the Quality Standards Subcommittee of the American Academy of Neurology and the European Federation of Neurological Societies. *Neurology* 2008; 71: 1183–1190.

Your personal notes:

....
....
....
....
....
....
....
....
....
....

Chapter 8: Tremor (Parkinson's Disease and Dystonia)

Problem 8-1:   Tremor and Parkinson's disease. How to manage a patient presenting with tremor?

Tremor and movement disorders are symptoms of other neurological disorders. The underlying pathology is often progressive and treatment is often symptomatic. Some of these disorders may respond to surgery.

Problem based tool box:

Tremor

Essential tremor

Rubral tremor

Parkinson's disease

Parkinsonism

PCS8-1-1:

A 75-year-old man presented with a two-year history of right-sided hand tremor and freezing of speech. His gait was satisfactory at that time and he was given Levodopa and benserazide hydrochloride. His symptoms gradually deteriorated and two and a half years after his initial presentation he developed right side leg tremor and bradykinesia (slowness of movement). Selegiline and propranolol were added to his medications.

He deteriorated gradually and three years after his initial presentation he underwent a left-sided deep brain stimulation (DBS) procedure. Postoperatively he developed dysphasia which was very brief and resolved spontaneously. One month after his DBS implantation he developed a moderate degree left sided tremor which was not apparent previously. His right sided tremor was under excellent control by the left sided DBS. One year after his DBS surgery his Parkinson's disease had progressed and his movements became slower although he still had very good control of the right sided tremor. One and a half years after his left side DBS, the tremor, rigidity and bradykinesia on the left had become worse so a right side DBS was inserted (Figure 8-1).

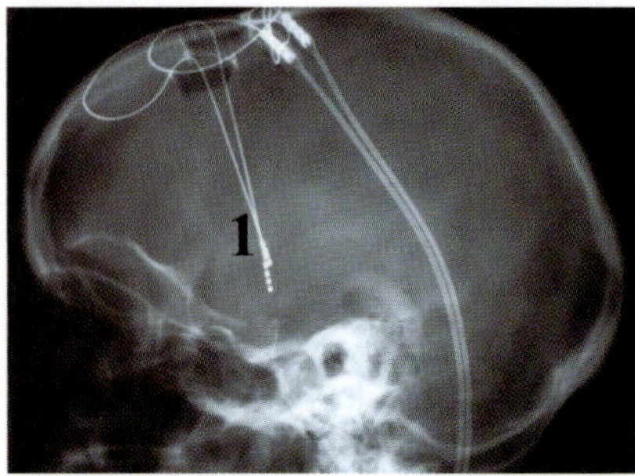

Figure 8-1: Plain radiograph of the skull demonstrating bilateral DBS (1). Note the DBS leads are connected at the scalp level to lead extenders tunneled subcutaneously in the neck to reach an implantable pulse generator (IPG) located in the left subclavicular region.

8-1-2 *What is the differential diagnosis of tremor?*

The differential diagnosis in a patient presenting with tremor includes:

- Tremor of Parkinson's disease (PD).
- Essential tremor (ET).
- Rubral tremor (RT).
- Dystonia.
- Other movement disorders.

8-1-3 *What is Parkinson's disease (PD) and Parkinsonism?*

PD is a movement disorder characterised by muscle rigidity, tremor, and bradykinesia and, in extreme cases, a loss of physical movement (akinesia). The primary symptoms are the results of decreased stimulation of the motor cortex by the basal ganglia, normally caused by insufficient formation and action of dopamine. Secondary symptoms may include high level cognitive dysfunction and subtle language problems. PD is the most common cause of chronic progressive Parkinsonism, a syndrome of tremor, rigidity, bradykinesia and postural instability. While many forms of parkinsonism are "idiopathic", "secondary" cases may result from drug side effects (metclopromide, chlorpromazine and haloperidol), head trauma, or other medical disorders. The disease is named after James Parkinson, who made a detailed description of PD in 1817.

PD prevalence is estimated at being from 120–180 per 100,000.

8-1-4 *How to treat PD?*

At present, there is no cure for PD, but medications or surgery can provide relief from symptoms.

The most widely used form of treatment is L-dopa in various forms. L-dopa is transformed into dopamine in the dopaminergic neurons by L-aromatic amino acid decarboxylase. However, only 1–5% of L-DOPA enters the dopaminergic neurons. The remaining L-DOPA is often metabolised to dopamine elsewhere, causing a wide variety of side effects. Due to feedback inhibition, L-dopa results in a reduction in the endogenous formation of L-dopa, and eventually becomes counterproductive. Carbidopa and benserazide are dopa decarboxylase inhibitors. They help prevent the metabolism of L-dopa before it reaches the dopaminergic neurons and are generally given as combination preparations of carbideopa/levodopa (Sinemet) and benserazide/levodopa (Madopar). There are also controlled release versions of Sinemet and Madopar that spread out the effect of the L-dopa. The second type of drug treatment includes COMT inhibitors: (Tolcapone) prolonging the effects of L-dopa, and so has been used to complement L-dopa. However, it can cause liver failure. Dopamine agonists are the second line anti-PD drug treatment. Bromocriptine, pergolide, pramipexole, ropinirole, piribedil, cabergoline, apomorphine, and lisuride are moderately effective. These have their own side effects including somnolence, hallucinations or insomnia. Several forms of dopamine agonists have been linked with a markedly increased risk of addictive gambling. Dopamine agonists initially act by stimulating some of the dopamine receptors. However, they cause the dopamine receptors to become progressively less sensitive; thereby increasing the symptoms of PD. Dopamine agonists can be useful for patients experiencing on-off fluctuations and dyskinesias as a result of high doses of L-dopa. Apomorphine can be administered via subcutaneous injection using a small pump which is carried by the patient. A low dose is automatically administered throughout the day, reducing the fluctuations of motor symptoms by providing a steady dose of dopaminergic stimulation. After an initial "apomorphine challenge" in hospital to test its effectiveness and educate the patient and primary caregiver it can be continued in the community. The injection site must be changed daily and rotated around the body to avoid the formation of granulation nodules and infection. MAO-B inhibitors such as selegiline and rasagiline reduce the symptoms by inhibiting monoamine oxidase-B (MAO-B). MAO-B breaks down dopamine secreted by the dopaminergic neurons, so inhibiting it will result in inhibition of the breakdown of dopamine. Metabolites of selegiline include L-amphetamine and L-methamphetamine that cause side effects such as insomnia.

8-1-5 *What is the surgical treatment of PD?*

Advanced PD patients may require deep brain stimulation (DBS). Several targets were used such as the ventral intermediate nucleus (VIM) of the thalamus, the internal segment of globus pallidus (Gpi) and subthalamic nucleus (STN). Initially lesions were used to treat PD (Figure 8-2) but DBS was found as effective, less risky and reversible.[1]

The preferred target of DBS in PD is STN (Figure 8-3). DBS controls tremor in up to 86% of patients and improves other symptoms by 60–80%.

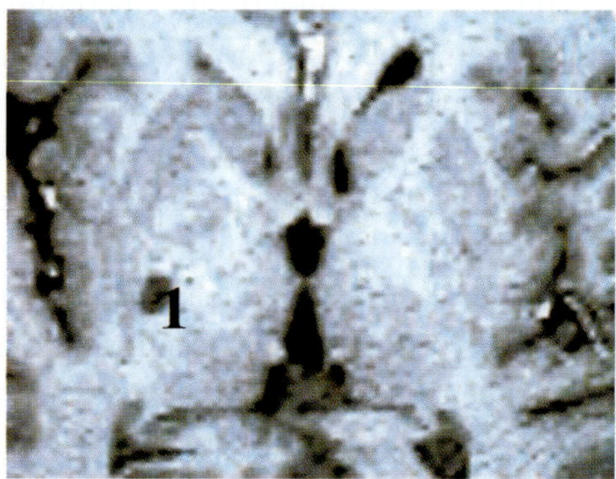

Figure 8-2: Axial MRI image demonstrating a lesion in the right Gpi (1).

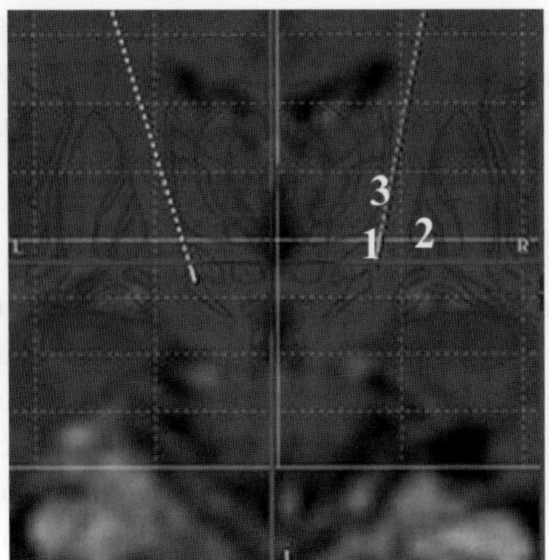

Figure 8-3: Coronal MRI image of basal ganglia with the stereotactic atlas superimposed demonstrating the STN (1), Gpi (2) and VIM (3).

8-1-6 *What are the indications for surgery in PD?*

The indications for surgery in PD are: advanced PD that failed medical treatment either because of side effects or lack of sustainable response, PD must be L-dopa responsive and the patient does not suffer from severe cognitive dysfunction, severe depression or uncorrectable bleeding disorder.

8-1-7 *What is essential tremor (ET)?*

ET is familial progressive neurological disorder manifesting with tremor of arms that is apparent during voluntary movements such as eating and writing. This type of tremor is often referred to as "kinetic tremor". The tremor may affect the head (neck), jaw, speech and other body regions. Women are more likely to develop head tremor than men. Other types of tremor: postural tremor of the outstretched arms, intentional tremor of the arms and rest tremor in the arms may also occur. Some patients may have unsteadiness and problems with gait and balance. Recent studies have demonstrated that old-onset ET may be associated with an increased risk of developing dementia.[2] ET is one of the most common neurological diseases and the second most common tremor after physiological tremor in the population, with a prevalence of approximately 4% of those over 40 years of age. Although ET is often mild, patients with severe tremor have difficulty performing many of their routine activities of daily living.

8-1-8 *How to treat ET?*

There are no effective drugs against ET, however patients often observed that the tremor is significantly reduced with drinking alcohol, and it can also be reduced by propranolol. Propranolol improves tremor in 50–60% of patients and 15–20% of responders develop tolerance. Primidone has also been used in ET with similar response as propranolol. However, as with propranolol, primidone is most beneficial for essential hand-tremor, and efficacy against head and speech tremor is variable. The duration of effect after a single dose is approximately 24 hours. As with propranolol, after 12 months of therapy approximately 10–15% of responders may develop tolerance to primidone.

8-1-9 *What is the surgical treatment of ET?*

Vim-DBS is effective against ET in 80–90% of patients (Figure 8-4). Patients should be considered for surgery if their tremor was severe enough to interfere with activities of daily living, and they do not suffer from severe cognitive decline, severe depression or uncorrectable bleeding disorders.

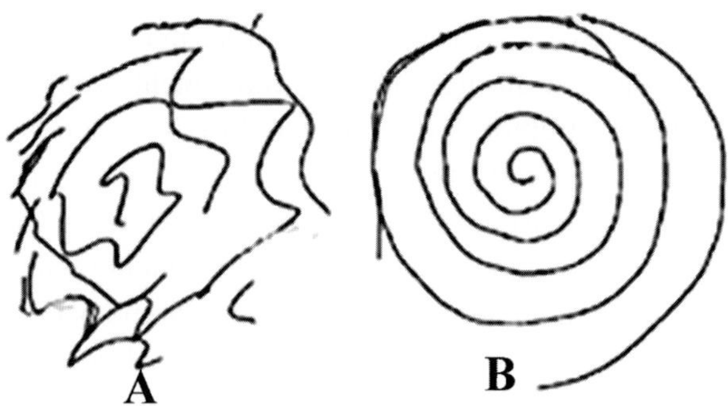

Figure 8-4: Photograph of Archimedes spiral in a patient with ET: (A) before the DBS was switched on and (B) after the DBS was switched on.

8-1-10 *What is rubral tremor (RT)?*

RT is characterised by a slow coarse tremor at rest that is exacerbated by postural adjustments and by guided voluntary movements. Lesions of the superior cerebellar peduncle, midbrain tegmentum or posterior part of the thalamus may cause this peculiar tremor, and it is probable that lesions of the red nucleus itself are not crucial for its production. RT often complicates MS and there is no effective drug treatment for it. The same medications used for ET can be used and VIM-DBS can also be used with some success.

Your personal notes:

....

....

....

....

....

....

....

....

....

....

Problem 8-2:   Movement disorders and dystonia. How to manage a patient with dystonia?

Dystonia should be distinguished from other movement disorders such as tremor, and dyskinesia as their management is different.

Problem based tool box:

Dystonia

Primary dystonia

Secondary dystonia

8-2-1 *What is dystonia?*

Dystonia is characterised by sustained muscle contractions causing twisting and repetitive movements or abnormal postures. The disorder may be hereditary or caused by other factors such as birth-related or other physical trauma, infection, poisoning (lead) or reaction to drugs.

8-2-2 *How to classify dystonia?*

Dystonia can be generalised (GD), focal (FD) or segmental (SD) in distribution. The incidence of GD is about one in 2,000,000. Examples of FD include:

1- Cervical dystonia causes the head to rotate to one side (spasmodic torticollis (ST)), to pull down towards the chest, or back (retrocollis), or a combination of these postures.
2- Blepharospasm causes rapid blinking of the eyes or even their forced closure.
3- Focal hand dystonia (also known as musician's or writer's cramp) interferes with writing or playing a musical instrument by causing involuntary muscular contractions.

8-2-3 *What causes dystonia?*

The causes of dystonia are not yet known or understood; however, they are categorised as follows:

- *Primary dystonia* is caused by pathology in the basal ganglia, and the GABA producing neurons. The precise cause of primary dystonia is unknown. In many cases it may involve genetic predisposition.

- *Secondary dystonia* is brought on by identified cause, usually involving brain injury, or chemical imbalance. Some cases of (focal) dystonia are brought on after trauma, are induced by certain drugs (tardive dystonia), or the result of (Wilson's disease).

Environmental and task-related factors are suspected to trigger the development of focal dystonias because they appear disproportionately in individuals who perform high precision hand movements such as musicians, engineers, architects and artists.

8-2-4 *How to treat dystonia?*

Treatment of dystonia has been limited to minimising the symptoms of the disorder as there is yet no successful treatment for its cause. Reducing movements that trigger or worsen dystonic symptoms provides some relief, as does reducing stress, getting plenty of rest, moderate exercise, and relaxation techniques. Various treatments focus on sedating brain functions or blocking nerve communications with the muscles by drugs, neuro-suppression or denervation. Drug treatment is often ineffective. Medications that have had positive results in some patients include: diphenhydramine, benzatropine, trihexyphenidyl, diazepam, benzatropine, and acetylcholine. Botulinum toxin injections into affected muscles have proved quite successful in providing some relief for around three to six months, depending on the kind of dystonia. Botox injections have the advantage of ready availability and the effects are not permanent. There is a risk of temporary paralysis of the muscles being injected or the leaking of the toxin into adjacent muscle groups causing weakness or paralysis. The injections have to be repeated as the effects wear off and around 15% of recipients will develop immunity to the toxin. There is a Type A and Type B toxin approved for treatment of dystonia. Dopamine-responsive dystonia, can be completely treated with regular doses of L-DOPA in a form such as Sinemet.

8-2-5 *What is the surgical treatment of dystonia?*

Baclofen intrathecal infusion pump has been used to treat patients of all ages exhibiting muscle spasticity along with dystonia. The pump delivers baclofen via a catheter into the spinal thecal sac. Surgical denervation of selected muscles may provide some relief; however, the destruction of nerves in the limbs or neck is not reversible and should only be considered in the most extreme cases. DBS has proven successful in a number of cases of severe generalised dystonia. The target in dystonia is bilateral Gpi DBS stimulation.

8-2-6 *What other surgical treatments for functional disorders?*

There are a number of established and emerging surgical techniques for the treatment of functional disorders. These interventions are not curative and should only be performed within specialist centres with appropriate infrastructure of multidisciplinary teams. They should only be performed in patients with treatment refractory disorders who are able to consent and have realistic understanding of the goals of therapy. These techniques include:

1- Vagus nerve stimulation (VNS) for treatment refractory epilepsy.
2- VNS for treatment refractory depression.
3- Subgenual cingulate DBS for treatment refractory depression.
4- Anterior capsular DBS for treatment refractory obsessive compulsive disorders (OCD).
5- Anterior capsulotomy for treatment refractory OCD.
6- Anterior cingulotomy for treatment refractory depression.
7- Anterior thalamic DBS for treatment refractory epilepsy.

References

1. Schuurman PR, Bosch DA, Bossuty PMM *et al*. A comparison of continuous thalamic stimulation and thalamotomy for suppression of severe tremor. *N Engl J Med* 2000; 342: 461–468.
2. Bermejo-Pareja F, Louis ED, Benito-Leon J. Risk of incident dementia in essential tremor: a population-based study. *Mov Disord* 2007; 22: 1573–1580.

Your personal notes:

....
....
....
....
....
....
....
....
....
....

Chapter 9: Para-/Tetraparesis (Spinal Compression)

Problem 9-1: Bilateral limb paresis (malignant spinal compression). How to manage suspected malignant spinal compression?

Patients suspected of malignant cord compression require immediate admission, investigations and appropriate management to prevent serious morbidity.

> **Problem based tool box:**
> **Malignant spinal compression**
> **Paraparesis** **Sensory level**
> **Tetraparesis**

PCS9-1-1:

A 64-year-old right-handed man presented with four days history of reduced mobility. The immobility began gradually and slowly progressed. He also complained of weakness in the right leg and reduced sensation on the left side of his body up to the waist. He had dull aching pain between the shoulder plates. He was able to feel when he wanted to pass urine and was able to control it until it was convenient. Physical examination revealed that he had weakness of all muscle groups in the left lower extremity grade 4, and 4+ on the right. His ankle and knee jerks were brisk compared to his biceps and triceps jerks and his planters were upgoing. He had impaired sensation to pain from T6 downwards on the right sparing the saddle area. There was no other significant history.

9-1-2 What is the differential diagnosis of bilateral leg weakness?

A patient presenting with acute gradual onset paraparesis with sensory level has spinal compression until proven otherwise. Abnormal lower limbs and normal upper limbs locate the lesion below T1 spinal cord segment. The presence of brisk reflexes and upgoing planters locate the lesion above the conus and a sensory level at T6 puts the lesion around the T6 segment. A unilateral sensory level on the right and more weakness on the left put the lesion on the left side of the spinal cord because the pain is transmitted in spinothalamic tracts that cross over to the contralateral side few segments above the level in the spinal cord and the descending motor fibres cross high up in the medulla oblongata. The pathological differential diagnosis would be;

- Malignant extradural spinal cord compression (MSC).
- Benign spinal cord compression (BSC).
- Other non-compressive causes, e.g. traverse myelitis.

9-1-3 *What investigations would you do in suspected MSC?*

1- Full blood count looking for anaemia or polycythemia that may be associated with malignancy. This was normal in this patient.
2- Chest X-ray looking for primary or secondary in the lungs. The chest X-ray was clear in PCS9-1-1 above.
3- C-reactive protein (CRP) and ESR/Plasma Viscosity (PV) to see if it was elevated indicating malignancy or infection. The CRP and PV were elevated in the patient (PCS91-1).
4- MRI spine covering the thoracic spine to confirm or rule out the suspected diagnosis (Figures 9-1 and 9-2) and the rest of the spine to rule out other metastases.
5- CT spine of the involved level to assess the integrity of the spine if internal fixation of the spine was planned.

PCS9-1-4:

A 78-year-old woman presented with low back pain radiating into both legs associated with urinary incontinence of seven days duration. When she was examined she had bilateral leg weakness with reduced reflexes and impaired sensation from S2 downward. The saddle area was also involved.

The differential diagnosis in this patient is the same as in problem case scenario PCS9-1-1. However, the fact that she had reduced reflexes bilaterally means the lesion's location is in the cauda equina rather than

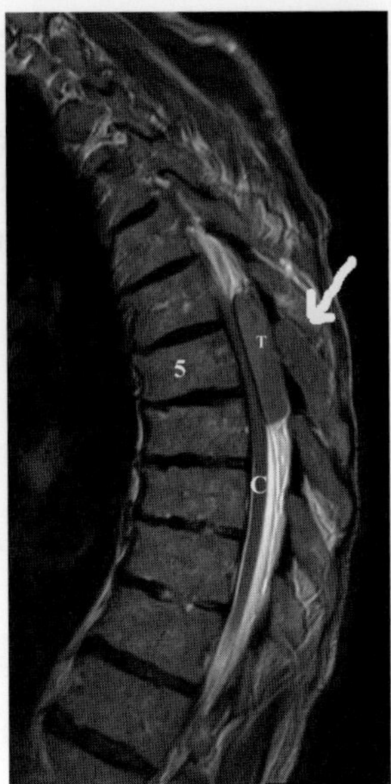

Figure 9-1: T2 sagittal MRI scan demonstrating epidural tumour (T), invading the posterior elements (arrow), and compressing spinal cord (C) at T4-6.

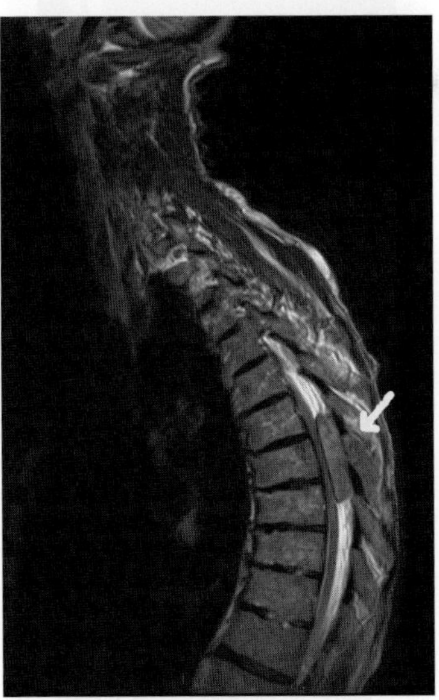

Figure 9-2: Sagittal T2 slice to the left demonstrating left-sided location of the tumour (arrow).

affecting the spinal cord. Similarly the sensory level and pain levels support this location.

Investigations required in this patient were the same as those in PCS9-1-1. The MRI of this patient (Figures 9-3 and 9-4) demonstrated malignant cord compression in the lumbo-sacral region.

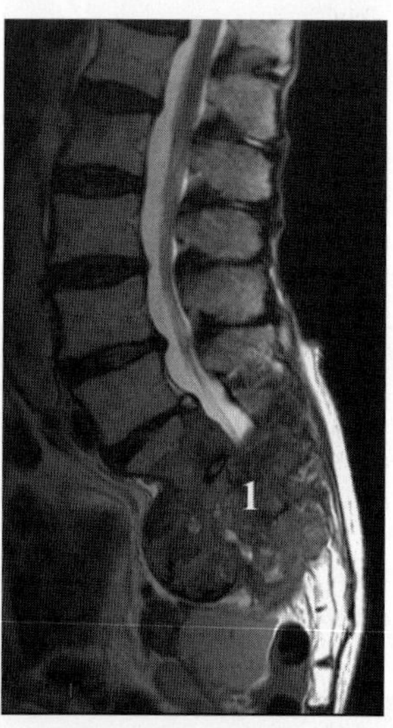

Figure 9-3: T2-MRI demonstrating a mass (1) destroying the sacral vertebrae and invading the spinal canal and posterior elements.

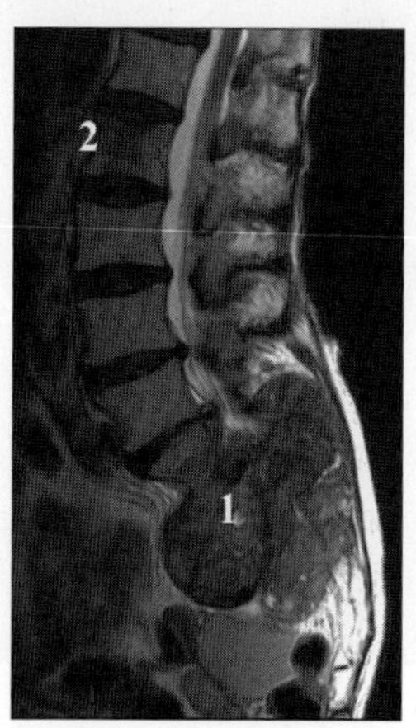

Figure 9-4: The same patient's T2-MRI demonstrating a second lesion (2).

9-1-5 *What is the incidence of malignant spinal compression?*

Malignant spinal compression (MSC) is a surgical emergency. Improved life expectancy of cancer patients increased the prevalence of spinal metastatic disease and the morbidity and mortality due to MSC had also increased. Five percent of all cancer patients develop spinal extradural metastases, and of these 20% develop symptoms of MSC. MSC requires early diagnosis and urgent treatment to avoid severe neurological disturbances. Therefore keeping a high index of suspicion and recognising early symptoms of MSC are paramount if patients are to have any chance of retaining the ability to walk and sphincter control. Urgent diagnostic investigations, access to MRI and immediate treatment are all part of maintaining good quality of life of these patients.

9-1-6 *How does MSC present?*

MSC presents with spinal pain associated with progressive neurological deficit. Neurological deficits often include progressive motor weakness of the limbs, progressive sensory impairment with a sensory level corresponding to the level of MSC and impaired bladder and bowel functions. Disorders of bladder and bowel control, and sexual function indicate decompensation and rapid deterioration of cord function. Decompensation occurs in the spine when the spinal cord is no longer able to deal with the presence of tumour to maintain function. There is dysfunction of the autonomic nervous system. Bladder function is particularly affected when the cauda equina or S2, 3, 4 nerve roots are involved, causing urgency and hesitancy as in PCS9-1-4. Bowel dysfunction also occurs with S2, 3, 4 nerve root involvement, but more often causes constipation rather than incontinence of faeces.

T12 and T6 are the most often affected spinal levels. The mode of onset can be insidious or acute depending upon whether bony collapse had occurred and occasionally MSC presents after minor trauma. Back pain is the commonest initial symptom and is present in virtually all patients at the time of diagnosis. Neurological symptoms usually present about six to eight weeks after the onset of spinal pain. Therefore a recent onset of spinal pain in a patient known to have malignant disease, e.g. breast cancer or a patient in the high risk for malignancy should be taken seriously to keep the patient ambulant. Spinal compression can be the initial presenting feature of malignant disease, e.g. lung cancer, prostate cancer, multiple myeloma, lymphoma or any other systemic malignancy.

9-1-7 *What are the stages of MSC?*

MSC can be divided into three stages:

a- **Neuralgic stage:** Characterised by pain and paraesthesia around the trunk at the level of compression and tight band-like sensations around the trunk (girdle pain), extensor plantar response, exaggeration of lower limb reflexes, and urinary urgency or hesitancy.

b- **Hemicord syndrome:** The clinical picture is atypical of Brown-Sequard Syndrome. Characterised by pain and temperature loss over affected dermatome and also the opposite side of the body below the lesion, dorsal column dysfunction below and ipsilateral to the lesion (dissociate anaesthesia), upper motor neuron picture on the side of the lesion and urinary urgency, incontinence and hesitancy.

c- **Transection stage:** Characterised by the loss of all motor and sensory functions below the level of the lesion and acute retention of urine.

These stages occur if the lesion is situated lateral to the spinal cord. Most metastatic tumours are situated laterally or anteriorly.

At the time of presentation, 80% of patients with metastases have weakness, 50% have sensory symptoms and 50% sphincter dysfunction. The main sites from which metastases occur are from lung, breast and prostate. Most of these cancers spread to the spine by haematogenous routes due to a system of valveless vertebral veins which communicate freely with the intercostal and lumbar veins. Involvement of posterior spinal elements by cancers is uncommon because the vascular networks are anteriorly located.

9-1-8 *How do metastases cause MSC?*

Tumours can cause MSC in a number of ways. The most important is by mechanical compression due to the expanding mass (Figure 9-4).

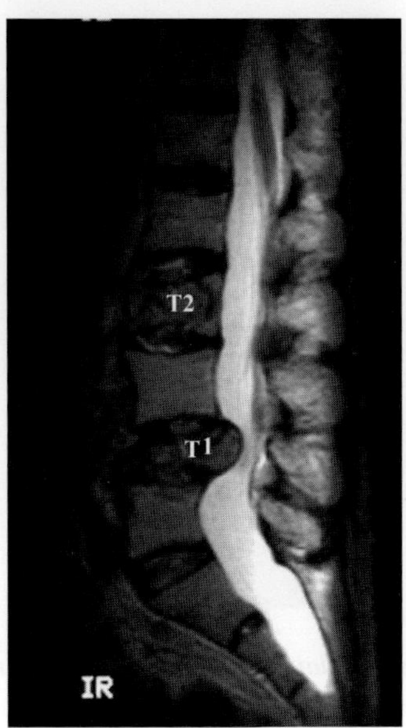

***Figure 9-5:** Malignant tumour caused collapse of L3 vertebra (T1) causing MSC at that level, there is also disease at L1 (T2).*

A malignancy can also cause vertebral collapse which allows fragments of bone to access the spinal canal causing MSC (Figure 9-5).

Compression of arterial blood supply can also lead to neural ischaemia, and venous occlusion can lead to congestion and infarction. Venous occlusion may be more relevant as venous drainage occurs via the extradural space, and this is where most malignant lesions occur. Slow growing tumours may allow for neural and vascular adaptation (compensation) and so may not present until further on in the disease process.

9-1-9 *How to investigate suspected MSC?*

Suspected MSC should be investigated on an urgent basis. These investigations include:

i) A spinal X-ray may reveal pathological collapse, lytic lesion or erosion of the pedicle. The hallmark of metastatic disease to the spine on

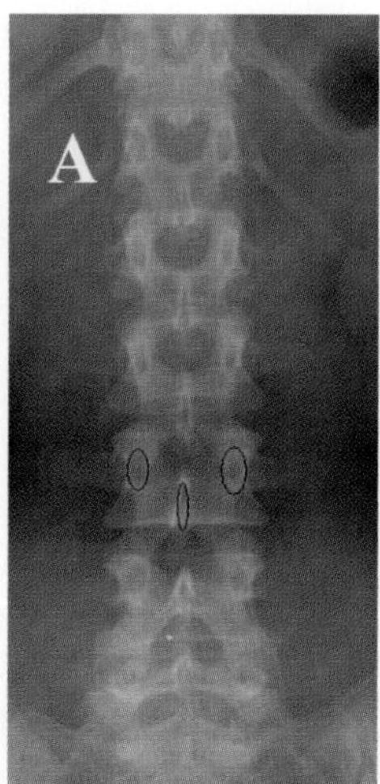

Figure 9-6: Anterior-posterior plain radiographs of the lumbar spine demonstrating normal pedicles and spinous process (A).

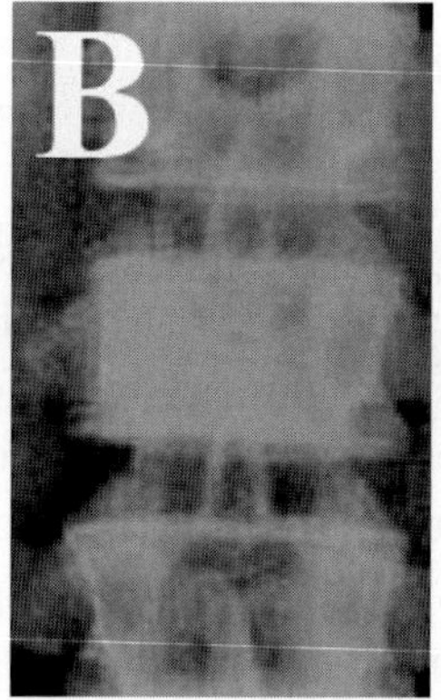

Figure 9-7: AP radiograph demonstrating eroded pedicle on the right (winking owl sign) (B).

X-ray is erosion of the pedicles (winking owl sign when one pedicle is eroded, Figures 9-6 and 9-7). Other non-specific features include multiple lytic, osseous deposits and angled end-plates. However, plain radiographs will pick up MSC only after 50% of trabecular bone is destroyed.

Metastatic lesions in the spine can be osteolytic or osteoplastic in nature. Different tumours produce different types of lesions (Table 9-1). A chest X-ray is also essential when dealing with metastatic disease.

ii) MRI is the gold standard for imaging the spine in a patient suspected to have MSC as it gives accurate anatomical details of anatomy, exact location of the tumour, state of the bone marrow and extent of disease (Figures 9-8 to 9-11).

Table 9-1: Lytic and plastic metastases

Lytic	Plastic
Lung	Breast
Breast	Prostate
Kidney	Lung
Thyroid	
Large bowel	

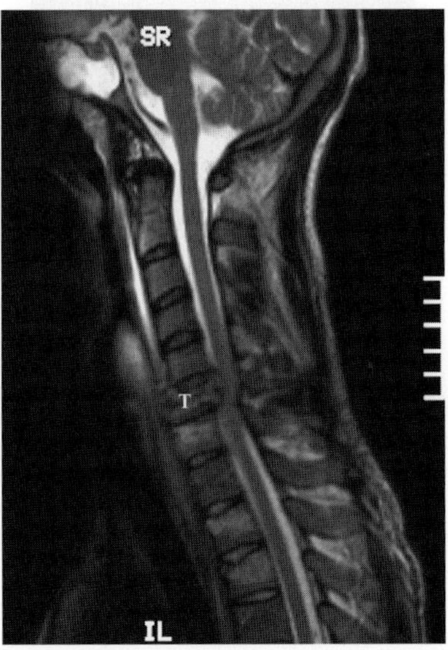

Figure 9-8: Sagittal T2 MRI scan of cervical spine of a 60-year-old woman with past history of breast cancer diagnosed five years ago who presented with neck pain and weakness of all four limbs of three weeks duration. The MRI demonstrated collapse of C6 vertebra and spinal cord compression at that level (T).

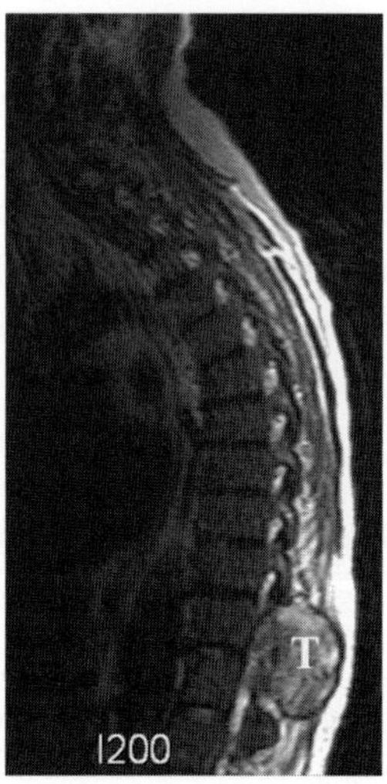

Figure 9-9: MRI scan demonstrates large tumour posteriorly causing MSC at T12 (T).

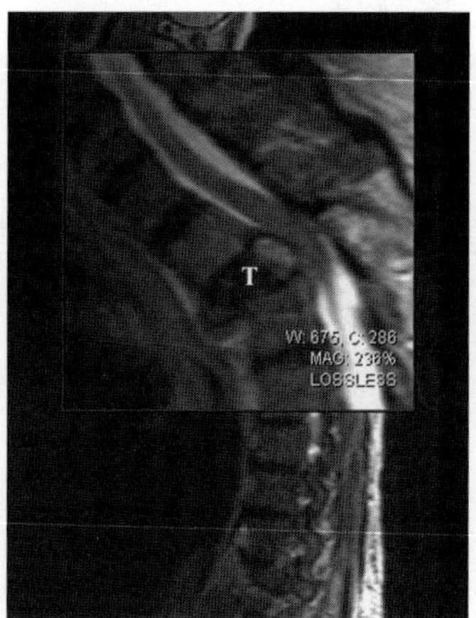

Figure 9-10: MRI demonstrating MSC at T4 (T) the tumour completely destroyed T4 leading to kyphotic deformity.

iii) Myelography shows block of contrast and is especially useful when used with CT scan (CT-myelogram). The pattern of contrast displacement will indicate the position of the tumour. The disadvantages of myelography include invasiveness and disturbance of the intraspinal

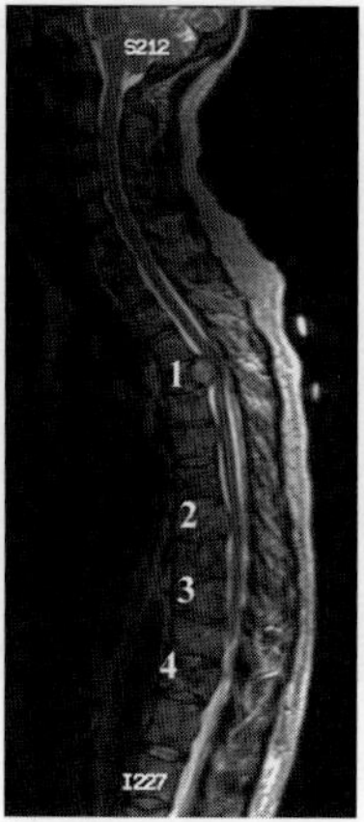

Figure 9-11: *MRI of the cervical and thoracic spine showing multiple metastatic lesions (1, 2, 3, and 4) with collapse at locations 1 and 4 and marrow infiltration at other vertebrae.*

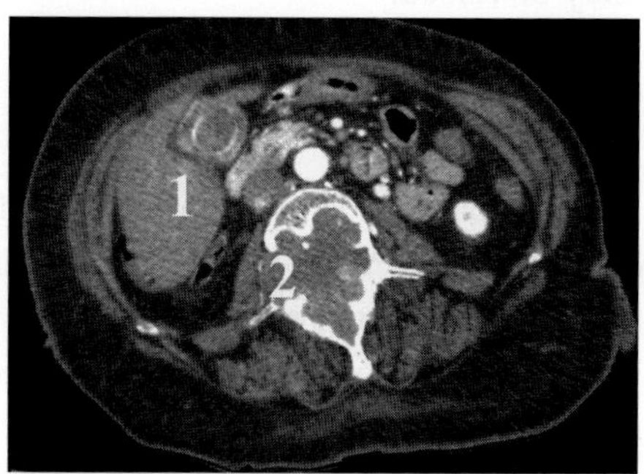

Figure 9-12: *Axial CT demonstrating spinal compression with a large tumour (2) scalloping the vertebra, 1 is the liver.*

CSF pressure that may lead to neurological deterioration in the presence of complete spinal block and may not show the upper or lower limits of the MSC if the contrast was injected from one side of a complete spinal block.

iv) CT scan of the chest, abdomen and pelvis are required for staging (Figures 9-12 and 9-13).

v) Other useful investigations include ESR which, when raised, indicates an inflammatory process or disseminated malignancy, serum protein

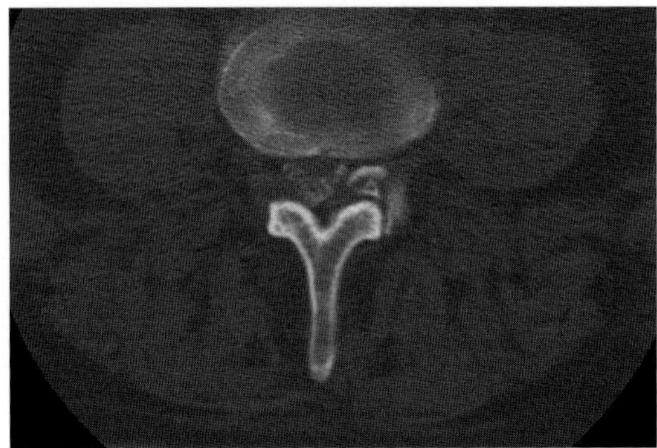

Figure 9-13: CT-myelogram demonstrating how useful the CT after myelogram in demonstrating the exact location of compression.

electrophoresis used to diagnose multiple myeloma, and serum acid phosophatase may be raised.

9-1-10 *How to manage patients diagnosed with MSC?*

The management of these patients is dependent on the following factors: Is the underlying cancer known? What is the state of cancer control at the primary site? What is the underlying pathology? What is the state of the patient? What is the state of the spine? Where is the MSC?

Management of each patient should be individualised as no jacket fits all. The decision about the best management plan should be agreed within a multidisciplinary team involving a surgeon with the appropriate expertise in spinal compression, an oncologist with the appropriate expertise in the underlying cancer and others as necessary, e.g. pain specialist and palliative care physicians. Histological diagnosis and biopsy may have to be obtained in patients where the primary was unknown. The technique of biopsy will vary from patient to patient, e.g. a patient with predominantly bony disease with good neurology may benefit from CT-guided core biopsy whilst another fit patient with spinal canal compromise and more severe neurology may benefit from surgical decompression at the same time as the biopsy. If the spine was unstable the patient will benefit from internal fixation at the same time as the decompression. Fixation may also be indicated in patients with a lot of spinal instability pain. If the diagnosis is confirmed or known and the neurology is minor and stable most patients will go for primary radiotherapy treatment with surgery as a backup for future deterioration. Fit patients with good prognosis, for example breast cancer, multiple myeloma and prostate cancer MSC often receive aggressive spinal surgery while unfit patients with a lot of co-morbidity and poor prognosis will receive symptomatic relief without surgery.

All patients with MSC should be discussed with a neurosurgeon for assessment as emergency neurosurgery may be needed. Diagnostic error is the main cause of delay of treatment, as well as poor neurological assessment. All physicians should be aware of the symptoms of MSC and know the importance of immediate referral. Back pain in a patient who is known to have cancer must always be urgently investigated. The patient must first be stabilised and pain should be controlled adequately. Pain is particularly severe in patients with extradural metastases and opiates may be required. Bed rest is important to avoid instability provoking symptoms or pathological fractures. If there is acute urine retention or dribbling incontinence, a urinary catheter should be inserted. Dexamethasone is used to give neurological stability until definitive treatment is carried out. It is used to reduce local oedema of the spinal cord which can cause further compression. Furthermore, very high doses of steroids increase the blood flow to the spine, reducing the effects of ischaemia.

The aims of treatment are to relieve pain, preserve function and restore mobility and normal sphincter function. The expected survival time is often short and will depend on the primary tumour. It is more important to maintain good quality of life rather than prolonging life. The best and most effective treatment of a spinal tumour is complete excision although this often cannot be obtained. The amount of excision depends on the location of the tumour and its relationship to adjacent neurological structures. How the surgery is approached also depends on these factors. Removing metastases involving the spinal cord is not possible. Posterior and lateral tumours can be approached by removal of the overlying spinal elements and the extradural component of the tumour. In principle if the tumour lies posterior causing posterior

MSC, the approach is via laminectomy, laterally located MSC is approached through the posterior-lateral approach, e.g. costo-transversectomy, while anteriorly located MSC is approached anteriorly via vertebrectomy.

Following surgical decompression, spinal stabilisation is essential. This can be done with pedicle screws posteriorly, vertebral replacement cage anteriorly and lateral plate when necessary or a combination of two of these techniques. Not all patients are suitable for surgery. The age and general medical condition of the patient are important when deciding on treatment. If a patient has complete cord transection, multiple levels of disease and those with advanced disseminated disease may benefit more from conservative symptomatic treatment. In these patients, pain control is of utmost importance. All treatment options for patients with MSC are palliative in nature and aimed at maintaining high quality of life. Apart from surgery, the other options are radiotherapy and chemotherapy.

Although surgery is the first option for treatment, several studies have shown that radiotherapy combined with steroids has a similar beneficial effect when the neurology is good and the MSC was diagnosed early.

In general, surgical decompression should be considered when the tumour is radio-resistant, if deterioration occurred during radiotherapy, if vertebral collapse caused cord compression, if compression recurred after maximum radiotherapy, and if single level disease with anterior cord compression. On the other hand, radiotherapy is indicated when the tumour is radiosensitive, in stable patients with minor neurological deficits, advanced generalised disease, refusal of, or unfit for surgery. Rehabilitation techniques can greatly improve the patient's health and quality of life by helping them to use their remaining abilities. This involves working closely with physiotherapists, occupational therapists and a palliative care team as required to optimise the effects of treatment and to allow the patient to return to as much normality as possible. The following flow diagram (Figure 9-14) explains how a patient with suspected MSC should be managed.[1,2]

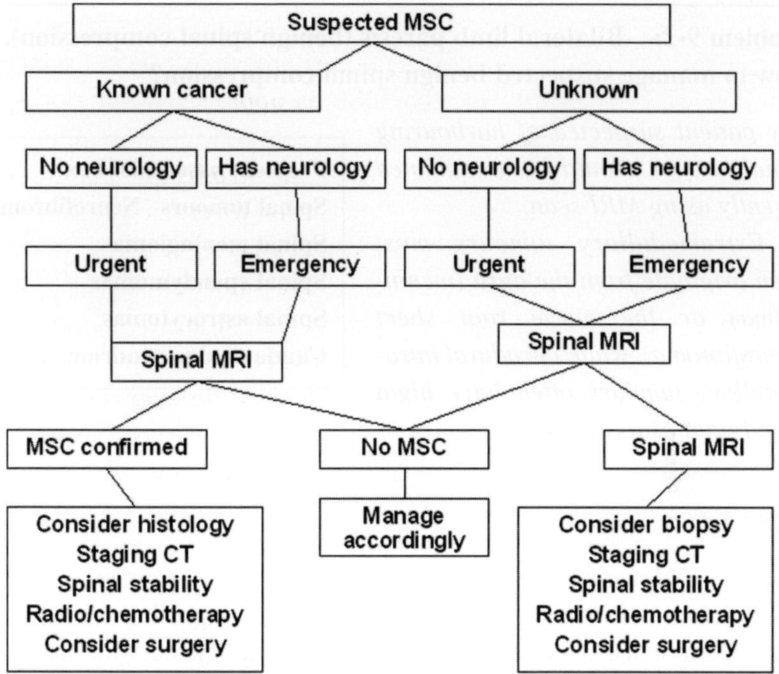

Figure 9-14: Flow chart of MSC management.

Your personal notes:

....

....

....

....

....

....

....

....

....

....

Problem 9-2:   Bilateral limb paresis (benign spinal compression). How to manage suspected benign spinal compression?

Any patient suspected of harbouring spinal tumour should be investigated urgently using MRI scan.

Extramedullary tumours most often originate from the dura (meningioma) or the nerve root sheet (neurofibroma), while intradural intramedullary tumours often have night spinal pain as a feature.

Problem based tool box:

Spinal tumours   Neurofibroma

Spinal meningioma

Spinal ependymomas

Spinal astrocytomas

Cauda equina syndrome

PCS9-2-1:

A 40-year-old marathon runner presented with bilateral leg pain in the sciatic nerves distribution associated with difficulty in passing urine for the last three months. It started gradually and was associated with back pain at night time. Previously he had been very well. Examination revealed bilateral leg weakness of 4 associated with sensory level at L1 including the saddle area.

9-2-2 *What is the differential diagnosis of cauda equina?*

A patient presenting with bilateral leg pain associated with urinary problems, paraparesis and sensory level at L1 means cauda equina compression, the differential diagnosis would be;

- Acute disc prolapse at L1/2 level, but this would be unlikely based on insidious onset and its rarity.
- Spinal infection: the lack of tenderness and normal temperature and CRP and ESR would be against this diagnosis.
- Malignant spinal compression (MSC).
- Benign spinal compression (BSC) particularly with the night pain due to spinal meningioma, neurofibroma, ependymoma or epidermoid cyst.

9-2-3 *How to investigate suspected cauda equina?*

This patient needed blood counts, urea and electrolytes, blood sugar and MRI of the spine. All results were normal except the MRI which demonstrated an intradural mass arising from the conus and compressing the cauda equina (Figures 9-15 to 9-17).

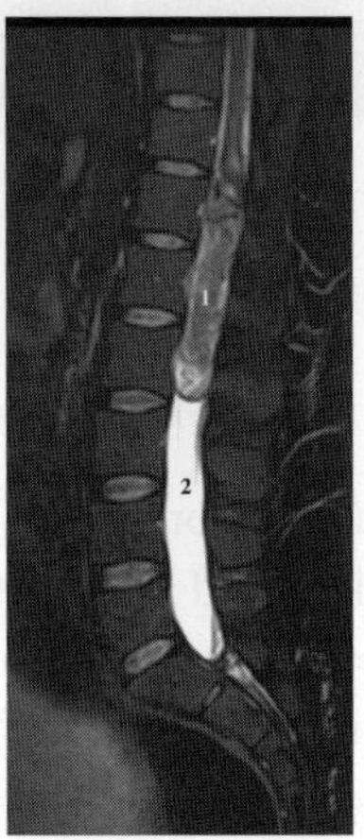

Figure 9-15: T2-weighted sagittal image demonstrating intradural tumour arising from the conus (1) from T12 to L3 and associated with distal cystic component (2).

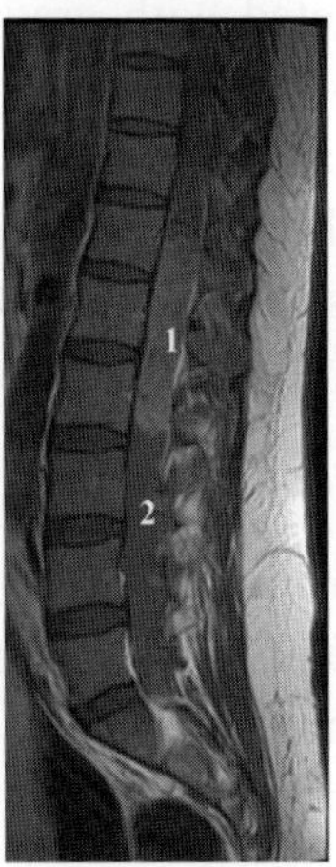

Figure 9-16: T1-weighted sagittal MRI scan demonstrating the tumour (1) enhanced with gadolinium.

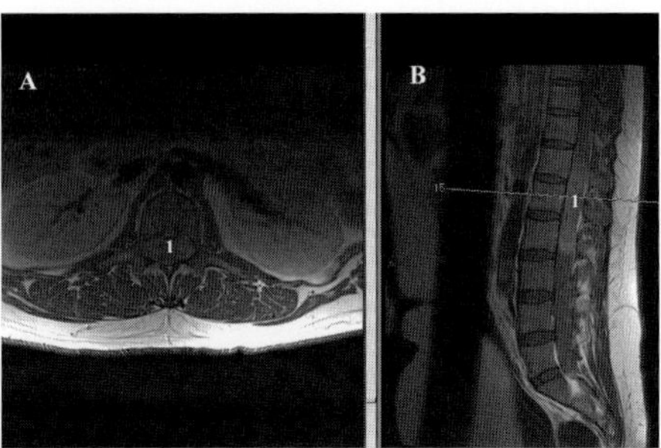

Figure 9-17: T1-weighted MRI of the tumour (1) axial (A) and sagittal with contrast (B).

9-2-4 *How to manage a patient with intradural spinal tumour?*

This patient was given dexamethasone 4 mg four times daily then underwent posterior decompression and near-total excision of the tumour, which turned to be myxopapillary ependymoma WHO grade I. He underwent whole spine and cranial MRI looking for other lesions. There were no other lesions. He underwent adjuvant radiotherapy.

PCS9-2-5:

A 58-year-old woman presented with gradual slowly progressive paraparesis with no sphincter disturbances. Her muscle tone in the legs was increased, power of hip flexors was 4+, knee extenders were 4 and ankle dorsiflexion was 3. The ankle and knee jerks were exacerbated with clonus. She had reduced sensation to L2 sparing the saddle area.

9-2-6 *What is the differential of paraparesis?*

A patient presenting with insidious progressive spastic paraparesis and sensory level at L1 means spinal cord compression in the lower thoracic region. The differential diagnosis would be:

- Thoracic disc prolapse.
- Spinal infection: The lack of tenderness and normal temperature and CRP and ESR would be against this diagnosis.

- Malignant spinal cord compression (MSC).
- Spinal AVM.
- Benign spinal cord compression (BSC) particularly with the night pain meningioma, neurofibroma, ependymoma or epidermoid cyst.

9-2-7 *How to investigate paraparesis?*

This patient needed blood counts, urea and electrolytes, blood sugar and MRI of the spine. All results were normal except the MRI which demonstrated an intradural extramedullary mass (Figures 9-18 to 9-21).

9-2-8 *How to manage intradural extramedullary spinal tumours?*

This patient was given dexamethasone 4 mg four times daily then underwent posterior decompression and total excision of the tumour, which turned out to be meningioma WHO grade I.

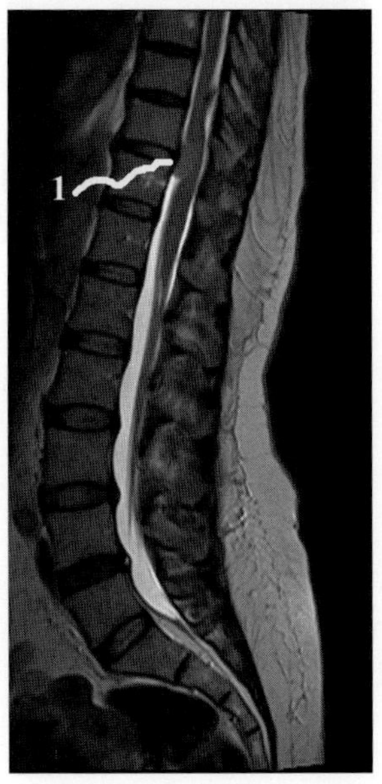

Figure 9-18: Sagittal T2-weighted MRI demonstrating intradural extramedullary lesion (1) at T12.

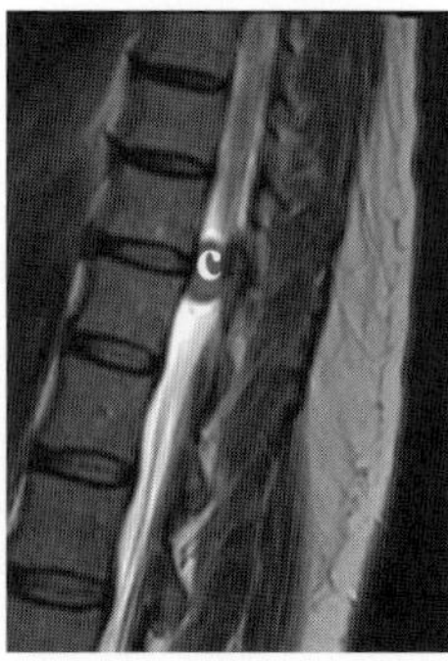

Figure 9-19: Magnified view of the tumour (c).

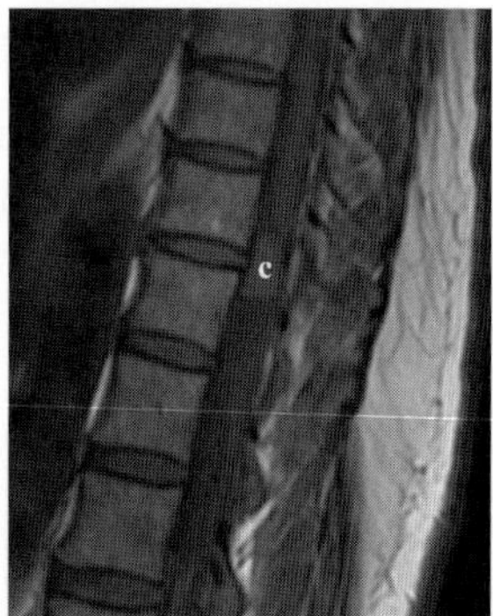

Figure 9-20: The tumour (c) enhances with gadolinium.

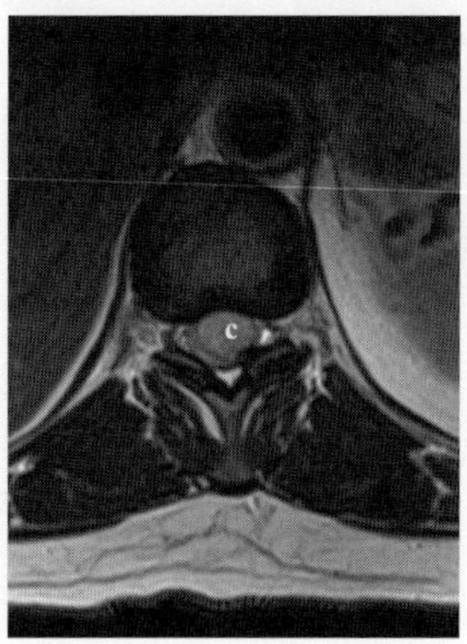

Figure 9-21: Axial T1 with contrast demonstrating the tumour (c) was located anteriorly and the spinal cord was compressed and pushed back and to the right.

9-2-9 *What are the different types of dural/intradual spinal tumours?*

1- **Spinal meningiomas:**

Epidemiology:

Spinal meningiomas are the second most common benign spinal tumours and account for 25% of all spinal tumours. Their incidence is about three per 100,000. The most common location is in the thoracic spine (60%) followed by the cervical spine (15%). Only 3% occur in the lumbar region and 2% around the foramen magnum. They are most common in women and in the fifth and sixth decades of life, with less than 6% occuring in children.[3,4]

Presentation:

Spinal meningiomas present with insidious onset of motor and sensory deficits depending on the location: spastic tetraparesis in cervical location, spastic paraparesis in thoracic location or Brown Sequard syndrome in laterally located tumour.

Diagnostic features:

On MRI scan spinal meningiomas appear as intradural extramedullary lesion with dural base and enhances with gadolinium (Figures 9-22 and 9-23).[5]

Management:

Surgery is the treatment of choice. Surgical excision is curative and the prognosis is excellent. After surgical resection patients are followed up to detect any recurrences.

2- **Spinal neurofibromas:**

Epidemiology:

Spinal neurofibromas or schwannomas are the commonest benign spinal tumour (30%). They affect men and women equally and are commonest during the fourth and fifth decades of life. They are mostly benign and

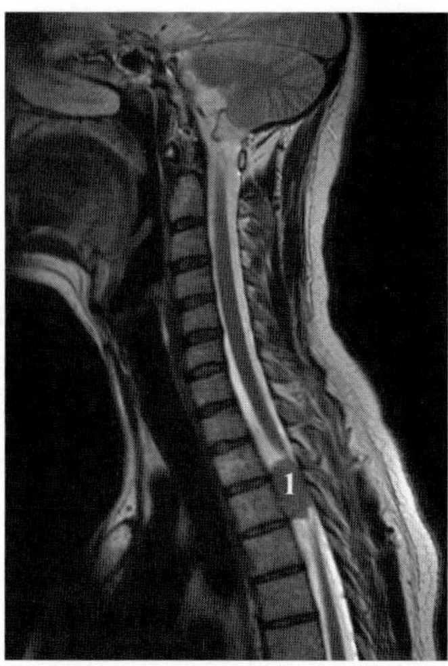

Figure 9-22: Sagittal T1-weighted MRI demonstrating spinal cord compression at T3 due to meningioma (1).

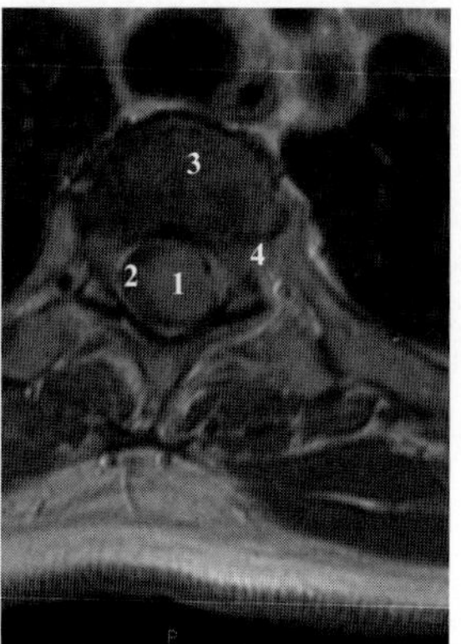

Figure 9-23: Axial T1-weighted MRI image of the same tumour (1) in Fig. 8 — 3 =disc, 2 =spinal cord, and 4 =inter-vertebral foramen.

only 2.5% are malignant. One third occur in association with neurofibromatosis, a hereditary genetic disorder divided into: neurofibromatosis type I (NFI) characterised by subcutaneous neurofibromas and café-au-lait spots, and NFII characterised by multiple meningiomas and central schwannomas.

Presentation:

Spinal schwannomas present with either radiculopathy with radicular pain, dermatomal sensory impairment, and myotomal weakness or myelopathy due to spinal cord compression or cauda equina.

Diagnostic features:

Spinal schwannoma often extends intradural and extradural in a dumbbell shape eroding and enlarging the intervertebral foramen (Figures 9-24 to 9-28). The tumour enhances with gadolinium and may be cystic in nature.

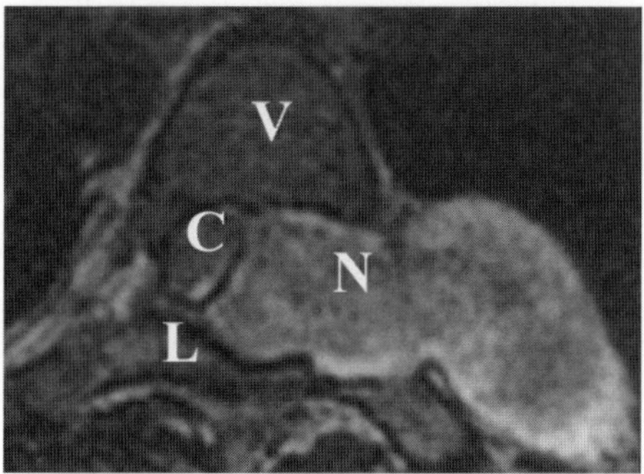

Figure 9-24: Axial T1 with gadolinium demonstrating a dumbbell lesion (N) expanding the foramen. V = vertebral body, L = lamina, and C = spinal cord compressed and pushed to the right.

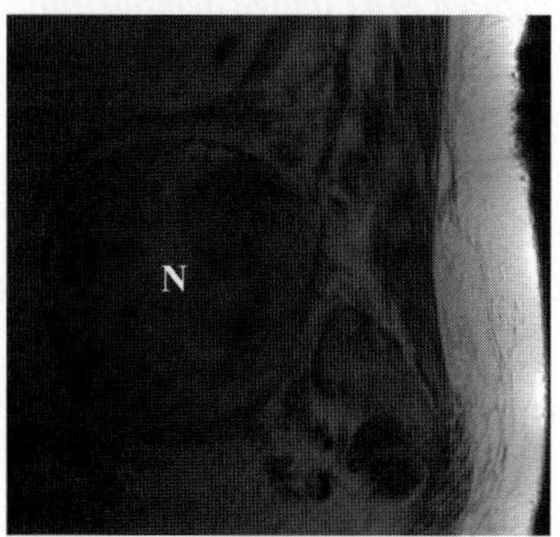

Figure 9-25: Large neurofibroma (N) arising in the lumbar intervertebral foramen and extending into the abdomen.

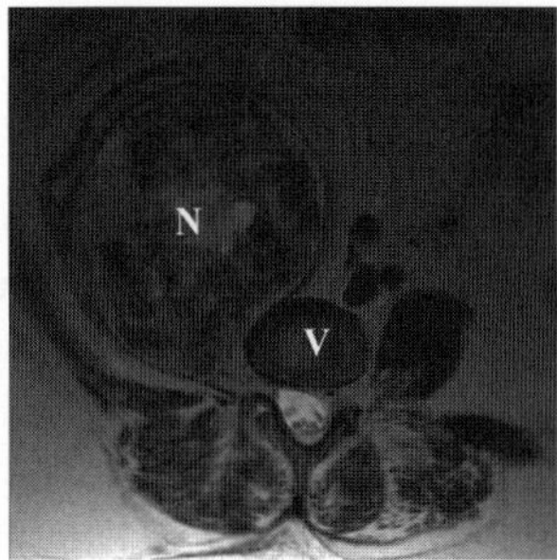

Figure 9-26: Large neurofibroma (N) demonstrated on axial T2-weighted MRI in the lumbar spine.

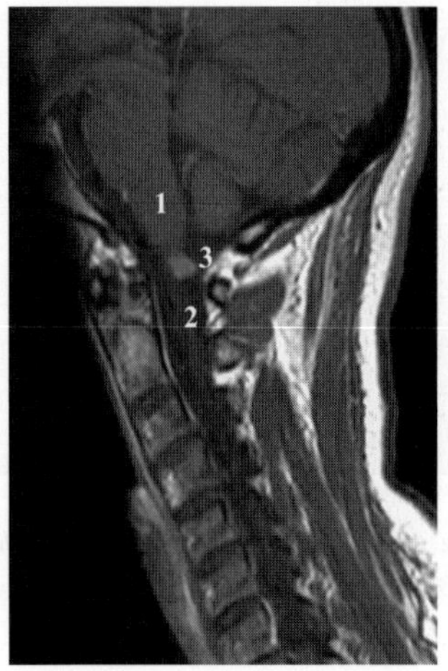

Figure 9-27: Sagittal T1-weighted MRI image demonstrating a neurofibroma (3) at the foramen magnum.

Management:

Surgical excision is the treatment of choice with good prognosis.

3- **Spinal ependymomas:**

Epidemiology:

Ependymomas represent 60% of all intramedullary spinal cord tumours. They are divided into intramedullary (IME), myxopapillary (MPE) and

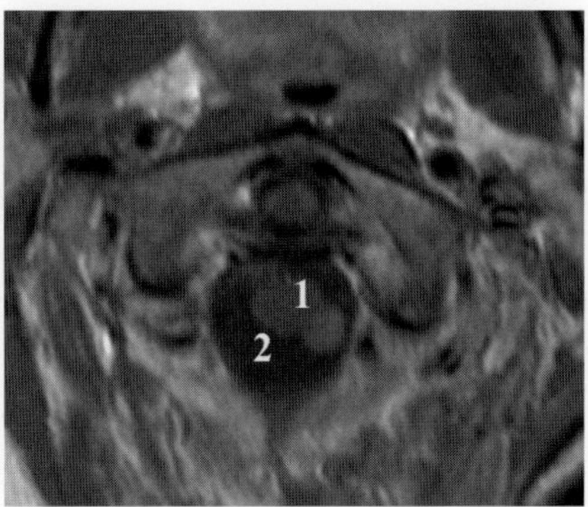

Figure 9-28: Axial T1-weighted MRI image of the same patient from in Figure 9-27. The neurofibroma (1) enhances with contrast and 2 is the spinal cord.

drop metastases from intracranial ependymomas. They are more common than intracranial location and MPE are more common in the young and in males whilst IME are more common in females. MPE almost exclusively occurs in the conus as in PCS9-1-1 above and represent 90% of tumours in this location compared to IME. IME are more common in the cervical and crevice-thoracic region.

Presentation:

They present with LBP especially at night time associated with spinal cord compression symptoms and signs, e.g. numbness, weakness and sphincter disturbance.

Diagnostic features:

MRI findings are of intramedullary or conal lesion which diffusely expands the spinal cord that enhances with contrast and with cystic formation (Figures 9-15 to 9-17).

Management:

Surgery is the treatment of choice and gross total resection is curative. However, adjuvant radiotherapy reduces recurrence rates in those incompletely resected.[6]

4- **Spinal astrocytomas:**

Epidemiology:

Eighty per cent of spinal cord astrocytomas are low grade and represent one-third of all intramedullary tumours. The incidence is about 1.1 per 100,000 and accounts for 4–10% of all CNS tumours. They occur at any age but peak between 30–60 years with slight male preponderance.[6]

Presentation:

These tumours present with back pain (70%) especially at night associated with numbness, weakness, sphincter disturbance or ataxia below the location of the tumour and can be unilateral or bilateral.

Diagnostic features:

On MRI these tumours are shown as intramedullary diffuse lesions associated with tumour cyst or syrinx. Enhancement is variable and dependent upon the grade of the tumour (Figure 9-29).

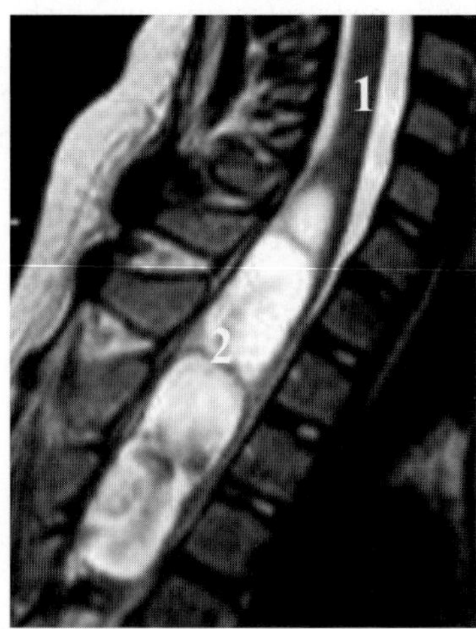

Figure 9-29: Sagittal T2-weighted MRI demonstrating large multiloculated intramedullary astrocytomas (2) arising in upper thoracic cord (1).

Management:

Gross total resection increases disease-free progression to 50% at five years in low grade astrocytomas. However, neurological deficit is not uncommon post-operatively. Adjuvant radiotherapy is recommended in higher grade tumours.

5- **Spinal haemangioblastoma:**

Epidemiology:

They represent 3% of all intramedullary tumours with 75% sporadic and 25% in association with Hipplet-Lindau disease. They affect the young, 30–40 years of age, with slight male predominance.[7]

Presentation:

Their presentation is similar to spinal ependymomas and astrocytomas.

Diagnostic features:

MRI is the investigation of choice and demonstrates the tumour as a cystic lesion with solid enhancing nodule or an enhancing nodule. Digital subtraction angiography demonstrates tumour blush.

Management:

Surgical excision is the treatment of choice and total surgical excision is curative.

6- **Spinal dermoid/epidermoid:**

Epidemiology:

These are inclusion cysts rather than tumours and account for 0.3% of all CNS tumours. They can be congenital associated with dermal sinus, tuft of hair or subcutaneous lump. Acquired dermoid/epidermoid cysts can be as a result of trauma or iatrogenic. They are most common in males and between 40–50 years of age. Their location is 50% intramedullary and 50% intradural extramedullary.

Presentation:

Their presentation is similar to that of other spinal intradural tumours.

Diagnostic features:

MRI is the best investigation; it demonstrates the exact location of the lesion in multiplanes with high spatial resolution. Fat droplets within these cysts appear high signal on T1 and T2 (Figure 9-30).

Management:

Symptomatic lesions are surgically treated to evacuate the cyst and remove the cystic capsule that can be removed safely without compromising neurological structures. The capsule is quite often adherent to the surrounding structures making its removal dangerous, risky and almost impossible.

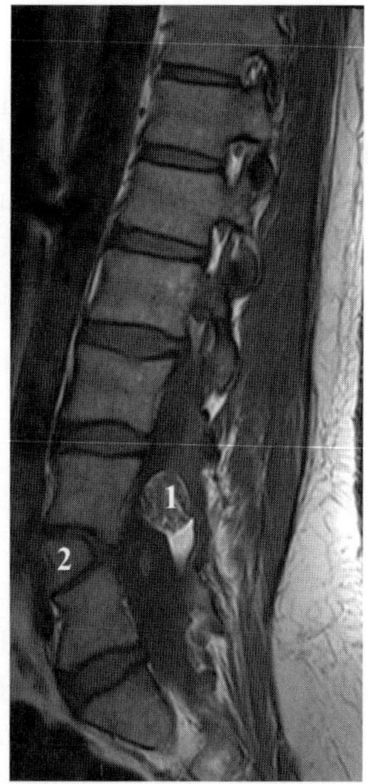

Figure 9-30: Sagittal T1-weighted MRI image demonstrating epidermoid cyst (1) associated with congenital vertebral anomaly (2).

Yours personal notes:

....
....
....
....
....
....
....
....
....
....

Problem 9-3:   Bilateral limb paresis (spinal infections). How to manage suspected spinal infection?

Any patient presenting with acute back pain and muscle weakness involving the limbs bilaterally should be considered to be suffering from spinal cord compression until proven otherwise. If there was fever, and severe bony tenderness spinal sepsis should be suspected.

Problem based toolkit:

Acute back pain Discitis

Osteomyelitis

Psoas abscess

Spinal tuberculosis

Spinal epidural abscess

Although some patients presenting with acute paraparesis or tetraparesis do not in fact have spinal cord compression, any patient presenting in this fashion should be managed as such to exclude spinal cord compression.

PCS9-3-1:

A 27-year-old man presented with three weeks history of gradually worsening lower cervical/upper thoracic back pain. The pain was constant and aching in character, radiating bilaterally to his shoulders. Increasing severity over the previous four days confining patient to bed, was followed by a 24-hour history of sudden bilateral lower limb numbness and numbness up to the level of the umbilicus. Back pain radiated to the base of the back. Patient described legs as "feeling heavy" on attempts to walk and was unsteady on his feet. Neither leg suffered from a feeling of tingling, temperature change or burning sensation. Patient remained continent — bladder and bowel were not affected. No complaint of headache, dizziness or changes in speech or vision. No history of trauma. No significant past medical history and was on Paracetamol and Ibuprofen as required. He had no allergies and works in a fast food chain while studying at college. He smoked four to five cigarettes per day and drank one to four units of alcohol per week. Examination revealed that his temperature was 36.1°C, BP 169/95 mmHg, pulse 96/min — regular, respiratory rate 14/min and he was alert and oriented. Muscle tone was normal in all limbs. Reflexes: SJ ++, BJ ++, TJ ++, KJ +/(present with reinforcement), AJ and plantar response was normal. Muscle power was 5 in all muscle groups in the upper limbs, hip flexion and extension was 4, knee flexion and extension was 4 and plantar and dorsi-flexion of the foot was also 4 bilaterally.

Sensory examination demonstrated normal light touch and pinprick (PP) in upper limbs and reduced from T10 downwards. Joint position and movement as well as vibration sensation were abnormal in the feet.

9-3-2 *What is the differential of acute backache with paraparesis?*

1) Malignant cord compression (MSC) due to extradural tumour arising from the vertebra, e.g. metastases from lung, prostate, or kidney, or myeloma or lymphoma. However the patient is only 27 years of age and MSC is unlikely.
2) Degenerative spinal pathology due to prolapsed intravertebral disc or spinal stenosis. Again the patient's young age is against this diagnosis.
3) Benign spinal tumour such as meningioma or neurofibroma is a consideration. Thoracic region is a common place for either, but meningioma is more common in females and neurofibromas in neurofibromatosis.
4) Spinal AVM but this is uncommon.
5) Guillain-Barré syndrome should also be considered but only made by excluding compressive lesion.
6) Infection due to discitis, osteomyelitis or epidural abscess.

9-3-3 *Where is the lesion in PCS9-3-1?*

The patient had paraparesis so the lesion is most likely to affect spinal cord segment T1 downwards (thoracic cord, conus, cauda equina, or peripheral nerves). The sensory level at T10 points to a lesion at T10 level, although one would expect to find hyperreflexia in the lower limbs and up-going planters (which was not the case in this patient).

9-3-4 *What investigations should this patient have?*

1- Plain radiographs of the thoracic spine may reveal a collapse or osteolytic lesion, but in this patient it was normal.

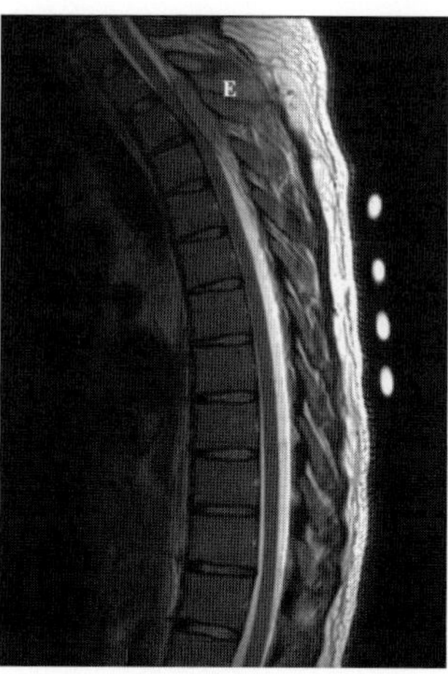

Figure 9-31: MRI thoracic spine demonstrating an epidural lesion (E).

2- Blood counts and blood chemistry demonstrated that he had a very high ESR, plasma viscosity and CRP.
3- MRI spine revealed an epidural lesion at T10 compressing the spinal cord posteriorly (Figure 9-31). It was thought initially to be a lymphoma.

This patient underwent decompressive laminectomy and the epidural mass was noted to have caseation material and intra-operative diagnosis of tuberculosis (TB) was therefore suspected and the patient was started on triple anti-TB treatment. TB was confirmed both on culture and histopathology. Although the patient was not infective, the public health department was informed and all his contacts were traced and screened for TB. Following decompression, the patient had made an excellent post-operative full recovery.

Anti-TB drug therapy is required for a long time and it carries significant side effects that need to be discussed with the patient and monitoring is required to detect these side effects. Liver function tests should be obtained regularly to ensure no lasting damage is being done to the liver when the drugs are being taken, particularly as the drug course can last at least six months and in some cases up to 18 months.

- Rifampicin — although its adverse effects are infrequent, they can be serious as it causes hepatotoxicity and certain "toxic syndromes". Orange discolouration of the urine is also a common side effect. It also has several drug interactions.
- Isoniazid — adverse effects occur in 5% of patients and include peripheral neuropathy, hepatotoxicity and may induce autoimmune conditions.
- Pyrazinamide — causes hepatotoxicity but also raises plasma urate levels that can lead to gout. Resistance to the drug unfortunately develops rapidly.
- Ethambutol — rarely causes adverse effects but is known to induce reversible optic neuritis.

Only 2% of cases involving TB affect the spine.[8] The risk of developing spinal TB is associated with certain risk factors including the patient's country of origin, socioeconomic status, HIV infection, alcoholism and intravenous drug abuse.[8] Spinal TB occurs most frequently in the thoracic spine[9–11] but may occur anywhere along the dura.[10] Most patients presenting with spinal TB are under the age of 30.[10] In comparison to other CNS infections, spinal cord compression resulting from an extradural abscess is more frequently seen in TB.[10] Diagnosis is regarded as difficult due to spinal TB's insidious onset with chronic progression culminating in a sudden deterioration to cause neurological deficits.[9,11] Most agree that early surgical intervention, particularly when focal neurological signs are present, reduces the risk of permanent spinal cord damage.[9] However, when focal neurological signs are not present it is regarded as safer to maintain pharmacological therapy and avoid surgery.[12]

9-3-5 *What are the types of spinal infections?*

The spine can be infected by numerous organisms including bacteria and fungi. The incidence of these pathogens varies and can present acutely, sub-acutely or chronically with an array of clinical features related to the anatomical site infected and the pathogen involved. Classification of CNS infections is made according to the main site infected, e.g. infection of meninges results in meningitis, spinal cord infection causes myelitis whilst infection of the disc space is called discitis and infection of the vertebrae is called osteomyelitis. An abscess may form in the epidural space or in front of the spine particularly in the region of the psoas muscle.

9-3-6 *How does the spine become infected?*

Bacterial infections enter the spine by the following routes:

1- Haematogenous spread from distal infection such as bacterial endocarditis or bronchiectasis that may result in septicaemia or produce septic emboli.
2- Iatrogenic infection may occur following procedures, e.g. after microdiscectomy, decompression or fixation of the spine — notably *Staphylococcus aureus* is the most common organism.
3- Direct spread can occur from an external source with an infection gaining access following trauma such as an open fracture.

PCS9-3-7:

A 35-year-old woman presented with severe low back pain (LBP) seven days after lumbar microdiscectomy. She had no root tension signs on examination and her previous severe sciatica resolved. She was slightly tender over the small of her back. Her bladder and bowel functions were normal. Her straight leg raising was restricted to ten degrees because of severe back pain. Her C-reactive protein (CRP), plasma viscosity (PV) and ESR were very elevated (CRP > 100).

9-3-8 *How to manage discitis?*

The differential diagnosis is either pure mechanical LBP or post-operative infection. As the inflammatory markers were elevated (CRP > 100) infection should be the working diagnosis in this patient. If the surgical wound healed with no obvious infection and she was not very tender, then discitis would be the most likely diagnosis.

Discitis is a low-grade infection that affects the disc space between two vertebrae. Although discitis is uncommon, post-disc surgery (all types of discectomy: open, micro, endoscopic, percutaneous, laser and even discography) can occur in <1% of patients. Post-operative discitis can be minimised by pre-operative antibiotic prophylaxis.[13] Spontaneous discitis is much rarer and children under ten are usually the ones affected. In adults, discitis is most common in those predisposed to infections, e.g. diabetics or IV drug users. The most common organism is *Staphylococcus aureus*. Discitis is characterised by the slow onset of severe back pain and may or may not be associated with fever, chills, sweats, feeling tired, loss of appetite or other systemic symptoms. The diagnosis is usually made by seeing narrowing of the disc space between two vertebrae on plain radiographs (Figure 9-32) and an isotope bone scan that shows the disc and adjacent vertebrae as "hot" spot. MRI scan shows the discitis well (Figure 9-33). Inflammatory markers (CRP, ESR and PV) are markedly elevated.

Discitis can be very painful and is often aggravated by any movement of the spine. The pain often radiates to other areas including the abdomen, hip, leg, or groin. It usually occurs in the lumbar and thoracic spine. The adjacent endplates of the infected disc become eroded, and the degree of erosion depends on the amount of destruction resulting from the infection. The areas of erosion become recalcified as the healing process occurs and eventually an interbody fusion is evidence of a successful resolution of the discitis.

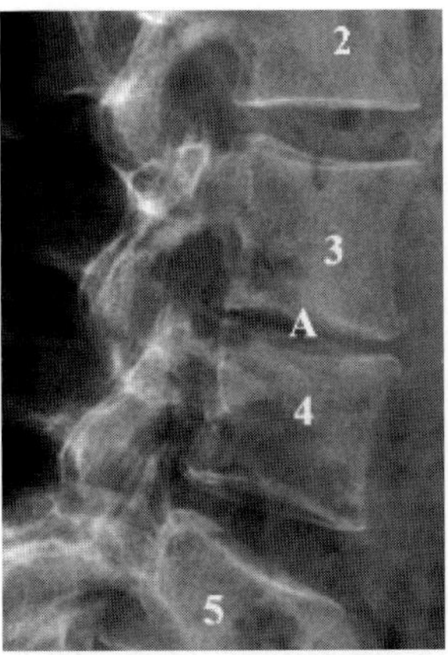

Figure 9-32: Plain radiographs demonstrating narrowing of disc space (L3/4) (A).

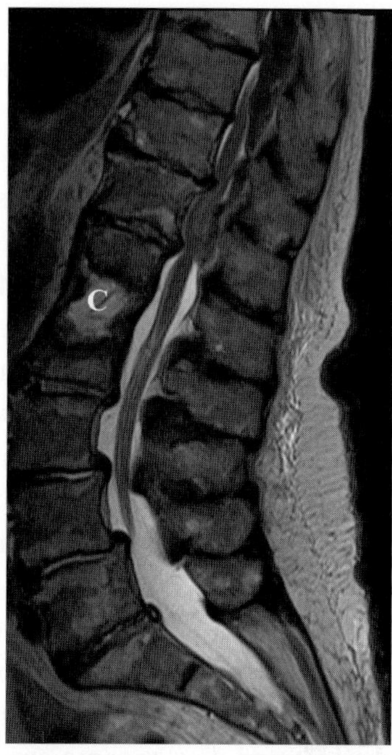

Figure 9-33: MRI demonstrating discitis at L1/2 disc (C). This patient was 88 years old who had recently had nephrostomy and urinary tract infection and came in with severe low back pain and elevated CRP and ESR.

Young children with this condition are usually irritable and uncomfortable and refuse to sit up, stand or walk. The treatment of discitis generally involves intravenous antibiotics, bed rest, and a brace and mobilisation when the infection is on the road to recovery. Surgery is rarely needed except in cases where there was doubt about the diagnosis where CT-guided aspiration may be required. Response to treatment is monitored by daily CRP measurements.

PCS9-3-9:

A 60-year-old diabetic patient was admitted with severe LPB in the mid-thoracic area of the spine. He quickly developed bilateral leg weakness and sensory level at the umbilicus area. This ascended very quickly upwards. He was extremely tender and would not allow anyone to touch his back. His diabetes was way out of control with blood sugars all over the place. The CRP, PV and ESR were all markedly elevated (CRP > 150).

9-3-10 *How to manage spinal epidural abscess?*

This clinical picture is classical for spinal epidural abscess. The key features are the ascending neurological deficit and the severe spinal tenderness. The neurological deficit ascends upwards and is only limited by the dural attachment to the foramen magnum. The other differential diagnosis of rapidly ascending neurological deficit is Guillain-Barré syndrome (GBS).

If an epidural abscess in the spine was suspected an emergency MRI scan is needed to clinch the diagnosis. In spinal vertebral infections the plain radiographs may be normal early on and involvement of the disc space helps to differentiate osteomyelitis from MSC (Figure 9-34).

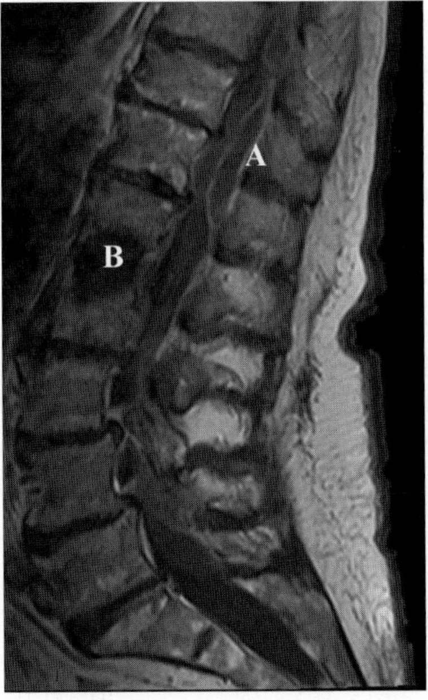

Figure 9-34: Osteomyelitis on MRI (B) note that the disc between the involved bones had been involved. There was also an epidural abscess (A) with enhancing edges.

Treatment with empirical antibiotics must include anti-*Staphylococcus aureus* antibiotics intravenously. Blood culture is used to grow the microorganism. The effectiveness of antibiotic therapy is monitored by measuring CRP and ESR. Bed rest is also implemented to minimise pain and promote resolution. If the patient presented with incomplete neurological deficit or deteriorating neurology, then emergency surgical decompression is the usual treatment of choice to drain the pus.

References

1. Levack P *et al.* A prospective audit of the diagnosis, management and outcome of malignant cord compression (CRAG 97/08). Edinburgh: CRAG, 2001.

2. Loblaw DA, Laperriere NJ, Mackillop WJ. A population-based study of malignant spinal cord compression in Ontario. *Clin Oncol* 2003; 15(4): 211–217.

3. Solero CL, Fornari M, Giombini S *et al.* Spinal meningiomas: review of 174 operated cases. *Neurosurgery* 1989; 25: 153–160.

4. Dillon WP, Norman D, Newton TH *et al.* Intradural spinal cord lesions: Gd-DTPA-enhanced MR imaging. *Radiology* 1989; 170: 229–237.

5. Matsumoto S, Hasuo K, Uchino A *et al.* MRI of intradural-extramedullary spinal neurinomas and meningiomas. *Clin Imaging* 1993; 17: 46–52.

6. Epstein FJ, Farmer JP, Freed D. Adult intramedullary astrocytomas of the spinal cord. *J Neurosurg* 1992; 77: 355–359.

7. Neumann HP, Eggert HR, Weigel K *et al.* Hemangioblastomas of the central nervous system. A 10-year study with special reference to von Hippel-Lindau syndrome. *J Neurosurg* 1989; 70: 24–30.

8. Mulleman D, Mammou S, Griffoul I *et al.* Characteristics of patients with spinal tuberculosis in a French Teaching Hospital. *Joint Bone Spine* 2006; 73: 424–427.

9. Nas K, Kemaloglu MS, Cevik R *et al.* The results of rehabilitation on motor and functional improvement on spinal tuberculosis. *Joint Bone Spine* 2004; 71: 312–316.

10. Almeida A. Tuberculosis of the spine and spinal cord. *Eur J Radiol* 2005; 55: 193–201.

11. Baleriaux DL, Neugroschl C. Spinal and spinal cord infection. *Eur Radiol* 2004; 14: 72–83.
12. Moon MS. Tuberculosis of spine — contemporary thoughts on current issues and perspective views. *Curr Orthop* 2007; 21: 364–379.
13. Mastronardi L, Rychlicki F, Tatta C *et al*. Spondylodiscitis after lumbar microdiscectomy: effectiveness of two protocols of intraoperative antibiotic prophylaxis in 1167 cases. *Neurosurg Rev* 2005; 28: 303–307.

Your personal notes:

....

....

....

....

....

....

....

....

....

....

Chapter 10: Pain, Weakness or Numbness in a Limb (Radiculopathy, Myelopathy and Peripheral Nerve Pathologies)

Problem 10-1:   Brachalgia, myelopathy and cervical disc prolapse. How to manage a patient presenting with arm pain or myelopathy?

Any patient presenting with neck pain radiating into the arm should be managed urgently if there are associated red flag signs such as neurological deficit, sphincter disturbance, bony tenderness, night spinal pain or history of or high risk of malignancy.

Problem based tool box:

Brachalgia   **Neck pain**

Radiculopathy

Cervical disc prolapse

Cervical spondylotic
   myelopathy

PCS10-1-1:

A 51-year-old right-handed man presented with two years history of neck pain associated with right shoulder and arm pain of two weeks duration. The pain in the right arm spreads to the thumb and index finger. It started overnight and did not get better. Over the last few days he began to feel pins and needles in the right thumb and index. He had no bladder or bowel problems and can walk without difficulties. When he coughed or strained the right arm pain was unbearable and he had to sleep in an upright position most of last week. In the past he was involved in a motorcycle accident and took painkillers (dihydrocodiene and diclofenac) for the last two years. He also had a history of hypertension and was on bendroflumethiazide and perindopril to control it. He had no other relevant past history and had no known allergies. He was married and lived with his wife and two children. He did not smoke and drank alcohol socially. He worked in a heavy manual job.

He generally looked well with an average built. His neck movements were restricted to the right and had an associated muscle spasm of the right trapezium. His right shoulder movements were normal. Right lateral flexion of the neck reproduced the paraesthesia and exacerbated his pain, whilst putting his right palm behind his occipital region relieved the pain (root tension signs). The power was reduced in his right biceps 4 and wrist extension 4 and had reduced sensation in the right thumb, index and radial aspect of the right forearm (C6). His biceps and brachioradialis reflexes were reduced. He had no signs of myelopathy.

10-1-2 *What is the differential diagnosis of brachalgia?*

A patient presenting with neck pain radiating in C6 distribution and associated with reduced biceps and brachioradialis reflexes and C6 sensory changes is consistent with right C6 radiculopathy. The absence of myelopathy indicates that the C6 nerve root on the right is compressed and the spinal cord is unaffected. The acute nature of the symptoms and the long history of neck pain make the diagnosis of acute cervical disc prolapse at C5/6 most likely. However, the differential diagnosis of cervical radiculopathy includes:

- Cervical disc prolapse.
- Cervical stenosis.
- Cervical subluxation.
- Cervical extradural malignant spinal compression (MSC).
- Cervical spinal infection.
- Cervical spinal neurofibroma.
- Cervical meningioma.

10-1-3 *How to investigate cervical radiculopathy?*

The most important investigation in this patient is MRI scan of the cervical spine. If the patient cannot have or did not tolerate an MRI scan then CT-myelography can be performed. If there was any suspicion that the neck was not aligned, flexion/extension radiographs of the cervical spine under doctor's supervision should be performed to assess stability. This

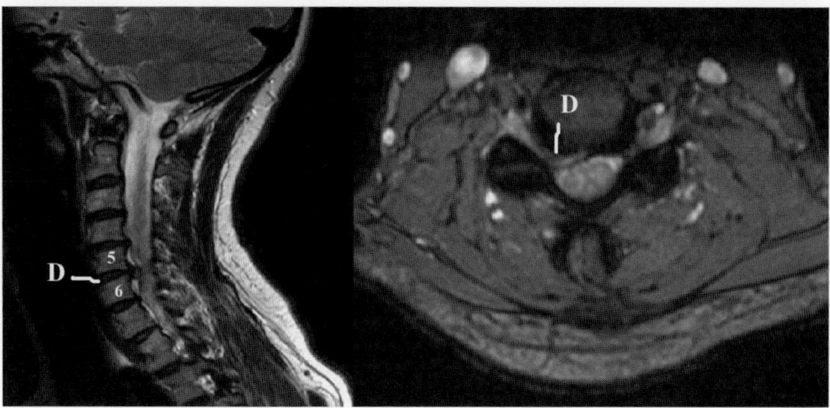

Figure 10-1: Sagittal and axial MRI scan T2-weighted demonstrating C5/6 disc (D).

patient had an MRI of the cervical spine that demonstrated acute disc prolapse at C5/6 (Figure 10-1).

PCS10-1-4:

A 65-year-old right-handed woman presented with three months history of gradual slowly progressive immobility and stiffness of the lower limbs associated with clumsiness of the hands. She was no longer able to button and unbutton her shirts and her mobility was very poor. She had no pain and no sensory or sphincter problems. In the past she had no significant past medical or surgical history. She was not on any medications and had no known allergies. She smoked 20 cigarettes per day and drank alcohol socially. She generally looked well. Her neck movements were normal. Muscle tone was increased in all four limbs with brisk reflexes and her planter responses were going up. She could not walk because of the stiffness but the muscle power was normal. She had no sensory deficit.

10-1-5 *What the differential diagnosis of cervical myelopathy?*

A patient presenting with spastic quadri-paresis without sensory loss means there was compression of the cervical spinal cord above C5 segment. The commonest cause of this clinical picture is cervical spondylotic myelopathy. However, the differential diagnosis of cervical myelopathy includes cervical:

1- Central disc prolapse.
2- Stenosis.
3- Subluxation.
4- Extradural malignant spinal cord compression (MSC).
5- Spinal infection.
6- Spinal neurofibroma.
7- Meningioma.

10-1-6 *How to investigate cervical myelopathy?*

The most important investigation in this patient is MRI scan of the cervical spine. This patient had an MRI of the cervical spine that demonstrated severe spinal canal stenosis at C4/5 (Figure 10-2).

10-1-7 *What is the pathophysiology of the cervical spondylosis?*

The vertebral bodies of C3 to C7 articulate via facet joints posteriorly and the lateral aspects of vertebral bodies articulate via uncovertebral joints. The uncovertebral joints can develop osteophytic spurs which can narrow the intervertebral foramina (Figure 10-3).

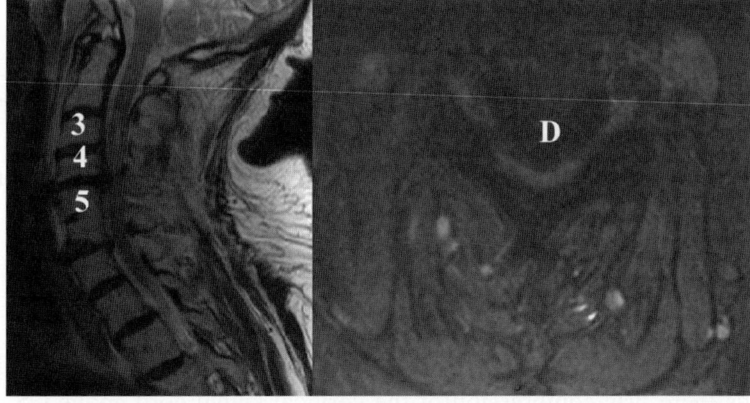

Figure 10-2: Sagittal and axial MRI scan T2-weighted demonstrating C4/5 stenosis (D).

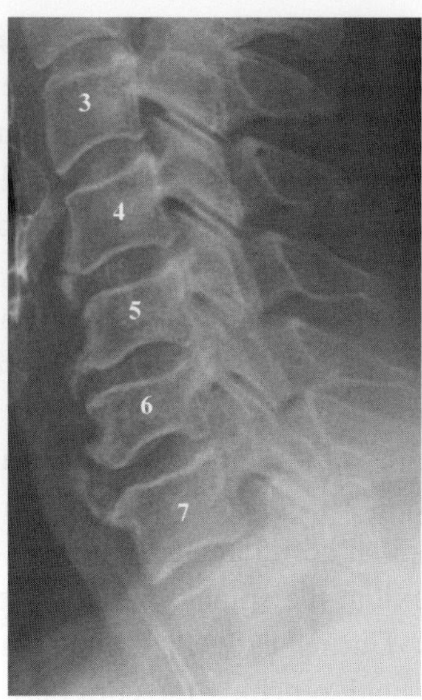

Figure 10-3: Plain X-ray of the neck demonstrating anterior osteophytes at C4, C5, C6 and C7.

The intervertebral discs (IVD) exist between adjacent vertebrae from C2/3 to C6/7. The IVD are composed of an outer annular fibrosis and an inner nucleus pulposus and serve as shock absorbers. The foramina are largest at C2/3 and progressively decrease in size to the C6/7. The nerve root occupies approximately 25% of the foraminal space. The neural foramen is bordered anteromedially by the uncovertebral joints, posterolaterally by the facet joints, superiorly by the pedicle of the vertebra above and inferiorly by the pedicle of the lower vertebra. Medially the foramina are formed by the edge of the end plates and the IVD. The nerve roots exit above their corresponding numbered vertebral body from C2 to C7. C1 exits between the occiput and the atlas and C8 exits below the pedicle of C7. C1 had no dermatomal supply, C2 supplies the skin of the occiput, C3 supplies the skin of the neck including a small area around the angle of lower jaw, C4 supplies the shoulder, and C5 to C8 supplies the upper limb. Degeneration of the structures that form the foramina can cause nerve root compression (radiculopathy). This compression can occur from osteophytes formation, disc herniation or a combination of the two. Cervical radiculopathy is more common in men than women and has a peak incidence in the fifth to sixth decades of life.

Cervical spondylotic myelopathy (CSM) occurs as a result of three important pathophysiologic factors: static-mechanical, dynamic-mechanical, and spinal cord ischaemia. A congenitally narrowed spinal canal (10–13 mm) is an important predisposing factor to CSM. As ventral osteophytosis occurs in a person with a congenitally narrowed canal, the space available to the spinal cord becomes further reduced. Age-related hypertrophy of the ligamentum flavum and thickening of bone may restrict the cord space further and cause buckling of these elements into the canal. Dynamic factors may also be important in that normal flexion and extension of the spine may aggravate spinal cord damage, initiated by static compression of the cord. During flexion, the spinal cord lengthens, which stretches it over osteophytic bars. During extension, the ligamentum flavum may buckle into the spinal canal, pinching the cord between the ligaments and anterior osteophytes. Spinal cord ischaemia is also involved in CSM. Histopathologic changes that are observed in CSM frequently involve gray matter with minimal white matter involvement (a pattern consistent with ischaemic insult). On T2 MRI the cord may appear high signal (Figure 10-4) and if this signal was low on T1 MRI sequences it indicates that irreversible spinal cord damage had occurred.

CSM is the most common cause of non-traumatic spastic paraparesis and quadriparesis. CSM represents 23.6% of patients presenting with non-traumatic myelopathic symptoms.[1] The prevalence of CSM in males was 13% in the third decade, rising to nearly 100% by the age of 70 years. In females, the prevalence ranged from 5% in the fourth decade to 96% in those older than 70 years.[2]

10-1-8 *How does cervical nerve root compression present?*

Clinically cervical root compression presents with pain, described as sharp, achy or burning in the neck, shoulder, arm or chest depending on the root or roots involved. Pain is displayed in a myotomal pattern whereas other sensory symptoms such as tingling follow a dermatomal pattern. Weakness of the arm and hand is reported less often than symptoms of pain and paraesthesia. Provocative tests may reproduce symptoms of radiculopathy. Holding

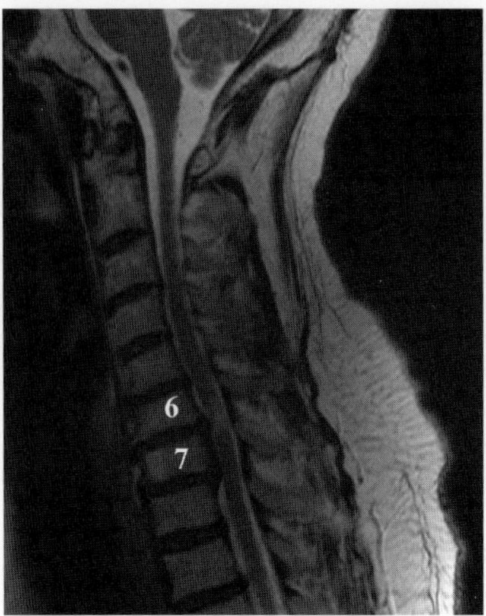

Figure 10-4: T2-weighted MRI sagittal of a patient presented with CSM demonstrating high signal at C6/7 level in the spinal cord.

the affected arm on top of the head or moving the head to look down and away from the symptomatic side often improves the pain, whereas rotation of the head or bending it towards the symptomatic side increases the pain (Spurling's test-observing a positive result from doing this test is helpful in differentiating cervical radiculopathy from other neurological disorders presenting with upper limb pain). Findings on physical examination vary depending on the level of the radiculopathy (Table 10-1). The nerve-root that is most frequently affected is the C7, followed by the C6.

10-1-9 *What are the indications for surgery?*

1- Failure of conservative therapy.
2- Patients who do not have the time to wait.
3- Progressive pain.
4- Progressive motor deficit.

The most widely used surgical operations to relieve symptoms and signs of cervical disc disease are anterior microdiscectomy, anterior cervical discectomy and fusion (ACDF) and formenotomy. The introduction of the

                                    Chapter 10

*Table 10-1: **Symptoms and signs of cervical nerve root compressions***

Nerve root (%)	Disc	Site of pain	Muscle affected (reflex)	Sensory change
C4	C3/4	Shoulder	Shoulder elevators	Shoulder area
C5 (2)	C4/5	Lateral arm	Deltoid (BJ)	Lateral arm
C6 (19)	C5/6	Lateral forearm	Biceps/wrist extension (SJ)	Thumb and Index
C7 (69)	C6/7	Back of arm/forearm	Triceps (TJ)	Middle finger
C8 (10)	C7T1	Ulnar side of arm/forearm	Intrinsic hand muscles	Little finger

surgical microscope provided better illumination and magnification of the surgical field leading to better teaching and less blood loss. Several techniques are used after disc removal to stabilise the level, e.g. artificial cages, plates and screws, and more recently disc replacement devices. The choice of procedure is governed by the pathology treated, the stability of the spine and the expertise and preferences of the surgeon. Recently, cervical IVD replacement has been instituted. However, its long-term results are still awaited and if the benefits prove to be excellent and reduces adjacent disc disease, it may become the procedure of choice in the future in some patients. The main reasons for performing disc replacement in the spine are to avoid adjacent disc disease and slow down spinal degeneration.

Your personal notes:

....

....

....

....

....

....

....

....

....

....

Problem 10-2: Sciatica, cauda equina and lumbar disc prolapse. How to manage a patient presenting with leg pain or cauda equina?

Any patient presenting with sudden low back pain (LBP) should be examined carefully to establish if (s)he has any of the red flags associated with LBP. Any patient who has LBP and any of the red flags should be investigated to rule out sinister aetiology that may cause irreversible nerve injury such as cauda equina syndrome (CES).

Problem based toolkit:	
Backache	**Discectomy**
Radiculopathy	**Laseque's**
Root tension	**SLR**
Sciatica	**Stenosis**
Spinal claudication	

PCS10-2-1:

A 41-year-old labourer presented with sudden onset sharp pain in his lower back and right leg, radiating down to his foot for six days. This followed lifting a sofa at home. The pain radiated from his back down the posterior aspect of his right thigh and calf to the foot. The pain had gradually decreased over the last five days, but was still bad and scored 80% on VAS and was not alleviated by analgesia. The pain was aggravated by lying on his left side and walking down stairs. He felt no noticeable weakness but he had episodes where the right leg could not support his weight and he tripped over a few times. He had constant numbness in the right foot. He knew when he wanted to pass urine and was able to hold it until it was convenient. He had left carpel tunnel decompression in 2008 and L2/3 lumbar microdiscectomy in 2007. He smoked 20 cigarettes a day for the last 25 years, and drank ten units of alcohol a week. He had no known allergies. Physical examination was normal apart from reduced straight leg raising (SLR) of 45 degrees on the right because of leg pain that was made worse by dorsiflexion (Lasègue's sign positive) and made better by bending the right hip and knee (bow-string sign). SLR on the left was 60 degrees because of pain in the right leg (cross-leg sign) He had impaired sensation in the lateral border of the right foot, absent right ankle jerk and globally reduced power in the right leg because of pain.

10-2-2 *What is the differential diagnosis of sciatica?*

1- Acute prolapsed lumbar disc most likely to be a right L5/S1 due to the sensory changes, reflex change and distribution of pain.
2- Extradural radicular nerve compression due to metastatic or primary bone lesion.
3- Extradural spinal infection, e.g. osteomyelitis.
4- Extradural benign radicular nerve compression due to neurofibroma, or epidural cyst.

10-2-3 *How to investigate a patient with sciatica?*

Full blood count, ESR and C-reactive protein were all normal excluding malignancy and spinal infections.

MRI scan of the spine demonstrated acute sequestrated disc at L5S1 level (Figures 10-5 and 10-6).

10-2-4 *How to manage a patient with lumbar radiculopathy?*

Management of patients with a prolapsed lumbar disc is initially conservative. If this fails surgery would be indicated.

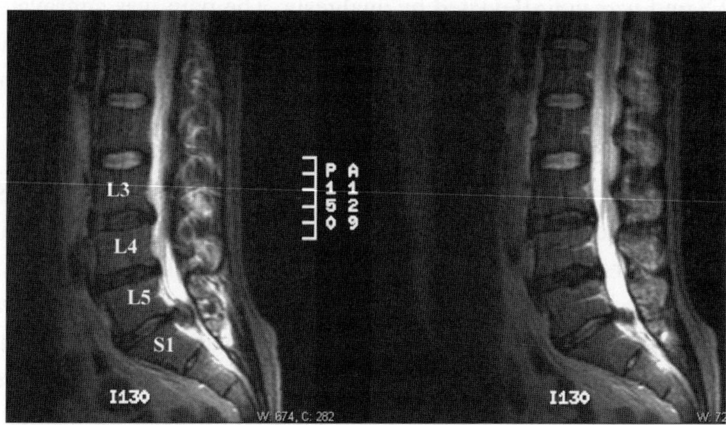

Figure 10-5: Sagittal MRI (T2) demonstrating disc prolapse at L5/S1. Note also that L4/5 and L3/4 discs are also degenerative, while discs above L3 look normal in appearance.

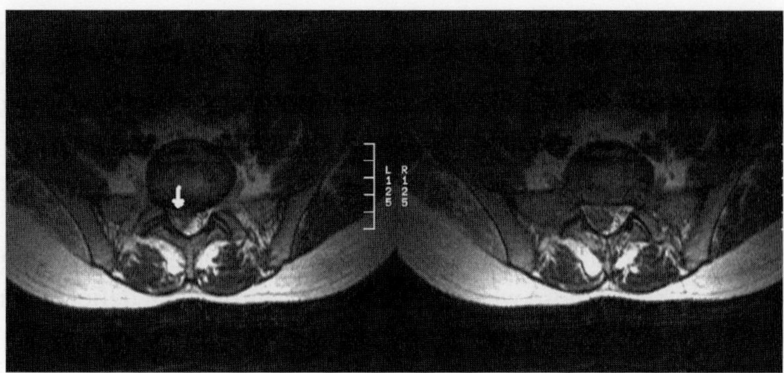

Figure 10-6: Axial MRI (T2) at the same level showing right-sided disc prolapse (arrow).

- **Conservative management:** This involves rest for one week with adequate analgesia and muscle relaxant if there was spasm of the back muscles. Once the pain is better, gentle back exercises would be recommended under the supervision of a physiotherapist. A second week of rest could be instituted if the pain was not getting worse and there was no significant neurological deficit. However, if the pain did not get better after two weeks of conservative therapy, or there was significant neurological deficit, or the pain was getting worse than better, then further investigation and surgery might become necessary. The reason for initial conservative therapy in all patients who do not have serious neurological deficit is that most patients in this category get better spontaneously (80% of patients in eight weeks from acute exacerbation) making surgery unnecessary in most patients. Historically patients with acute back pain were advised bed rest to avoid excessive strain on the spine. The initial thinking of the benefit of resting supine was based on the observation of symptom alleviation in this position. Further study of the intradiscal pressure showed significant reduction of intradiscal pressure in the horizontal position.[3] However more recent studies showed that staying active had a beneficial effect on pain and reduced sick leave in the long run. Thus, current advice for patients with acute LBP is to avoid complete bed rest and remain active within the limits of pain.[4]

- **Surgical management:** The indications for surgery include failure of conservative therapy, as in this case scenario PCS10-1-1, focal neurological deficit such as foot drop or sphincter disturbance or in some cases patient's preference. Discectomy including microdisectomy and percutaneous techniques are effective in 80% of patients. The risks of this procedure include infection in 2% of patients, discitis in < 1%, CSF leakage due to unintended durotomy, worsening neurological deficit in 8% of those who present with a neurological deficit and new neurological deficit such as cauda equina in one in 400.

10-2-5 *What is the pathophysiology of lumbar disc prolapse?*

Lumbar disc prolapse is a common presentation in middle-aged patients. Intervertebral discs consist of an annulus fibrosis, a tough outer layer analogous to onion skin, and a central soft nucleus pulposus, analogous to crab meat (Figure 10-7).

The disc acts as a shock absorber between the adjacent vertebral bodies. However, over time the disc is susceptible to degenerative changes with the annulus fibrosis weakening due to multiple tears occurring as a result of the frequent flexion/extension manoeuvres of activities of daily living and the nucleus pulposus drying out due to pressure. Figure 10-5

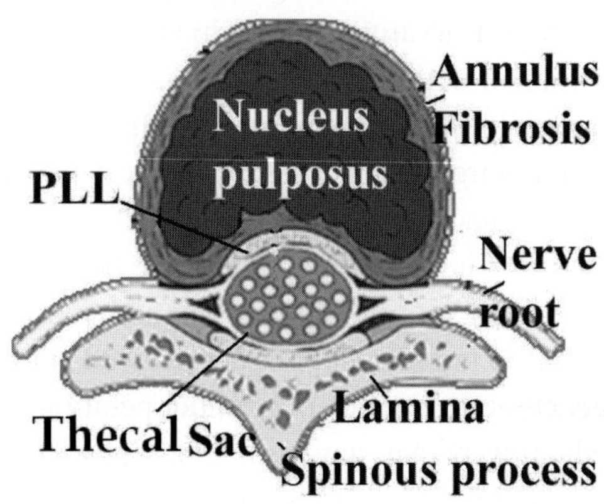

Figure 10-7: Schematic representation of intervertebral disc: PLL = posterior longitudinal ligament.

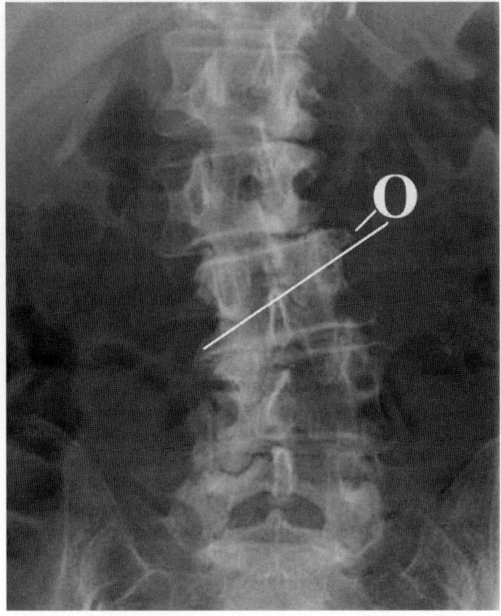

Figure 10-8: X-ray lumbar spine demonstrating osteophytes (O).

demonstrates disc degeneration in L3/4, L4/5 and L5/S1. These changes occur because the human spine was designed to be in the horizontal position and as humans adopted the upright posture with frequent flexion, the spine undergoes spinal degeneration of the discs, hypertrophy of the posterior elements (ligamentum flavum and facet joints) and development of osteophytes (spur of bones from the edges of the vertebrae) (Figure 10-8).

10-2-6 *What are the types of disc prolapse?*

Spinal degeneration follows the following steps:[3,4]

1- **Disc degeneration:** The discs become dehydrated resulting in weakening and reduction of the disc height, without herniation (L3/4 and L4/5 in Figure 10-5).

2- **Disc prolapse:** The annulus might stretch out like a balloon and the disc bulges causing slight narrowing of the spinal canal. This is

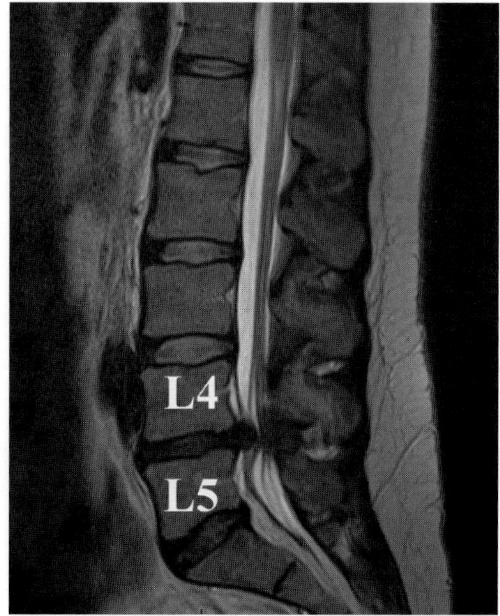

Figure 10-9: Contained disc hernia at L4/5.

called disc protrusion, diffuse disc bulge or contained disc herniation (Figure 10-9).

3- **Disc extrusion:** The soft nucleus pulposus ruptures through the annulus fibrosus but remains in continuity with the disc space (L5/S1 disc prolapse in Figure 10-5).

4- **Disc sequestration (sequestered disc):** The nucleus pulposus is squeezed out and is separated from the main part of the disc (Figure 10-10). A fragment of the nucleus pulposus therefore lies outside the disc and within the spinal canal. In some instances the fragment is sequestrated into the foramen and at a distance from the actual rupture, referred to as a free disc fragment (Figure 10-11).

The vast majority of intervertebral disc prolapses (IVDP) occur at L4/5 and L5/S1 levels and posterior lateral (Figure 10-5) because the central part of the annulus is supported by the posterior longitudinal ligament which is less formed laterally (Figure 10-7).

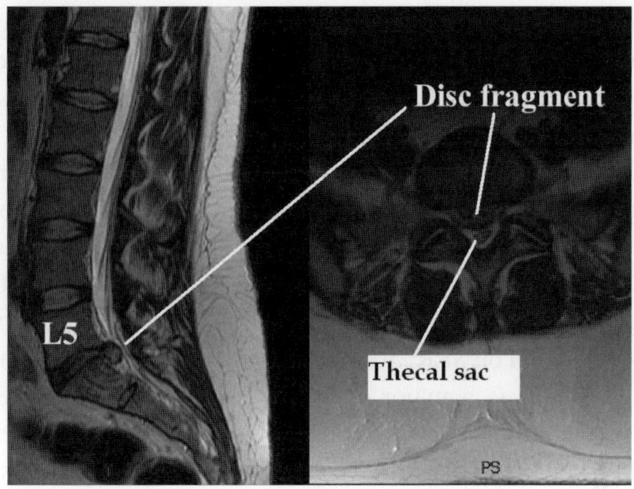

Figure 10-10: Sequestrated disc at L5/S1.

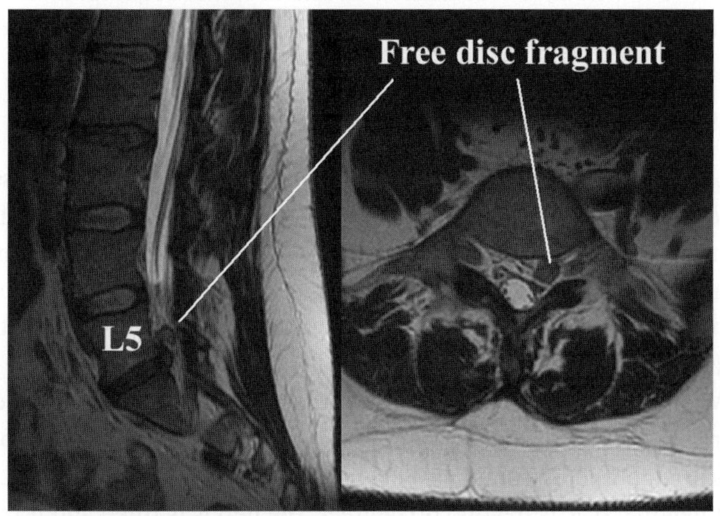

Figure 10-11: Free disc fragment.

10-2-7 *How does lumbar IVDP present and what are the signs?*

Lumbar IVDP often presents with pain radiating down the nerve root: L5 and S1 at the back of the thigh and leg down to the foot in a sciatic distribution, L3 and L4 down the lateral side of the thigh or sometimes anteriorly in femoral nerve distribution, while L1 and L2 radiate into the groin. Absence of sciatica in lumbar IVDP is found in less than 0.1%. Motor weakness occurs in 28%; sensory disturbance in the form of paraesthesia or impaired sensation or pins and needles in a dermatomal distribution occurs in 45%; reflex changes occurs in 51%; root tension signs are found in the majority of cases; positive cough effect occurs in 87% and bladder symptoms occur in a very small number of patients.

In high lumbar region L1/2, L2/3 and L3/4, 40% of patients will have positive root tension on SLR, 50% will have reduced knee jerk and in 51% of cases, trauma was a major factor in causation. Although each disc prolapse in the lumbar region compresses the descending nerve root, e.g. L5/S1 compresses S1 and L4/5 compresses L5, 3–10% of discs are more laterally located and compress the upper nerve root, e.g. a lateral L5/S1 disc will compress the L5. In these cases, 90% will have positive SLR root tension, 75% will have root tension on lateral spinal bending, in 60% will have free fragment (Figure 10-11) and double IVDP in 15% of patients.

10-2-8 *What are the root tension signs in lumbar spine?*

1- **Lasègue's sign:** SLR is restricted because of pain along the sciatic nerve between 30 and 60 degrees and made worse by dorsiflexion of the foot. When the leg is raised in a straight line without bending the knee from the supine position: during the first 30 degrees the lumbar lordosis is reversed and if the SLR was restricted at this range, it indicates mechanical LBP or an overlay sign due to secondary gain. When the SLR is 30–60 degrees, the sciatic nerve is stretched and any restriction due to leg pain at this range, indicates nerve root tension sign and is found in 83% of IVDP at L3/4, L4/5 and L5/S1. When the SLR is beyond 60 degrees, the pelvis is tilted and if restriction at this range then the sacro-iliac joints (SIJ) might be responsible (Figure 10-12).

2- **Cram test:** Some patients, particularly those who have free fragment and those who have high lumbar IVDP affecting the femoral nerve, patients are most comfortable with their knees and hip flexed; if the leg is straightened down, severe leg pain ensues.

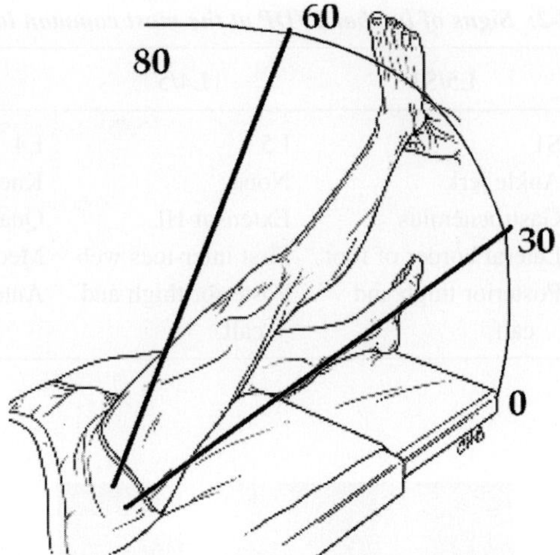

Figure 10-12: SLR and its interpretations; 0–30 degrees reversal of lumbar lordosis, 30–60 degrees stretching of the sciatic nerve and beyond 60 degrees pelvic tilt occurs.

3- **Fajersztajn's sign:** Present in free disc fragment and sequestrated discs, it is elicited by doing the SLR on the opposite leg and triggering leg pain in the symptomatic leg.

4- **Femoral stretch test:** Elicited by extending the hip in the prone position and would be positive if the L2, L3, or L4 are affected. Most of these patients are comfortable sitting up with their painful leg elevated with the knee extended and the hip flexed to 90 degrees.

5- **Bowstring sign:** Elicited by flexing the knee and hip from the SLR to relief root tension in the sciatic nerve.

6- **FABER test:** Femoral abduction and external rotation is a useful test to differentiate between hip joint problems and sciatica. In lumbar IVDP FABER is negative.

10-2-9 *How to clinically identify which nerve roots are affected?*

The most common locations for lumbar IVDP is L5/S1 representing 50%, the L4/5 is the second most common at 45%, the L3/4 represents 3.6%, the L2/3 1.8% and L1/2 0.28%. The following table lists the signs for each of the common locations (Table 10-2).

Table 10-2: Signs of lumbar IVDP at the most common locations

IVDP level	L5/S1	L4/5	L3/4
Nerve root	S1	L5	L4
Reflex affected	Ankle jerk	None	Knee jerk
Muscle affected	Gastrocnemius	Extensor HL	Quadriceps
Sensory change	Lateral border of foot	First inter-toes web	Medial malleolus area
Location of pain	Posterior thigh and calf	Posterior thigh and calf	Anterior lateral thigh

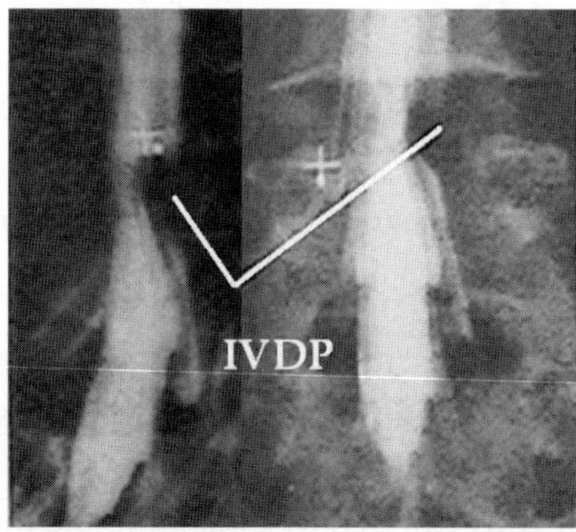

Figure 10-13: Myelogram demonstrating thumb impression sign indicating posterior-lateral lumbar IVDP.

10-2-10 *What imaging can be performed in lumbar IVDP?*

The investigation of choice is MRI scan as demonstrated in the example patient in this section, because MRI provides soft tissue high resolution images in multiple planes (Figures 10-5 and 10-6) and it does not expose the patient to ionising radiation. However, certain patients cannot have an MRI scan, these include: patients with cardiac pacemakers, metallic heart valves, intracranial aneurysm clips, neurostimulators and claustrophobics. In these circumstances it might be possible to reach the diagnosis by performing myelography or CT scan of the spine (Figure 10-13).

10-2-11 *What are the indications for surgery?*

1- Failure of conservative therapy.
2- Patients who do not have the time to wait.
3- Progressive pain.
4- Progressive motor deficit.
5- Cauda equina syndrome.

The most widely used surgical operation to relieve symptoms and signs of lumbar IVDP is microdiscectomy. It differs from naked eye discectomy in that it can be performed through a much smaller incision, the microscope provides better illumination and magnification of the surgical field leading to better teaching, less blood loss and less post-operative pain and earlier hospital discharge.[5] Several percutaneous procedures have been developed over the years including nucleotomy, endoscopy, laser, and chemonucleolysis. All these techniques achieve pain relief in the right patient: the right patient would be a patient with contained disc hernia with favourable trajectory, e.g. L4/5. Chemonucleolysis for example, was first used in 1963 by injecting the enzyme chymopapain derived from papaya skin, directly into the intervertebral disc. The enzyme degrades the nucleus pulposus relieving symptoms of IVDP. Studies comparing its efficacy with microdiscectomy showed conflicting results and highlighted how important patients' selection was.

Recently, lumbar IVD replacement has been instituted. However, its long-term results are still awaited and if the benefits prove to be excellent compared to the magnitude and risks of the procedure, it may become the procedure of choice in the future in some patients. The main reasons for performing disc replacement in the spine are to avoid adjacent disc disease and slow down spinal degeneration. In a recent randomised controlled trial (SPORT) comparing surgery to non-operative management of lumbar IVDP, of the 743 patients enrolled in the observational cohort, 528 patients received surgery and 191 received usual non-operative care. At three months, patients who chose surgery had greater improvement in the primary outcome measures of bodily pain (mean change: surgery, 40.9 vs. non-operative care, 26.0; treatment effect, 14.8; 95% confidence interval (CI), 10.8–18.9), physical function (mean change: surgery, 40.7 vs. non-operative care, 25.3; treatment effect, 15.4; 95% CI, 11.6–19.2), and Oswestry Disability Index (mean change: surgery, –36.1 vs. non-operative care, –20.9; treatment effect, –15.2; 95% CI, –18.5 to –11.8). These differences narrowed somewhat at two years: bodily pain (mean change: surgery, 42.6 vs. non-operative care, 32.4; treatment effect, 10.2; 95% CI, 5.9–14.5), physical function (mean change: surgery, 43.9 vs. non-operative care, 31.9; treatment effect, 12.0; 95% CI, 7.9–16.1), and Oswestry Disability Index (mean change: surgery, –37.6 vs. non-operative care, –24.2; treatment effect, –13.4; 95% CI, –17.0 to –9.7). In conclusion, the SPORT trial had shown that patients with persistent sciatica from lumbar IVDP improved in both operated and usual care groups. Those who chose operative intervention reported greater improvements than patients who elected non-operative care.[6]

10-2-11 *What is cauda equina syndrome (CES)?*

CES is compression of the nerve roots of the cauda equina in the lumbar region, it manifests with urinary retention in over 90% of patients, associated with reduced anal tone in 70% and impaired sensation of the saddle area in over 98% with or without motor weakness and bilateral leg pain.

10-2-12 *What is the outcome and risks of lumbar IVDP surgery?*

The leg pain relief rate at one year is 73% and for LBP is 63%. At ten years, 86% of patients are better and 5% develop failed back surgery syndrome (FBSS). In randomised controlled studies, patients who went for surgery upfront were better in the first year, but at four and ten years there was no difference and about 30% of patients developed neck problems by ten years. If patients presented with reflex changes, the reflex remains abnormal in 35–43%, motor deficit improved in 80% and worsened in 3%, sensory impairment improved in 69% and worsened in 15%. The risks of surgery include 2% risk of superficial wound infection, <1% risk of discitis, motor deficit in 1–8%, dural tear in 5% and very rarely other injuries.

10-2-13 *How do red flags work in patients with LBP?*

Red flags were established by LBP guidelines development groups to help doctors and other health care workers to identify those patients at risk of sinister pathologies as LBP is very common in the community with more than 80% of the population experienced LBP sometime in their lives. Red flags associated with LBP can help identify which patients should be investigated (Figure 10-14). However, if you are in doubt, it is better to

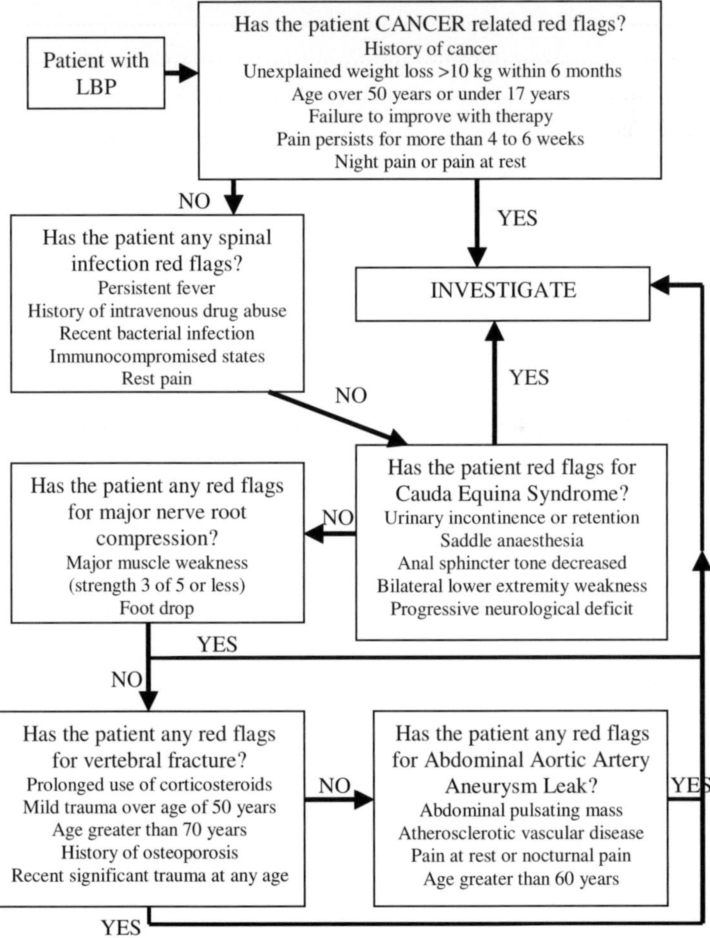

Figure 10-14: LBP and red flags.

investigate the patient with MRI scan of the spine to make sure that you do not miss a critical diagnosis.

Your personal notes:

....

....

....

....

....

....

....

....

....

....

Problem 10-3:   Hands and feet numbness and peripheral nerves. How to manage a patient presenting with hand or foot numbness?

Patients presenting with sensory symptoms in the arms and legs most likely to be suffering from peripheral nerve or nerve root disorder. Common problems of peripheral nerves include carpal tunnel syndrome (CTS), ulnar nerve compression (UNC), peripheral neuropathy (PN) and Guillain-Barre syndrome (GBS).

Problem based tool box:	
Paraesthesia	**Numbness**
CTS	**UNC**
Neuropathy	**GBS**

PCS10-3-1:

A 45-year-old woman presented with several weeks history of pins and needles in the radial three fingers. She tended to wake up in the middle of the night because of these symptoms. She often gets rid of the symptoms by shaking her hand, but lately she wakes up with difficulty gripping objects first thing in the morning. Examination revealed that she had altered sensation in the radial three and the half fingers and palm and she had some difficulty in thumb opposition. Her sensation was normal at the wrist and in the forearms.

10-3-2 *What is the differential diagnosis of numb index and thumb?*

You should suspect the following in any patient presenting with sensory symptoms in the radial aspect of the hand:

1- Carpal Tunnel Syndrome (CTS).
2- C6–C7 radiculopathy.
3- Peripheral neuropathy (PN).

PCS10-3-3:

A 56-year-old man presented with several months history of pins and nee-dles in the little finger. He tended to wake up in the morning with difficulty in straightening his little and ring fingers. Examination revealed that he had altered sensation in the little and ring fingers and the ulnar side of his palm and had normal sensation at the wrist and in the forearms.

10-3-4 *What is the differential diagnosis of the numb little finger?*

You should suspect the following in any patient presenting with sensory symptoms in the ulnar aspect of the hand:

1- Ulnar nerve compression at the elbow (UNC).
2- C8 radiculopathy.
3- Peripheral neuropathy (PN).

PCS10-3-5:

A 60-year-old diabetic woman presented with several months history of pins and needles in both hands and feet. She was an insulin-dependent diabetic for 20 years. Examination revealed that she had altered sensation in both hands up to 4 cm above the wrists and in both feet up to the level of the knees (gloves and stocking).

10-3-6 *What is the differential diagnosis of numb hands and feet?*

You should suspect the following in any patient presenting with bilateral sensory symptoms in hands and feet:

1- Peripheral polyneuropathy (PPN).
2- Chronic inflammatory demylinating polyneuropathy (CIDP).
3- Guillain-Barre Syndrome (GBS).

10-3-7 *How to manage carpal tunnel syndrome (CTS)?*

CTS is median neuropathy at the wrist, in which the median nerve is compressed at the wrist, leading to paraesthesia, numbness and weakness in the hand. Night symptoms and waking up at night is a characteristic of established CTS. CTS symptoms can be managed effectively with night-time wrist splint in most patients. However, some patients may require carpal tunnel release surgery. This is effective in relieving symptoms and preventing further median nerve damage, but established nerve dysfunction in the form of static (constant) numbness, atrophy, or weakness are usually permanent and do not respond to surgery. Compression of the median nerve as it runs deep to the transverse carpal ligament (TCL) causes wasting of the thenar eminence, weakness of the flexor pollicis brevis (FPB), opponens pollicis (OP), abductor pollicis brevis (APB), as well as sensory loss in the distribution of the median nerve distal to the TCL. There is a superficial sensory branch of the median nerve, which branches proximal to the TCL and travels superficial to it. This branch is therefore spared, and it innervates the palm towards the thumb.

The most important risk factor for CTS is structural and biological rather than environmental or activity-related. The strongest risk factor is genetic predisposition.[7] However, CTS is sometimes associated with other diseases; **M**yxoedema, **E**dema, **D**iabetes mellitus, **I**diopathic, **A**cromegaly, **N**eoplasm, **T**rauma, **R**heumatoid arthritis, **A**myloidosis and **P**regnancy (MEDIAN TRAP).

10-3-8 *How to diagnose CTS?*

If a patient presented with numbness in the median nerve include CTS in the differential. However, if pain was the predominant feature it would be unlikely that CTS is the cause of pain. You can also carry out the following tests:

1- Phalen's manoeuvre is performed by flexing the wrist gently as far as possible, then holding this position and awaiting symptoms. If numbness starts within one minute of holding the wrist in this position, Phalen's test is considered positive for CTS. The quicker the numbness starts, the more advanced the condition.

2- Tinel's sign is a way to detect irritated nerves. Tinel's is performed by lightly tapping the skin over the TCL to elicit a sensation of tingling or "pins and needles" in the median nerve. Tinel's sign is less specific in CTS.

3- Durkan test, carpal compression test, or applying firm pressure to the palm over the nerve for up to 30 seconds to elicit symptoms has also been proposed.

4- NCS is the main diagnostic test to confirm CTS by demonstrating slowness of conduction velocity across the wrist joint. Normal sensory conduction velocity (SCV) across the wrist to index finger is less than 3.7 m/sec and motor conduction velocity (MCV) across the wrist to APB muscle is less than 4.5 m/sec. Mild CTS is diagnosed when SCV and MCV were 3.7–4 and 4.4–6.9 m/sec respectively. Moderate CTS is diagnosed when SCV and MCV were 4.1–5 and 7–9.9 m/sec respectively. Severe CTS is diagnosed when SCV and MCV were >5 and >10 m/sec respectively.

10-3-9 *How to manage cubital tunnel syndrome (UNC)?*

UNC is the effect of pressure on the ulnar nerve, as it passes behind the medial epicondyle at the elbow. It can result in a variety of problems, including pain, swelling, weakness or clumsiness of the hand and tingling or numbness of the ring and little fingers. It also often results in elbow pain on the ulnar side of the arm. The ulnar nerve is positioned right next to the bone and has very little padding over it, so pressure on this can put pressure on the nerve, e.g. leaning the elbow against a table. In some patients, the ulnar nerve at the elbow clicks back and forth over the medial epicondyle as the elbow is bent and extended. If this occurs repetitively, the nerve may be significantly irritated. Additionally, pressure on the ulnar nerve can occur from holding the elbow in a bent position for a long time, which stretches the nerve across the medial epicondyle. Such sustained bending of the elbow tends to occur during sleep. Sometimes the connective tissue over the nerve becomes thicker, or there may be variations of the muscle structure over the nerve at the elbow that causes pressure on the nerve. UNC occurs when the pressure on the nerve is significant enough, and sustained enough, to disturb the way the ulnar nerve works.

UNC symptoms usually include pain, numbness, and tingling. The numbness or tingling most often occurs in the ring and little fingers. The symptoms are usually felt when there is pressure on the nerve, such as sitting with the elbow on an arm rest, or with repetitive elbow bending and straightening. Often symptoms will be felt when the elbow is held in a bent position for a period of time, such as when holding the phone, or while sleeping. Some patients may notice weakness while pinching, occasional clumsiness, or a tendency to drop things. In severe cases, sensation may be lost and the muscles in the hand may lose bulk and strength, particularly the first dorsal interosseous muscle.

The majority of UNC cases are idiopathic and a small number may be associated with trauma, pregnancy, rheumatoid arthritis or hypothyroidism.

10-3-10 *How to diagnose UNC?*

The diagnosis of UNC should be suspected in any patient presenting with numbness, paraesthesia and pain in the little and ring fingers, wasting of the interosseous muscles of the hand or clawing of the ulnar fingers. Other tests that may help in the diagnosis include:

1- Sensory loss restricted to the ulnar side of the palm and little and ring fingers with no sensory loss above the wrist joint.
2- Wartenberg's sign is abducted little finger due to weakness of the third palmer interosseous muscle.
3- Froment's prehensile thumb sign is elicited by asking the patient to hold on to a sheet of paper between the thumb and index fingers. A positive Froment's sign when the patient flexes the proximal phalanx of the thumb and flexes the distal phalanx as he uses the flexor pollicus longus to hold the paper instead of the weak first dorsal interosseous muscle.
4- Claw deformity of the hand.
5- NCS confirms the diagnosis by demonstrating slowness of SCV and MCV of the ulnar nerve across the elbow joint slower than 48 m/sec or more than 10 m/sec slower at the elbow than above or below the elbow.

Non-operative therapy such as painkillers and splints might help mild symptoms, but the majority of patients with troublesome symptoms require surgical treatment to decompress the ulnar nerve or transpose it away from the cubital tunnel.

10-3-11 *How to manage peripheral neuropathy (PN)?*

PN is dysfunction or damage of peripheral nerves as a result of disease or side effect of systemic illness or therapy. There are four main types; polyneuropathy (PPN), mononeuropathy (PMN), mononeuritis multiplex (MNM) and autonomic neuropathy (AN). The most common form is PPN that can be divided into small or large fibre PPN. In the majority of cases no cause could be identified (idiopathic).

Sensory symptoms include tingling, numbness, burning sensation or pain. Motor symptoms include weakness, twitching, cramps and spasms. Autonomic symptoms include abnormal blood pressure, abnormal heart rate, constipation, incontinence and impotence.

Although in many patients the cause of PPN cannot be ascertained the causes of PPN can be divided into:

1- Genetic diseases: Friedreich's ataxia, Charcot-Marie-Tooth syndrome.
2- Metabolic/endocrine: Diabetes mellitus, chronic renal failure, porphyria, amyloidosis, liver failure, hypothyroidism.
3- Toxic causes: Alcoholism, drugs [vincristine, phenytoin, nitrofurantoin, isoniazid, organic metals, heavy metals, excess intake of Vitamin B_6 (Pyridoxine)].
4- Fluoroquinolone toxicity: Irreversible neuropathy is a serious adverse reaction of Fluoroquinolone drugs.
5- Inflammatory diseases: Guillain-Barré syndrome, systemic lupus erythematosis (SLE), leprosy, Sjögren's syndrome.
6- Vitamin deficiency states: Vitamin B_{12} (Cyanocobalamin), Vitamin A, Vitamin E, Vitamin B_1 (Thiamin).
7- Physical trauma: Compression, pinching, cutting, projectile injuries (gunshot wound), strokes including prolonged occlusion of blood flow.
8- Others: Shingles, malignant disease, HIV, radiation, chemotherapy.

MNM is characterised by multifocal sensory motor axonal neuropathy on NCS and often associated with diabetes mellitus, polyarteritis nodosa, Wagner's granulomatosis, Chrug-Srauss syndrome, rheumatoid arthritis,

SLE, sarcoidosis, leprosy, HIV, Lyme disease, amyloidosis, ceyoglobuli-naemia, trichloroethylene and dapsone.

PPN can be divided into:

1- Distal axonopathy where the cell bodies remain intact while the axons are damaged commonly seen in diabetes mellitus.
2- Demyelinating neuropathy where the axons remain intact while the myelin sheath is damaged, e.g. in GBS and CIDP.
3- Ganglionopathy, the least common type.

Negative (loss of function) symptoms of PN include impaired sensation, muscle weakness, imbalance, tiredness and gait disturbance. Positive (gain) symptoms include tingling, itchiness, pain, burning sensation, pins and needles, cramps, tremor and fasciculations.

References

1. Moore AP, Blumhardt LD. A prospective survey of the causes of non-traumatic spastic paraparesis and tetraparesis in 585 patients. *Spinal Cord* 1997; 35: 361–367.
2. Irvine D, Foster J *et al.* Prevalence of cervical spondylosis in a general practice. *Lancet* 1965; 14: 1089–1092.
3. Scannell J, McGull S. Disc prolapse: evidence of reversal with repeated extension. *Spine* 2009; 34: 344–350.
4. Hofstee DJ, Gijtenbeek JM, Hoogland PH *et al.* Westeinde sciatica trial: randomized controlled study of bed rest and physiotherapy for acute sciatica. *J Neurosurg Spine* 2002; 96: 45–49.
5. Gibson JNA, Waddell G. Surgical interventions for lumbar disc prolapse. *Cochrane Database Syst Rev* 2007; (2): CD001350. DOI: 10.1002/14651858.CD001350.pub4.
6. Weinstein JN, Tosteson TD, Lurie JD *et al.* Surgical vs nonoperative treatment for lumbar disk herniation: the Spine Patient Outcomes Research Trial (SPORT): a randomized trial. *J Am Med Assoc* 2006; 296: 2451–2459.
7. Hakim AJ, Cherkas L, El Zayat S *et al.* The genetic contribution to carpal tunnel syndrome in women: a twin study. *Arthr Rheum* 2002; 47(3): 275–279.

Your personal notes:

....

....

....

....

....

....

....

....

....

....

Appendices

Appendix I: Scales and classifications in neurosurgery. How best to use these scales and grades?

Scales and grades used in neurosurgery to assist decision making, predict prognosis and compare results.

1-1 *The Glasgow coma scale (GCS): used to assess levels of consciousness:*

Score	EOR	BVR	BMR	Definitions
1	None	None	None	Any patient within
2	To speech	Sounds	Extension to pain	this shaded area
3	To pain	Words	Abnormal flexion to pain	is in **COMA**
4	Spontaneous	Confused	Flexion to pain	
5		Orientated	Localising pain	
6			Obeys simple commands	Not in coma

1-2 *The WFNS grades of SAH and the outcome of SAH:*

Grade	GCS	Hemi-/monoparesis or dysphasia	Prognosis odds ratio for poor outcome (95% CI)
I	15	Absent	
II	13–14	Absent	2.3 (1.3 to 4.1)
III	13–14	Present	6.1 (2.9 to 12.8)
IV	7–12	With or without	7.7 (4.3 to 13.7)
V	3–6	With or without	69.2 (30.6 to 156.3)

1-3 *Fisher grades of SAH on CT:*

Grade	Description	Signs of vasospasm
I	No blood detected on CT	0
II	Diffuse or vertical layers <1 mm thick	0
III	Localised clot or vertical layer of 1 mm or thicker	96%
IV	Intra-ventricular or intra-cerebral clot and diffuse SAH	0

1-4 *Spetzler-Martin AVM classifications:*

Grade	Size of nidus	Site	Venous drainage
I	<3 cm	Non-eloquent	Superficial
II	<3 cm	Eloquent location	Superficial
	<3 cm	Non-eloquent	Deep
	3–6 cm	Non-eloquent	Superficial
III	<3 cm	Eloquent	Deep
	3–6 cm	Eloquent	Superficial
	3–6 cm	Non-eloquent	Deep
	>6 cm	Non-eloquent	Superficial
IV	3–6 cm	Eloquent	Deep
	>6 cm	Eloquent	Superficial
	>6 cm	Non-eloquent	Deep
V	>6 cm	Eloquent	Deep

1-5 *Engel grades of epilepsy surgery outcome:*

Grade	Descriptor
I	Seizure free
II	Occasional seizures controlled on medications
III	Worthwhile improvement
IV	No improvement

1-6 *Gardner Robertson hearing grades (outcome of hearing preservation):*

Grade	Description	Audiogram	Speech discrimination
I	Good hearing	0–30 dB	70–100%
II	Serviceable	31–50 dB	50–69%
III	Non-serviceable	51–90 dB	5–49%
IV	Poor	91–max	1–4%
V	None	None	0

1-7 *House Brackmann grades of facial nerve function outcome:*

Grade	Facial nerve function	Description
1	Normal	Normal function in all areas
2	Slight dysfunction	Weakness noticeable on close examination
3	Moderate dysfunction	Noticeable but not disfiguring
4	Moderate to severe	Disfiguring facial asymmetry
5	Severe dysfunction	Barely facial movement
6	Total paralysis	No movement in the face

1-8 *Modified MRC grades of muscle power:*

Grade	Description
5	Full power against maximum resistance — difficult to overcome
4+	Movement against strong resistance — can be overcomed
4	Movement against moderate resistance that can be easily overcome
4-	Movement against mild resistance — easily overcomed
3	Movement against gravity
2	Movement with gravity eliminated
1	Flicker of movement
0	No movement — total paralysis

1-9 *Karnofsky performance status score (KPS) for physical function:*

Score	Description
100	Normal, no symptoms or signs of disease
90	Able to carry on normal activities, minor complaints
80	Able to carry on normal activities with effort, some symptoms
70	Self caring but unable to carry on with normal activities
60	Caters for most needs, requires occasional assistance
50	Requires frequent assistance and frequent care
40	Disabled requires special care and assistance
30	Severely disabled, requires hospitalisation
20	Very ill, requires active supportive care
10	Moribund progressing to death rapidly

1-10 *Glasgow outcome scale (GOS):*

Score	Description
5	Good recovery, resumption of normal activities despite minor disability
4	Moderate disability but independent, able to use public transport
3	Severe disability, dependent for daily support
2	Persistent vegetative state, unresponsive and speechless
1	Death

1-11 *Ashworth grades of spasticity:*

Score	Description
1	Normal tone
2	Slight increase "a catch"
3	More marked increase in tone, passive movement easy
4	Considerable increase in tone, passive movement with effort
5	Rigid in flexion or extension

1-12 *ASIA spinal injury scale: each function graded 0–5:*

Right	Segment	Muscles	Tested function	Left
	C5	Deltoid/Biceps	Shoulder abduction elbow flex	
	C6	Wrist extenders	Wrist extension	
	C7	Triceps	Elbow extension	
	C8	Finger flexors	Finger flexion	
	T1	Hand intrinsic	Finger abduction	
	L2	Iliopsoas	Hip flexion	
	L3	Quadriceps	Knee extension	
	L4	Tibialis anterior	Dorsiflexion foot	
	L5	EHL	Dorsiflexion big toe	
	S1	Gastrocnemius	Plantar flexion	
50			Maximum score on each side	50

1-13 *Astrocytoma grading system:*

Grade	Kernohan's	WHO	Description
Low	I	I	Minimal hypercellularity and pleomorphism
Low	II	II	Moderate hypercellularity and pleomorphism
High	III	III (AA)	Marked hypercellularity and pleomorphism
High	IV	IV (GBM)	Same as III plus neovascularization + necrosis

1-14 *Modified Brice and MacKissock spinal cord function with spinal metastasis:*

Grade	Weakness	Description
0	None	Normal power and sensation
1	Mild	Able to walk unaided
2	Moderate	Can mobilise against gravity for transfer
3	Severe	Unable to transfer but some movement and sensation
4	Very severe	Very slight residual or sensory function
5	Profound	No motor or sensory function

1-15 *Simpson grading for meningioma excision:*

Grade	Description	Risk of recurrence
I	Complete removal including dural origin	9% in 5 years
II	Complete excision cauterisation of origin	19% in 5 years
III	Gross excision only	29% in 5 years
IV	Partial removal	100%
V	Biopsy or decompression	100%

1-16 *NIH stroke score (NIHSS):*

Score	Function	Descriptions (Score 0 = Normal)
0–3	LOC	1 = easy to arouse, 2 = difficult to arouse, 3 = coma
0–2	Orientation	1 = partially oriented, 2 = disoriented
0–2	Commands	1 = intermittently obeys, 2 = not obeying commands
0–2	Gaze	1 = partial gaze palsy, 2 = forced gaze palsy
0–3	Visual	1 = scotoma, 2 = hemianopsia, 3 = bilateral hemianopsia
0–3	Face	1 = minor, 2 = partial, 3 = complete facial palsy
0–4*	Motor arm	1 = drift, 2 = against gravity, 3 = gravity eliminated, 4 = none
0–4*	Motor leg	1 = drift, 2 = against gravity, 3 = gravity eliminated, 4 = none
0–2*	Ataxia	1 = one limb, 2 = present in two limbs
0–2	Sensory	1 = mild to moderate, 2 = severe sensory loss
0–3	Speech	1 = mild to moderate, 2 = severe dysphasia, 3 = mute
0–2**	Dysarthria	1 = mild to moderate, 2 = severe
0–2	Attention	1 = neglect in one area, 2 = hemi neglect

1-17 *Smith grading of oligodendrogliomas:*

Descriptor	Grade A	B	C	D
Nucleus: cytoplasm ratio	Decreased	*	Increased	Increased
Cell density	Decreased	*	Increased	Increased
Pleomorphism	Absent	*	Present	Present
Endothelial proliferation	Absent	Absent	Present	Present
Necrosis	Absent	Absent	Absent	Present

* If one of these present, oligo is classified as B.

1-18 *ECOG/WHO/Zubrod score*

The ECOG score, also called the WHO or Zubrod score (after C. Gordon
Zubrod) runs from 0 to 5, with 0 denoting perfect health and 5 death

- 0 — Asymptomatic (fully active, able to carry on all pre-disease activities without restriction).
- 1 — Symptomatic but completely ambulatory (restricted in physically strenuous activity but ambulatory and able to carry out work of a light or sedentary nature. For example, light housework, office work).
- 2 — Symptomatic, <50% in bed during the day (ambulatory and capable of all self care but unable to carry out any work activities. Up and about more than 50% of waking hours).
- 3 — Symptomatic, >50% in bed, but not bedbound (capable of only limited self care, confined to bed or chair 50% or more of waking hours).
- 4 — Bedbound (completely disabled. Cannot carry on any self care. Totally confined to bed or chair).
- 5 — Death.

1-19 *Lansky score*

Children, who might have more trouble expressing their experienced
quality of life, require a somewhat more observational scoring system
suggested and validated by Lansky *et al.* in 1987.

- 100 — fully active, normal.
- 90 — minor restrictions in strenuous physical activity.
- 80 — active, but tired more quickly.
- 70 — greater restriction of play *and* less time spent in play activity.
- 60 — up and around, but active play minimal; keeps busy by being involved in quieter activities.
- 50 — lying around much of the day, but gets dressed; no active playing participates in all quiet play and activities.
- 40 — mainly in bed; participates in quiet activities.
- 30 — bedbound; needing assistance even for quiet play.

- 20 — sleeping often; play entirely limited to very passive activities.
- 10 — doesn't play; does not get out of bed.
- 0 — unresponsive.

Comparison

A comparison between the Zubrod and Karnofsky scales has been validated in a large sample of patients

- Zubrod 0 equals Karnofsky 100; 90–100.
- Zubrod 1 equals Karnofsky 80–90; 70–80.
- Zubrod 2 equals Karnofsky 60–70; 50–60.
- Zubrod 3 equals Karnofsky 40–50; 30–40.
- Zubrod 4 equals Karnofsky 20–30; 10–20.

1-20 *Modified Rankin Scale*

SCORE	DESCRIPTION
0	No symptoms at all.
1	No significant disability despite symptoms; able to carry out all usual duties and activities.
2	Slight disability; unable to carry out all previous activities, but able to look after own affairs without assistance.
3	Moderate disability; requiring some help, but able to walk without assistance.
4	Moderately severe disability; unable to walk without assistance and unable to attend to own bodily needs without assistance.
5	Severe disability; bedridden, incontinent and requiring constant nursing care and attention.
6	Dead.

- TOTAL (0–6): _______

1-21 *Menimental state examination (MMSE):*

Orientation:

What is the year, season, month, day, date?	1 point each
Where are we (state, country, city, hospital floor)?	1 point each

Registration:

Name 3 objects taking one second to say each. Ask pt to repeat all   1 point each
   3 immediately after you say them. Repeat until he/she learns
   all three.

Attention & Calculation:

Serial 7's (stop after 5 correct), or spell "world" backwards.   1 point each up to 5

Recall:

Ask pt to name the three objects named above.   1 point each

Language:

Name 2 objects that you show (i.e. pencil, pen, cup).   1 point each
Repeat "no ifs, ands or buts".   1 point
Have pt read sentence "Close your eyes" and have them do what   1 point
   it says.
Follow a three-step command (i.e. take the piece of paper, fold   1 point each step
   it in half, and toss it on the floor).
Write a sentence.   1 point
Copy a complex polygon.   1 point

Appendix II: Syndromes in neurosurgery

2-1 *Adie's tonic pupil:*

Pathology with unknown aetiology, which determines pupil alterations probably secondary to damage at the level of post-ganglion fibres. As the fibres innervating both the pupillary sphincter muscle and the ciliary muscle are involved, both pupil reflexes and accommodation are compromised. The pathology is characterised by an irregular and dilated pupil, with scarce or absent reaction to light. It is often associated with hypo- or areflexia.

2-2 *Argyll Robertson's pupil:*

Found in neurosyphilis, small-sized (< 2 mm) and often irregular pupils. Near dissociation is present, and pupils show scarce dilation after instillation of mydriatic eye drops. Similar features, for the presence of near dissociation, are present in diabetes (probably due to a peripheral autonomic neuropathy), chronic alcoholism, encephalitis and some degenerative diseases.

2-3 *Benedikt's syndrome:*

Ipsilateral third nerve palsy and contralateral hemiparesis and tremor due to a lesion involving the third nerve fibres, the red nucleus, cerebellothalamic fibres and the corticospinal tract.

2-4 *Cavernous sinus syndrome (CSS):*

Will result into complete ophthalmoplegia associated with trigeminal nerve dysfunction in V1 and V2 and often associated with propotosis due to obstruction of venous drainage of the orbit. The eye may be pulsatile and the eye is red in carotid-cavernous fistula (CCF).

2-5 *False localising sign (FLS):*

A sign that cannot be relied on to localise the neurological lesion, e.g. hemiparesis and sixth nerve palsy in raised intracranial pressure and C8 radiculopthy in cervical spinal cord compression.

2-6 *Foville's syndrome:*

Ipsilateral sixth and seventh nerve palsies and contralateral hemiparesis due to a lesion involving the corticospinal tract, the sixth nucleus and the fibres of the facial nerve.

2-7 *Gerstman's syndrome:*

Means dyscalculia, dysgraphia and finger agnosia found in lesions in the dominant parietal lobe.

2-8 *Gradenigo's syndrome:*

Gradenigo's syndrome, also called Gradenigo-Lannois syndrome and petrous apicitis, is a complication of otitis media and mastoiditis involving the apex of the petrous temporal bone. Symptoms of the syndrome include: otalgia due to pain in the area supplied by the ophthalmic branch of the trigeminal nerve (fifth cranial nerve), ipsilateral paralysis of the abducens nerve (sixth cranial nerve), and otitis media.

2-9 *Millard-Gubler's syndrome:*

Ipsilateral lower motor neuron facial weakness and contralateral hemiparesis due to a lesion in the pons involving the facial nucleus and corticospinal tract.

2-10 *Parinaud's syndrome:*

Or dorsal mesencephalus syndrome. Pupils in medium mydriasis (4–5 mm), round and regular. Dissociation between light reflex, which is scarce or absent, and near reflex, which is normal. A consequence of: involvement of afferent pupillary fibres at the pretectal level, that is the fibres which, once leaving the visual pathways, direct towards the pretectal nuclei. This syndrome can be associated with proptosis or compressive optic neuropathy. The signs are: paralysis of the upwards gaze and nystagmus *(convergence-retraction)* eyelid retraction (Collier's sign). The most frequent causes of Parinaud's syndrome are: tumours of the pineal gland region, multiple sclerosis, ischaemic lesions and hydrocephalus with ventricular dilation.

2-11 *Raymond's syndrome:*

Ipsilateral sixth nerve palsy and contralateral hemiparesis due to a lesion involving the sixth nerve nucleus and the corticospinal tract.

2-12 *Superior orbital fissure syndrome (SOFS):*

Means complete ophthalmoplegia and ophthalmic trigeminal neuropathy as the third, fourth, sixth and the ophthalmic division of the trigeminal nerve (V1) enter the orbit at the superior orbital fissure. Tumours, either primary or secondary, are the primary causes of SOFS and depending on the size and extent of the lesion.

2-13 *True localising sign (TLS):*

A sign indicating the location of an expanding intracranial lesion such as the third nerve palsy indicating that the side of the lesion is on the same side of the third nerve palsy.

2-14 *Uncal herniation syndrome (UHS):*

Third nerve palsy due to uncal herniation that may be associated with ipsilateral hemiparesis.

2-15 *Weber's syndrome:*

Iipsilateral third nerve palsy and contralateral hemiparesis due to a lesion involving the third nerve fibres and the corticospinal tract.

Appendix III: A–Z symptoms of body systems

- Abdominal Cramps, Abdominal Discomfort, Abdominal Pain
- Abnormal Taste (Loss of Appetite)
- Abnormal Vaginal Bleeding, Discharge (Vaginal Discharge)
- Abnormally Rapid Breathing (Hyperventilation)
- Absent Periods (Missed Menstrual Period), Amenorrhea
- Ache, Back (Back Pain), Ache, Ear (Earache), Ache, Tooth (Toothache)
- Acid Indigestion (Heartburn), Acid Reflux (Heartburn)
- Agitation (Anxiety)
- Alopecia (Hair Loss)
- Amnesia (Memory Loss)
- Anal Itching
- Anaemia
- Anorexia (Loss of Appetite)
- Anxiety
- Appetite, Loss of (Loss of Appetite)
- Apprehension (Anxiety)
- Arm Weakness (Weakness)
- Arthralgia (Joint Pain)
- Arthralgia, Elbow (Elbow Pain)
- Arthralgia, Knee (Knee Pain)
- Arthralgia, Shoulder (Shoulder Pain)

- Back Pain, Backache (Back Pain)
- Balance (Dizziness)
- Baldness (Hair Loss)
- Beat (Fatigue and Tiredness)
- Belching (Gas)
- Belly Ache (Abdominal Pain), Belly Pain (Abdominal Pain)
- Black Nails (Nail Discolouration)
- Black Stools (Stool Colour and Texture Changes)
- Blackout (Fainting)
- Bladder Incontinence (Incontinence, Urine)
- Bloating (Gas)

- Blood in Semen
- Blood in Spit (Bloody Sputum)
- Blood in Stool (Rectal Bleeding)
- Blood in Urine
- Blood in Vomit (Vomiting Blood)
- Bloodshot Eye (Pink Eye)
- Bloody Mucus (Bloody Sputum)
- Bloody Nose
- Blurred Thinking (Confusion)
- Bottom Itch (Anal Itching)
- Bottom Pain (Buttock Pain)
- Breast Discharge
- Breast Lumps
- Breast Mass (Breast Lumps)
- Breast Pain
- Breathing Shortness
- Breathlessness (Hyperventilation)
- Brown Vaginal Discharge (Vaginal Discharge)
- Bruising, Easy (Easy Bruising)
- Bumps on Skin
- Burning Eyes (Eye Pain)
- Burning in Throat (Sore Throat)
- Burning Urination
- Butt Pain (Buttock Pain)
- Buttock Pain

- Cachexia (Weight Loss)
- Can't Sleep (Insomnia)
- Cervical Pain (Neck Pain)
- Chest Pain
- Chest Pain with Breathing (Pleurisy)
- Chronic Cough (Cough)
- Chronic Pain
- Cloudy Thoughts (Confusion)
- Cold Feet
- Cold Fingers

- Confusion
- Constipation
- Convulsions (Seizures)
- Cotton Mouth (Dry Mouth)
- Cough
- Coughing Up Blood (Bloody Sputum)
- Cramps, Abdominal (Abdominal Pain)
- Cramps, Menstrual (Menstrual Cramps)
- Cramps, Muscle (Muscle Cramps)

- Dandruff (Flaky Scalp)
- Dark Stools (Stool Colour and Texture Changes)
- Deafness (Hearing Loss)
- Dental Pain (Toothache)
- Depigmentation of Skin
- Depression
- Diarrhea
- Difficulty Breathing (Shortness of Breath)
- Difficulty Sleeping (Insomnia)
- Difficulty Swallowing (Sore Throat)
- Discharge, Breast (Breast Discharge)
- Disorientation (Confusion)
- Dizziness
- Drowsiness (Fatigue and Tiredness)
- Dry Eye
- Dry Flaky Scalp (Flaky Scalp)
- Dry Heaves (Nausea)
- Dry Mouth
- Dry Vagina (Vaginal Dryness)
- Dyspepsia
- Dyspnea (Shortness of Breath)
- Dysuria (Burning Urination)

- Ear Ache (Earache)
- Ear Ringing (Ringing in Ears)
- Earache

- Easy Bruising
- Ecchymosis (Easy Bruising)
- Eczema (Rash)
- Edema (Leg Swelling)
- Elbow Pain
- Epilepsy (Seizures)
- Epistaxis (Bloody Nose)
- Erectile Dysfunction (Impotence)
- Erythema (Rash)
- Exhaustion (Fatigue and Tiredness)
- Eye Pain
- Eye Redness (Pink Eye)
- Eye, Watery (Watery Eye)

- Fainting
- Farting (Gas)
- Fatigue and Tiredness
- Fear Syndrome (Anxiety)
- Faeces Colour Changes (Stool Colour and Texture Changes)
- Feeling Tired (Fatigue and Tiredness)
- Feeling Uptight (Anxiety)
- Fever
- Finger Numbness (Numbness Fingers)
- Finger Tingling (Numbness Fingers)
- Fingers, Cold (Cold Fingers)
- Flaky Scalp
- Flatulence (Gas)
- Fluid Retention (Weight Gain)
- Food Aversion (Loss of Appetite)
- Foot Pain
- Forgetfulness (Memory Loss)
- Frequent Bowel Movements (Diarrhea)
- Frequent Urination
- Fuzzy Thinking (Confusion)

- Gas
- Genital Itching (Female) (Vaginal Itching)
- Gland Swelling (Swollen Lymph Nodes)
- Green Nails (Nail Discolouration)
- Green Stools (Stool Colour and Texture Changes)
- Green Vaginal Discharge (Vaginal Discharge)
- Gut Pain (Abdominal Pain)

- Hair Loss
- Headache
- Hearing Loss
- Heart Palpitations (Palpitations)
- Heartbeat Sensations (Palpitations)
- Heartburn
- Heat Rash (Rash)
- Heavy, Prolonged, Irregular Periods (Vaginal Bleeding)
- Haematemesis (Vomiting Blood)
- Haematochezia (Rectal Bleeding)
- Haematospaemia (Blood in Semen)
- Haematuria (Blood in Urine)
- Haemoptysis (Bloody Sputum)
- Hives (Rash)
- Hoarseness
- Hot Flashes
- Hyperventilation

- Icterus (Jaundice)
- Impotence
- Inability to Think Clearly (Confusion)
- Inablity to Think Quickly (Confusion)
- Incontinence, Urine
- Increased Respiratory Rate (Hyperventilation)
- Indigestion (Dyspepsia)
- Indigestion, Acid (Heartburn)

- Infertility
- Ingrown Fingernail (Nail Discolouration)
- Ingrown Nail (Nail Discolouration)
- Ingrown Toenail (Nail Discolouration)
- Insomnia
- Intention Tremor (Tremor)
- Itch

- Jaundice
- Joint Aches (Joint Pain)
- Joint Pain

- Knee Pain

- Lack of Energy (Fatigue and Tiredness)
- Lack of Sleep (Insomnia)
- Lacrimation (Watery Eye)
- Laryngeal Voice (Hoarseness)
- Leg Cramps (Muscle Cramps)
- Leg Swelling
- Leg Weakness (Weakness)
- Leg, Restless (Restless Leg Syndrome)
- Lethargy (Fatigue and Tiredness)
- Lightening of Skin (Depigmentation of Skin)
- Lightheadedness (Fainting)
- Long-Term Memory Loss (Memory Loss)
- Loose Bowel Movements (Diarrhea)
- Loose Stool (Diarrhea)
- Loss of Appetite
- Loss of Balance (Dizziness)
- Loss of Bladder Control (Incontinence, Urine)
- Loss of Hair (Hair Loss)
- Loss of Hearing (Hearing Loss)
- Loss of Memory (Confusion)
- Loss of Memory (Memory Loss)

- Loss of Orientation (Confusion)
- Loss of Skin Pigment (Depigmentation of Skin)
- Loss of Sleep (Insomnia)
- Loss of Strength (Weakness)
- Loss of Weight (Weight Loss)
- Lower (Low) Back Pain (Back Pain)
- Lumbar Pain (Back Pain)
- Lump in Breast (Breast Lumps)
- Lupus Rash (Rash)

- Melena (Stool Colour and Texture Changes)
- Memory Loss
- Memory Loss (Confusion)
- Men's Snoring (Snoring)
- Mennorrhagia (Vaginal Bleeding)
- Menorrhea (Vaginal Bleeding)
- Menstrual Cramps
- Missed Menstrual Period
- Muscle Cramps
- Muscle Pain and Weakness (Weakness)
- Muscle Weakness (Weakness)

- Nail Discolouration
- Nausea
- Neck Pain
- Nipple Discharge (Breast Discharge)
- Noise, Ear (Ringing in Ears)
- Non-Acid Dyspepsia (Dyspepsia)
- Non-Cardiac Chest Pain (Heartburn)
- Nosebleed (Bloody Nose)
- Numbness Fingers
- Numbness Toes

- Obesity (Weight Gain)
- Odour, Vagina (Vaginal Odour)

- Overactive Bladder (Incontinence, Urine)
- Overbreathing (Hyperventilation)
- Overweight (Weight Gain)

- Pain (Chronic Pain)
- Pain in the Butt (Buttock Pain)
- Palpitations
- Paresthesia, Fingers (Numbness Fingers)
- Paresthesia, Toes (Numbness Toes)
- Pharyngitis (Sore Throat)
- Pink Eye
- Pleurisy
- Poor Appetite (Loss of Appetite)
- Problems Sleeping (Insomnia)
- Pruritic (Itch)

- Rapid Breathing (Hyperventilation)
- Rash
- Rectal Bleeding
- Red Eye (Pink Eye)
- Red Stools (Stool Colour and Texture Changes)
- Reflux, Acid (Heartburn)
- Restless Leg Syndrome
- Ringing in Ears
- Ringworm of the Nails (Nail Discolouration)
- Runny Nose

- Seizures
- Shakes (Tremor)
- Shaky Feet (Tremor)
- Shaky Hands (Tremor)
- Short-Term Memory Loss (Memory Loss)
- Shortness of Breath
- Sick to Stomach (Nausea)
- Skin Depigmentation (Depigmentation of Skin)
- Skin Eruption (Rash)

- Skin Rash (Rash)
- Skin Redness (Rash)
- Sleep Difficulty (Insomnia)
- Sleep Disturbances (Snoring)
- Sleeplessness (Insomnia)
- Sleepy (Fatigue and Tiredness)
- Smelly Vagina (Vaginal Odour)
- Snoring
- Sore Throat
- Spitting up Blood (Bloody Sputum)
- Sterility (Infertility)
- Stomach Ache (Abdominal Pain)
- Stomach Cramps (Abdominal Pain)
- Stomach Pain (Abdominal Pain)
- Stomach Upset (Dyspepsia)
- Stress (Anxiety)
- Sudden Memory Loss (Memory Loss)
- Suicide
- Swollen Ankles and/or Swollen Feet
- Swollen Legs (Leg Swelling)
- Swollen Lymph Nodes
- Syncope (Fainting)

- Tachypnea (Hyperventilation)
- Tailbone Pain (Coccydynia)
- Teary Eye (Watery Eye)
- Tennis Elbow (Elbow Pain)
- Throat Pain (Sore Throat)
- Tingling Fingers (Numbness Fingers)
- Tingling Toes (Numbness Toes)
- Tinnitus (Ringing in Ears)
- Tiredness (Fatigue and Tiredness)
- Toothache
- Trembling (Tremor)
- Tremor

- Unclear Thinking (Confusion)
- Uncontrollable Bladder (Incontinence, Urine)
- Unsteadiness (Dizziness)
- Upset Stomach (Dyspepsia)
- Urinary Frequency (Frequent Urination)
- Urinary Incontinence (Incontinence, Urine)

- Vaginal Bleeding
- Vaginal Discharge
- Vaginal Dryness
- Vaginal Itching
- Vaginal Odour
- Vaginal Pain
- Vertigo (Dizziness)
- Vomiting (Nausea)
- Vomiting Blood

- Watery Eye
- Watery Stool (Diarrhea)
- Weakness
- Weakness in Arms (Weakness)
- Weakness in Legs (Weakness)
- Weariness (Fatigue and Tiredness)
- Weight Gain
- Weight Loss
- Wheezing (Shortness of Breath)
- White Nails (Nail Discolouration)
- White Spots on the Nails (Nail Discolouration)
- White Vaginal Discharge (Vaginal Discharge)
- Woozy (Dizziness)